Ethics in Child Health

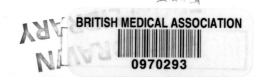

Ethics in Child Health
Principles and Cases in Neurodisability

Edited by Peter L. Rosenbaum, Gabriel M. Ronen,
Eric Racine, Jennifer Johannesen
and Bernard Dan

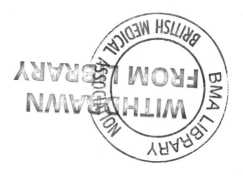

2016
Mac Keith Press

Managing Director: Ann-Marie Halligan
Production Manager/Commissioning Editor: Udoka Ohuonu
Project Management: Riverside Publishing Solutions Ltd

First published in this edition in 2016 by Mac Keith Press
6 Market Road, London, N7 9PW

British Library Cataloguing-in-Publication data
A catalogue record for this book is available from the British Library

Cover design: Hannah Rogers

ISBN: 978-1-909962-63-7

Typeset by Riverside Publishing Solutions Ltd

Printed by Hobbs the Printers Ltd, Totton, Hampshire, UK
Mac Keith Press is supported by Scope.

Contents

The editors were very fortunate to engage as a co-editor Jennifer Johannesen, the parent of Owen (*No Ordinary Boy*), who was born with profound impairments and died at age 12 years. She offers insights, as someone with training in ethics, to share her personal experiences.

Johannesen provides three vignettes she and her family experienced in their journey with Owen into the world of the clinician. Each story provides invaluable perspectives that reflect the good intentions of the healthcare providers and systems with which their family worked. At the same time, as she describes the actions of medical professionals, it becomes apparent that there were unrecognized implications and consequences to these encounters.

The co-editors address, among other themes, current insights and beliefs about children, families, disability issues, rights, policies and the conceptual and clinical underpinnings of work in childhood neurodisability. They reflect on how the current era has been enormously influenced by developments in, for example, public health (survival of children with impairments);

concepts about 'health' (such as the World Health Organization's International Classification of Functioning, Health and Disability); and movements to enshrine the rights of children and the rights of people with disabilities in international conventions.

Co-editor Eric Racine is an ethicist with a major interest in child neurodisability. His informative, context-setting chapter was written as the book was being completed, and brings together a number of themes and approaches to ethical analysis. We believe that this chapter will help readers frame their understanding of the cases that populate the book as well as their own real-life professional encounters. It explains and discusses the importance and complexity of the methods by which ethical deliberation processes are engaged. While one chapter can scarcely do more than sketch the outlines of this multifaceted and evolving field, readers may well find themselves returning to this essay as they delve into individual chapters.

SECTION B: EARLY DAYS, THE START OF THE DIFFERENT DEVELOPMENTAL JOURNEY

A recurring theme in this book concerns the ways in which advances in modern technology challenge service providers and families to confront 'new' issues. For example, prenatal assessments provide 'information' at earlier and earlier stages of fetal development. Before the availability of our current early detection capacities, infants were usually first identified as having a developmental issue at birth or in infancy. Today, detection of impairment at a prenatal stage makes the level of uncertainty faced by counselors, and of course by families, proportionally greater. In this chapter Kett and colleagues present a clear interface between what can be considered 'good clinical practice' and what are emerging as the ethical imperatives that must explicitly guide these practices. In a pair of contrasting scenarios, they illustrate these issues and the ethical considerations that flow from them.

Despite scores of trials, the best 'evidence' for the management of a specific clinical dilemma is often lacking, although decisions still need to be made and prognoses still need to be given in the individual situation. In the case scenario presented in this chapter, Chouinard and colleagues demonstrate the complexity of prognostication and end-of-life decision-making for newborn infants with an apparently very poor neurological prognosis, particularly when evidence is not clear and/or is conflicting. The case also highlights the type of evidence that weighs more heavily when there is biomedical uncertainty. The authors discuss both the limits of 'evidence' from best studies when such evidence is to be applied to the individual, and the reality that for many of the important questions that parents and practitioners face there is simply no good evidence available. This issue is also discussed in Chapter 6.

6 **The importance of beliefs and relationships in the decision-making process** 75
Howard Needelman and David Sweeney

In many clinical situations in the field of developmental impairment, knowledge of the facts may be limited or conflicting, and the decisions clouded by emotion, time pressures and alternate, often competing, views among the protagonists. Needelman and Sweeney bring these issues clearly into focus in this chapter, with a scenario covering the need to make decisions about the care and prognosis of a high-risk preterm neonate. By identifying the 'cast' and the 'roles' of the major players, the authors show us that this kind of drama unfolds without a pre-set script, and cannot be presented as a story that is 'typical' or formulaic. They remind us of the essentially personal nature of each story, and of the challenge and thus of the limitations of using 'the literature' appropriately in the specific case.

7 **Humanism in the practice of neurodevelopmental disability: examples of challenges and opportunities** 85
Garey Noritz

Noritz's chapter provides reflections from an academically trained clinician working in both a hospital clinic and a community-based disability practice. While related situations are also reported and discussed by other authors (see, e.g. Chapter 4), it is Noritz's particular vantage point that allows him to raise these issues and consider them from the perspective of 'the community'. The author uses an ethical framework, language and thinking to provide context and opportunities for discussion of the challenges he describes so clearly and compellingly within this framework. As such, the chapter offers readers a way to think about the many common challenges we experience in our work in developmental disability – and to refract these issues through the lens of an ethical framework.

Contents

Communicating bad news to parents and carers must be recognized as a process rather than a one-time event. When this process is done ineptly or insensitively it can add a considerable burden to the suffering experienced by families new to the 'career' of parents of a child with a chronic problem. In this sensitive and also practical chapter, Novak and colleagues discuss the communication of bad news by exploring the processes through an ethical framework, and present comments from several parents to illustrate the impact that this process can have. The authors then provide an evidence-based approach to sharing 'bad news', developed in the field of cancer care (the six steps of the SPIKES framework) as a guide to this challenging but essential step in building a relationship with families.

SECTION C: ETHICAL ISSUES IN ADDRESSING FAMILIES' PRIORITIES

Reddihough and Tracy's chapter tells the moving story of an adolescent and her family who come to the attention of clinical services for the first time when the young woman is 14 years old. The authors use this story to explore the issues associated with the process of engaging with an adolescent. They report on the challenges they experienced, the distress and upset they felt and the process of developing a relationship between the healthcare team and the family over a period of time. Rather than engaging child services, the clinical team took the time and effort to build a trusting rapport with the family that eventually led to a satisfactory resolution of many of the issues that could easily have been addressed punitively. Variations on this theme are also discussed in Chapter 18.

This chapter explores the intersection of medical capability and families' personal narratives. The authors remind us of the essential responsibility to understand the perspectives and stories of the patients and their families. They present, analyze and follow the story of a 15-year-old girl with cerebral palsy and her widowed mother across time and crises, outlining how the many people in this young woman's life worked together in this complex situation, and considered the potential benefits and costs of various courses of action. By applying a systematic process of case analysis and reflective practice the care team – including the family and their support – reached what appears to have been an appropriate decision for all concerned.

There are clearly times when all health professionals – as advocates for children and families – face the dilemma about whether it is right to bend the truth on behalf of the people we serve. Tervo and Wojda have produced a fascinating chapter about the ethics of deception. They cite authorities, both ancient and contemporary, who have reflected on these issues in considerable philosophical detail. Their analysis is likely to support some readers' views and challenge others'.

With the advent of two modern developments – the democratization of knowledge through the availability of the Internet, and the expectation of patient engagement in the management of their own conditions – there appears to be an acceleration of requests from consumers for service providers to know about, and perhaps to endorse and support, the use of 'complementary and alternative' therapies. In their desire to do the best for their children, parents are often susceptible to the lure of interventions that promise more than they can provide. Hurvitz and Noritz explore these issues thoughtfully and sensitively. They offer sensible and useful ways for service providers to consider the challenges of working openly and honestly with families. To illustrate their approach consideration is given to the challenges associated with a specific contemporary 'alternative' therapy that is growing in popularity and complexity.

Parents of children and young people with complex and incurable neurodisabilities sometimes request support and endorsement from their service providers for interventions that are outside the scope of conventional practice. In some circumstances these requests can generate considerable discomfort for the practitioners. Clinicians can be caught between wanting to respect parent/patient autonomy (in the service of family-centeredness), and being concerned about issues of safety, legality or probity of these alternative approaches. The more complex the child's issues and the less we have to offer from conventional management, the more ethically challenging the parents' demands might become. Mann, Saneto and Gospe explore a case scenario where medical marijuana is the perceived complementary and alternative medicine for a child with uncontrolled seizures.

SECTION D: RESPECTING SOCIAL AND CULTURAL VALUES

It might seem unusual to include a chapter on language and terminology in a discussion of ethical issues in childhood disability. However, the way we talk reflects the way we think and at times clinicians may fail to think about the meaning and impact of our words. Drawing on an extensive personal narrative, Samson-Fang probes the use of words and explores issues of stereotyping and stigma – issues she believes should be front of mind for professionals working in neurodevelopmental disability.

In this sensitive and deeply personal chapter, the authors describe the complexities and ethical challenges faced by healthcare workers in an under-resourced community with a horrific history that rocked their country and the world only 20 years ago. While the resource limitations in Rwanda make the clinical practice of child healthcare very difficult, the chapter reflects particularly on the personal and ethical dilemmas experienced by healthcare professionals, including the threat of burnout. The authors discuss the potential for professionals to withdraw into fatalism and to lose the humanism that drew them to the healthcare field in the first place.

Many of the families we meet have come to our communities from cultures in which 'disability' carries meaning quite different from our understanding.

As a result, cultural clashes can arise and be daunting for everyone. This chapter discusses the story of a young teenager with significant impairments, whose family's values and actions contrasted with those the care team were recommending as important. These differences created tensions for everyone involved with the young lady's care. Funkhouser and Linett offer a thoughtful analysis of the approaches to these differences, in which good clinical practice includes listening, trying to understand and being attuned to others' realities. They also point out how important it is to maintain contact with families facing these kinds of predicaments, especially when situations change and what might have been difficult might become feasible. The issues discussed here have echoes of those discussed in Chapter 9 and Chapter 18.

17 Service provision for hard-to-reach families: what are our responsibilities? 193
Michelle Phoenix

Ethical challenges can emerge when clinical policies within an agency with decision-making responsibility – such as a community-based facility or government-run program – appear to conflict with the best intentions of the front-line service providers. Phoenix addresses these issues in a compelling story of the conflict created for her and her colleagues when a standard policy about families' missed appointments came up against the clinicians' awareness of and sensitivity to the stresses on a family that accounted for this apparent delinquency. The clinicians were caught in a dilemma that led to a no-win situation – at least for the immediate issue – and caused discomfort for most of the players.

18 The obligation to report child abuse/neglect is more complex than it seems 203
Lucyna M. Lach and Rachel Birnbaum

In most jurisdictions, professionals who work in child health have a legal responsibility to report suspected child abuse. This mandate can abut against the advocacy roles we fulfill in working with families of children with neurodisabilities as we lean towards 'tolerating' and 'understanding' parental behaviors or attitudes that would not otherwise be considered acceptable. We may also believe that by reporting a family to child welfare authorities we risk doing more harm than good for the child and family. In this chapter, Lach and Birnbaum address this issue in the context of social work teaching and practice, with discipline-specific frameworks and principles. Similar themes are identified in Chapter 9, though the language may be somewhat different.

In this chapter, Blasco explores the issues of an able-bodied, but possibly
troubled, sibling of a child with significant impairments who is the focus of
the clinical attention. In recognizing the sibling's issues he explores the conflicts
inherent in deciding the clinicians' roles and responsibilities to the patient and
their family; the importance to the child of a family's well-being; the limits of our
time and resources with which to address the sibling issues; and the potential for
intervention to appear to overstep the narrow bounds of our clinical mandate.
In the next chapter, Reddihough and Davis show how the same challenges arise
when working with the parents of children with impairments.

It is increasingly recognized that the physical and mental health of parents
raising children with complex needs is at substantially greater risk than
the health of comparable parents of well children. For these reasons it is
essential that professionals learn to be able both to identify parental distress
and to help parents receive support for their own social and mental health
issues as part of a family-centered care program. In the scenario that runs
through this chapter the authors illustrate how, without specific attention
to parental and family well-being, issues can fester and negatively affect
everyone in the family.

SECTION E: THERAPIES, REHABILITATION AND INTERVENTIONS

Therapists are often on the front lines of service provision for children and
young people with neurodisabilities. In this role they can be caught between
the competing views, philosophies and practical realities of families, young
people with impairments, community colleagues and of course the service
systems within which they work. In this chapter, Woo and her colleagues discuss
three scenarios, each of which poses ethical as well as 'political' dilemmas. They
use the Occupational Therapy Code of Ethics and Ethics Standards from the
American Occupational Therapy Association (AOTA), and the Code of Ethics for
the Physical Therapist from the American Physical Therapy Association (APTA)
to analyse the scenarios. In the cases presented here, the authors could have

arrived at a variety of alternative solutions that were reasonable and defensible, and equally valid.

In their compelling vignette, the authors present a story that illustrates the potential ethical dilemmas associated with continuing to provide therapy for a 15-year-old with significant impairment for whom functional improvement is an illusory goal, but for whom hard-to-measure comfort care may be achievable at a cost. They identify both the professional guidelines by which they are constrained and the human dilemmas faced by the family of the young woman whose story is the focus of the chapter, as well as the expectations of the community-based physician seeking to advocate for their patient. They describe the approach they took to reconcile these disparate needs.

When children and young people have chronic conditions or are in situations in which therapies provide at best partial 'success', families may choose to adopt additional therapies in the community. These may be pursued outside the conventional community-based public services their child is attending. This can create challenges, conflicts and ethical dilemmas for professionals. Wright and her colleagues provide and work though a decision-making framework that can help service providers approach dilemmas like these in a thoughtful and organized way.

In our work with children with complex needs, the greater the level of uncertainty about a course of action (as discussed, e.g. in Chapters 5 and 6), the more challenging the issues become and the greater the chance of conflict, distress and dissatisfaction. This chapter illustrates these challenges clearly as the author considers the process of family and clinical team weighing the options for high-risk scoliosis corrective surgery in a teenager with severe impairments. The author presents the issues as they might be experienced by the child, the family and the healthcare team. The child and family's prior experience of surgeries and the intensive care unit weigh heavily on them, while the healthcare team must face the reality of the limitations of being 'evidence-based' when the facts are simply unavailable to guide their advice to families.

This chapter poses the provocative question about whether our Western focus on the value of an individual's autonomy might at times clash with our uncertainty about an individual's capacity for independent thought and action. This in turn raises questions about parental (or other proxy) decision-making, and the potential for clashes between professionals' values and perceptions of the limited 'personhood' of people with significant impairments, in contrast to the values that parents might hold even in the face of their child's severe impairments. Clarke's account of the story of Charlie, a significantly impaired adolescent, brings together and contrasts the notions of 'quality of life' (an essentially personal 'existential' perspective) and 'value of a life' (judged from the outside and often considered to be very low in people with significant functional challenges).

The fact that we often have the technological capacity to extend life can easily create considerable discomfort for practitioners as well as families, and can be the focal point for conflicts both between families and service providers, and more broadly within the health and social care teams. In their analysis of two cases, Newman and Zurbrugg discuss the impact of these challenges as they might concern the child, the family, the service providers and their teams, and the broader society in which these dramas play out. These dilemmas expose people's personal values, and bring into focus universal values such as those enshrined in United Nations' conventions on the rights of children and of disabled persons. (These issues are also addressed in Chapter 5.)

Reese and Pearl raise and explore the complexity of discussing sudden unexpected death in epilepsy (SUDEP). What makes this issue so unusual are features such as the variability of the risks of the condition from one form of epilepsy to another, the variable degrees of uncertainty in even beginning to try to predict it, and the potential to create considerable distress and perhaps suffering in people faced with this rare but obviously catastrophic event. The authors build their approach to these challenges using a combination of descriptive and research-based literature and a thoughtful analysis of the ethical as well as clinical considerations that can be brought to bear in the specific clinical situation.

This chapter raises fascinating issues related to both the politics and ethical implications of certain diagnoses, in this case the challenges associated with a diagnosis of fetal alcohol spectrum disorder. It covers a wide range of implications of this diagnosis, including the moral and ethical responsibilities of professionals in some jurisdictions to make and report the diagnosis; the responsibility to the young persons themselves when they are old enough to ask about their condition; and of course the responsibilities to the family to deal honestly with what remains in many places a stigmatizing label for both the child and the mother.

SECTION G: EMERGING INDEPENDENCE AND PREPARING FOR ADULTHOOD

One of the dilemmas associated with 21st-century Western medicine is the possibility to engage in interventions that in earlier times might not even have been imagined, and were in any case usually technically impossible. Samaan considers this dilemma in the context of the possibility to manipulate physical and pubertal growth in a young person with significant permanent functional limitations. Whose needs and wishes are being served, and to whom are we as professionals accountable? Drawing on the highly publicized story of Ashley, a child in Seattle, USA, he explores the considerations that can and should be brought to bear on whether this 'treatment' is indicated, appropriate and ethical.

Whereas typically developing young people have opportunities to take risks, make their own decisions, and learn from life, many young people with impairments have limited possiblities to do this, and can be thought of as being 'deprived'.

Gorter and Gibson apply ethical frameworks and processes to explore the many, often complex, challenges associated with our work as service providers striving to support the individuation of young people toward autonomy and seamless healthcare transition. They reflect on the possibility that some of our well-intentioned goals and activities may in fact be counter-productive. They also identify the very real challenges posed by environmental limitations and barriers that can interfere with even the best-laid plans for transition.

Chambers, a pediatric orthopedic surgeon and parent of a young man with complex needs, brings to readers' attention the legal dimensions (often challenges) that may arise as young people enter the 'adult' world and continue to require support from family or other designated caregivers.

The final chapter of the book, by co-editor Bernard Dan, provides a thoughtful summative reflection of the issues the book has covered, and how readers might use these issues as a basis for discussion and consideration of future situations and action. This integration was done after a full reading of all the chapters. It offers an important perspective on the ways that people may consider the integration of the themes, issues, analyses and ideas of how to achieve potential resolutions of the many dilemmas described by the authors whose work appears in this book. The chapter also identifies challenges on the road ahead, and encourages all of us to keep reflecting and communication about the issues that this book addresses.

Authors' Appointments

Ilona Autti-Rämö
Medical Director, Insurance Medicine Unit, The Social Insurance Institute, Health Benefits, Helsinki; Adjunct Professor, Department of Child Neurology, University of Helsinki, Finland

Nadia Badawi
Chair of Cerebral Palsy, Cerebral Palsy Alliance, Discipline of Child and Adolescent Health, The University of Sydney; Grace Centre for Newborn Care, Children's Hospital at Westmead, Discipline of Child and Adolescent Health, The University of Sydney, Australia

Rachel Birnbaum
Professor, Cross-Appointed with Childhood Studies (Interdisciplinary Programs) & Social Work, King's University College, Western, Ontario, Canada

Peter Blasco
Director, Neurodevelopmental Programs, Institutue on Development and Disability, Oregon Health and Science University, Portland, Oregon, USA

Henry G. Chambers
Professor of Clinical Orthopedic Surgery, University of California, San Diego, USA

Isabelle Chouinard
Medical Student, University of Calgary Alberta; PhD Candidate, Université de Montréal, Quebec, Canada

Michael A. Clarke
Consultant Paediatric Neurologist, Leeds Teaching Hospitals NHS Trust, UK

Barbara J. Cunningham
PhD Candidate, School of Rehabilitation Science, McMaster University, Hamilton, Ontario, Canada

Bernard Dan
Professor of Neuroscience, Université libre de Bruxelles (ULB), Brussels; Director of Rehabilitation, Rehabilitation Hospital Inkendaal, Vlezenbeek, Belgium

Elise Davis
Associate Director, Jack Brockhoff Child Health and Wellbeing Program, Melbourne School of Population and Global Health, The University of Melbourne, Australia

Kathleen Dekker
Speech-Language Pathology Profession Lead, Developmental Paediatrics and Rehabilitation, McMaster Children's Hospital, Hamilton, Ontario, Canada

Dan Doherty
Associate Professor, Department of Pediatrics, University of Washington, USA

Emily Esmaili
Graduate Student (Candidate for M.A. in Bioethics and Science Policy), Department of Science and Society, Duke University, Durham, North Carolina; Pediatrician, Lincoln Community Health Center, Durham, North Carolina, USA

Harriet Fain-Tvedt
Chief, Medical Therapy Program, County of Orange-California Children's Services, USA

Janey McGeary Farber
Pediatric Physical Therapist; Supervisor, Inpatient Therapies, Gillette Children's Speciality Healthcare, Minnesota, USA

Laura S. Funkhouser
Assistant Clinical Professor, Department of Pediatrics, School of Medicine, Loma Linda University, California, USA

Sandra Gaik
Occupational Therapy Profession Lead, Developmental Paediatrics and Rehabilitation, McMaster Children's Hospital; Assistant Clinical Professor (Adjunct), Faculty of Health Sciences, McMaster University, Hamilton, Ontario, Canada

Barbara E. Gibson
Senior Scientist, Bloorview Research Institute, Holland Bloorview Kids Rehabilitation Hospital, Toronto, Ontario; Associate Professor, Department of Physical Therapy, University of Toronto, Ontario, Canada

Jan Willem Gorter
Professor of Paediatrics, McMaster University, Hamilton, Ontario, Canada

Sidney M. Gospe, Jr
Herman and Faye Sarkowsky Endowed Chair; Professor, Neurology and Pediatrics; Head, Division of Pedatric Neurology, University of Washington; Head, Division of Neurology, Seattle Children's Hospital, Washington, USA

Edward A. Hurvitz
Professor and Chair, Department of Physical Medicine and Rehabilitation, University of Michigan, USA

Jennifer Johannesen
Author and Patient Advocate, Toronto, Ontario, Canada

Petra Karlsson
Research Fellow, Cerebral Palsy Alliance, Discipline of Child and Adolescent Health, The University of Sydney, Australia

Jennifer Cobelli Kett
Pediatric Palliative Care Physician, Mary Bridge Children's Hospital, Tacoma, Washington, USA

Lucyna M. Lach
Associate Professor, School of Social Work, McGill University, Montreal, Quebec, Canada

Suzanne Linett
Licensed Occupational Therapist, Private Practice, USA

Paul C. Mann
Assistant Professor of Pediatrics, Division of Neonatology, University of Washington; Faculty Member, Treuman Katz Center for Pediatric Bioethics, Seattle Children's Hospital, Washington, USA

Cathy Morgan
Research Fellow, Cerebral Palsy Alliance, Discipline of Child and Adolescent Health, The University of Sydney, Australia

Howard Needelman
Associate Professor of Pediatrics, Munroe Meyer Institute, University of Nebraska Medical Center, Omaha, Nebraska, USA

Christopher J. Newman
Consultant, Senior Lecturer, Paediatric Neurology and Neurorehabilitation Unit, Lausanne University Hospital, Switzerland

Garey Noritz
Associate Professor of Pediatrics, Nationwide Children's Hospital and The Ohio State University, USA

Iona Novak
Professor, Cerebral Palsy Alliance, Discipline of Child and Adolescent Health, The University of Sydney, Australia

Christian Ntizimira
Palliative Care Expert and Educator, Advocacy and Research Division, Rwanda Palliative Care and Hospice Organisation, Kigali, Rwanda

Phillip L. Pearl
Director of Epilepsy and Clinical Neurophysiology, Boston Children's Hospital; William G. Lennox Chair and Professor of Neurology, Harvard Medical School, Boston, Massachusetts, USA

Michelle Phoenix
PhD Candidate, School of Rehabilitation Science, McMaster University, Hamilton, Ontario, Canada

Eric Racine
Director, Neuroethics Research Unit, Institut de recherches cliniques de Montréal (IRCM); Full Research Professor, IRCM; Associate Director, Academic Affairs, IRCM; Associate Research Professor, Department of Medicine, Université de Montréal; Adjunct Professor, Department of Neurology and Neurosurgery, McGill University; Affiliate Member, Department of Medicine, Division of Experimental Medicine, and Biomedical Ethics Unit, McGill University, Montreal, Quebec, Canada

Dinah S. Reddihough
Paediatrician, Royal Children's Hospital, Melbourne; Honorary Professorial Fellow, The University of Melbourne; Group Leader, Developmental Disability & Rehabilitation Research, Murdoch Childrens Research Institute, Melbourne, Australia

James J. Reese, Jr
Assistant Professor of Neurology, University of New Mexico, Albuquerque, New Mexico, USA

Gabriel M. Ronen
Professor of Paediatrics, McMaster University, Hamilton, Ontario, Canada

Peter L. Rosenbaum
Professor of Paediatrics, McMaster University, Hamilton, Ontario, Canada

Elizabeth Russel
Research and Program Outcomes Coordinator, California Children's Services, Medical Therapy Program, Children's Medical Services, Department of Public Health, County of Los Angeles, California, USA

M. Constantine Samaan
Assistant Professor, Department of Pediatrics, McMaster University, Hamilton, Ontario, Canada

Lisa Samson-Fang
Pediatrician, Intermountain Medical Group, Salt Lake City, Utah, USA

Russell P. Saneto
Professor of Neurology and Adjunct Professor of Pediatrics, University of Washington; Attending Physician, Division of Neurology, Seattle Children's Hospital, Washington, USA

Scott Schwantes
Associate Medical Director of Pediatrics, Gillette Children's Specialty Healthcare, Minnesota; Associate Professor, University of Minnesota, USA

Eunice Shen
Physical Therapy Education Coordinator, California Children's Services, Medical Therapy Program, Children's Medical Services, Department of Public Health, County of Los Angeles, California, USA

M. Wade Shrader
Professor and Chief, Pediatric Orthopedic Surgery, Children's of Mississippi, University of Mississippi Medical Center, USA

Hayley Smithers-Sheedy
Research Fellow, Cerebral Palsy Alliance, Discipline of Child and Adolescent Health, The University of Sydney, Australia

Jean C. Kunz Stansbury
Certified Pediatric Nurse Practitioner, Gillette Children's Speciality Healthcare, Minnesota, USA

David Sweeney
Staff Chaplain and Ethics Consultation Service, Nebraska Medicine, Omaha, Nebraska, USA

Raymond Tervo
Professor of Pediatrics, Mayo Clinic, Minnesota, USA

Marelle Thornton
Former President of the Board and Parent, Cerebral Palsy Alliance, Discipline of Child and Adolescent Health, The University of Sydney, Australia

Jane Tracy
Director, Centre for Developmental Disability Health Victoria, Monash Health, Clayton, Victoria; Adjunct Associate Professor, Living with Disability Research Centre, LaTrobe University, Bundoora, Victoria; Adjunct Senior Lecturer, School of Primary Health Care, Faculty of Medicine Nursing and Health Sciences, Monash University, Victoria, Australia

Hannah M. Tully
Acting Assistant Professor, Division of Pediatric Neurology, Department of Neurology, University of Washington, USA

Pia Wintermark
Assistant Professor of Pediatrics, McGill University, Montreal, Quebec, Canada

Paul J. Wojda
Associate Professor, Theology Department, University of St. Thomas, Minnesota, USA

Lora Woo
Occupational Therapy Education Coordinator, California Children's Services, Medical Therapy Program, Children's Medical Services, Department of Public Health, County of Los Angeles, California, USA

Marilyn Wright
Physical Therapy Profession Lead, Developmental Paediatrics and Rehabilitation, McMaster Children's Hospital; Assistant Clinical Professor, Faculty of Health Sciences, McMaster University, Hamilton, Ontario, Canada

Eric B. Zurbrugg
Affiliated Staff (Neuroscience), Children's Healthcare of Atlanta, Georgia, USA

Foreword

Considering ethical issues is fundamental to the 'art' of clinical practice, complementing the 'science' of making diagnoses and understanding body structure and functions. Clinicians must apply to ethical consideration their knowledge, informed by the best possible evidence, their experience, intuition, integrity, clinical judgement and compassion. They must share in decision-making with children, young people and their families about aspects of individual healthcare. They must also share with healthcare provider organisations and funders how health services can be most efficiently and effectively designed. This book provides insight into how a structured approach to the application of ethical theory can underpin sound clinical practice. Many of the ethical dilemmas presented have more than one 'right' answer; the expert discussions in each chapter help the reader to understand the range of possible ethical arguments and considerations, so that when they face a similar scenario themselves they can adopt a structured approach to arriving at the best conclusion for the unique situations of their patients.

Opening with the family perspective, the reader is immediately drawn in and cannot help reflecting on the stories shared and how these relate to their own experience. The context is then set, with an account of how the conceptual framework of disability has evolved over time and how the rights of disabled people have come to be better protected in law. The language and frameworks of ethical theory are then explained. The book follows the developmental journey on a timeline from early days, through sharing difficult new information, to many examples and perspectives on a range of ethical issues. A person-centred/family-centred approach runs as a thread through the book, emphasising how ethical issues are best considered in partnership, underpinned by excellent communication between professionals and families with a shared understanding of the issues. Careful consideration is given to the ethical issues arising from the language we use to describe conditions and situations, to variations in ethical issues that arise due to differences in geography or culture and the ethical challenges in the field of safeguarding and child protection. There are clearly indexed separate sections for those wanting to home in on ethical issues relating to specific conditions, different therapies or interventions. The developmental journey continues to adulthood, with issues associated with emerging independence and preparing for adulthood explored in the book's final section.

The editors and authors have together made a hugely important contribution to the childhood disability literature here, with a volume that will sit comfortably on the shelves of practicing clinicians and clinicians in training, nurses, therapists, and policy makers across the globe. It is a book with great potential to change practices for the better, encouraging reflection and improvement in ethical considerations and decision-making. These aspects of 'art' within our clinical practice don't always get the time and attention they deserve in our continuing professional development, but are vital if we are to effectively apply our scientific knowledge in a way that leads to the best outcomes for disabled children, young people and their families.

This, therefore, is a must-have book for everyone who works in the field of clinical childhood disability. There is something for all clinicians, nurses, doctors and therapists, whether in training or established in clinical practice for many years. It 'works' because it is full of real stories of the situations we will all recognise from our own practice, written and edited by internationally renowned and respected clinicians and others with direct experience, who share their 'workings out' of the ethical issues discussed.

I highly commend this book and warmly thank the editors and authors for sharing their wealth of experience with such honesty and compassion.

Dr Karen Horridge
Disability Paediatrician, Sunderland, UK
Chair, British Academy of Childhood Disability

Acknowledgements

Creating a book like this on ethics can only be done as a collaborative effort among many people – and indeed there are many contributors to whom we owe a great debt. Without the enthusiasm and dedication of everyone involved in this project, this book would be very different, if it existed at all!

It will be obvious that we owe a huge debt of gratitude to all the people who contributed to this project. These include members of the American Academy for Cerebral Palsy and Developmental Medicine, the British Academy of Childhood Disability, the European Academy of Childhood Disability, the International Cerebral Palsy Society, Child-Neuro E-Mail List for Child Neurologists and HemiHelp, UK who responded to our survey. People who influenced the creation of this book include both those whose work appears within these covers, and the colleagues who offered us suggestions, potential topics, and drafts of work that did not quite 'fit' the mandate we established with increasing clarity as the process unfolded. Everyone who has written for this book has had the courage and honesty to expose themselves – their thinking and reflections – and to share issues they have actually experienced within the world of child health. As will be recognized, many of these issues may at times be discussed among colleagues, but they are much less often presented publicly with such clarity and openness in this thoughtful and humanistic way.

We want to thank our colleagues at Mac Keith Press for their confidence in us as this project unfolded, and for their unwavering support and wise counsel. They allowed us to fly into a new territory, to exercise our collective skills, and to engage colleagues around the world in this effort. They offered feedback, advice and perspectives on so many aspects of the book – from how best to frame the issues to approaches to promoting it across the world. Their extensive experience in this 'world' of creating books taught us a great deal.

Peter Rosenbaum and Gabriel Ronen also offer very special thanks to our three co-editors. All of us read, commented on and edited every chapter, but these three colleagues offered unique perspectives to expand the scope of this book. Jennifer Johannesen (Chapter 1) is a parent, a gifted communicator and an articulate writer, who shared her personal stories and insights in a way none of the clinical editors could ever do. Eric Racine's experience as an academically trained ethicist enabled him with his pragmatic approach to offer wise insights to our authors and fellow editors as their chapters evolved. His understanding of the clinical situations and dilemmas that are shared herein provided him the material around which to craft Chapter 3. Finally, after the chapters had been accepted, edited and assembled in the order in which they appear, Bernard Dan wrote the Epilogue. Like Jennifer's parental views and Eric's ethicist perspectives, Bernard's chapter provides a summative overview and ideas for how to move forward with the essential responsibilities to address the singularities of our patients' and families' issues with compassion, humility and humanity.

To all of these people, we and our readers owe a special thanks.

PLR and GMR

Chapter 3

Eric Racine acknowledges funding from an FRQ-S senior researcher career award and support from NeuroDevNet. Thanks go to Natalie Zizzo for comments on a previous version of this chapter and to Roxanne Caron and Simon Rousseau-Lesage for editorial assistance.

Introduction

Peter L. Rosenbaum and Gabriel M. Ronen

As a health professional, has this ever happened to you?

- *A family repeatedly fails to keep clinic appointments. Institutional policy indicates that they should be discharged from the program as 'hard to serve'. However, you are uncomfortable with this plan as you sense that there may be extenuating circumstances.*

- *A family demands extra therapy for their child, when the evidence (or the available resources) make this an 'unreasonable' request.*

- *Members of a family disagree with one another about a recommended approach to a clinical management issue, making further action difficult.*

- *Professionals working with a child and family disagree amongst themselves about a proposed course of action.*

- *Your center has a long waiting list, so a family of a 1-year-old with a suspected health or developmental problem will have to wait many months for assessment, and perhaps longer for intervention services.*

- *Professionals often are in a position to need to deliver 'bad news' to a family, and are unsure what the best processes should be.*

- *There are frequently times when people may feel that treatment becomes ineffectual. It is not clear how decisions about this situation should be decided.*

- *You are aware of issues and challenges like the ideas above, and wonder whether there are ethical approaches and algorithms that can help in complex decision-making.*

These brief questions are offered as but a few examples of what we all recognize as everyday realities experienced by healthcare providers in the field of child health, including childhood neurodevelopmental disability. Such challenges are very common, and each can provoke in service providers a mixture of anger, frustration, confusion, fatigue and a wish that there were easy answers to these predicaments experienced by families and by us! We all value and embrace the duty to care that our fields expect of us, but also identify frequent misalignments between that duty and the many complex realities of resources – families' and ours – such as time, human capital, community supports and the many layers of decision-making trajectories that can interfere with best – and ethical – services. Although we value, endorse and try our best to apply principles of 'evidence-based medicine' and to practice within a 'family-centered service' philosophy, neither of these important approaches explicitly provides guidance on how to address the issues outlined above.

This book has been developed with and written by people from a wide range of disciplines and populations who are in the forefront of childhood neurodisability. The goal is to present and discuss case scenarios that describe quotidian clinical issues and challenges, in order to consider them through the lens of ethical principles and practices.[1] We hope to encourage colleagues across the child health spectrum to add ethical perspectives and reflections to the clinical, administrative, fiscal, 'evidence-based medicine' and 'family-centered service' frameworks by which such problems are usually discussed and managed. The book aims to offer to clinicians and other professionals a set of guiding principles that overlap with and complement principles of 'best practice' and practical clinical wisdom.

Goals of the book

- To identify and discuss briefly a number of ethical challenges that arise in everyday practice and are part of the fabric of clinical and policy-making practice in all areas of child health practice. This will allow us to shine a light on the ethical dimensions of issues that we, and others, have often either not recognized, or have ignored, or have been unsure how to address.

- To offer pragmatic principles, frameworks and approaches that underlie sound ethical thinking and practice, and that we hope readers will find useful in their respective spheres of practice and influence.

- To provide approaches to the formulation and analysis of ethical questions in our field.

---

1   The cases presented and discussed in this book represent real people, insofar as the authors are telling stories of their experiences, but all the children and families depicted have been anonymized.

- To explore the intersections between good clinical practice, morality and ethics.
- To help professionals to develop practical ethical thinking that can also be shared with learners.
- To offer the book as a primer for students in the field.

This book is *not* meant to be

- A text on medical ethics
- A recipe book or formula for resolving ethical dilemmas
- A book of 'answers'
- A comprehensive resource for every possible issue or dilemma that can arise in our field
- A philosophical or theoretical treatise
- An account of the ethics of human research
- A compilation of monodisciplinary ethics perspectives

Background: the history of this book

For many years the editorial leadership of Mac Keith Press has been discussing its keen interest to publish a book on the broad topic of 'ethics in childhood neurodisability'. There has never been a shortage of issues with which to explore what we have identified as a wide range of realities in everyday practice. Rather, the challenge for this book was how to settle on an approach, situated within clinical practice, that expands upon the focus commonly placed on these complex issues in child health while taking into account the literature from pragmatic ethicists and philosophers. We hope to illustrate with this book that there are myriad challenging issues in *all* aspects of child health – including but of course not limited to neurodevelopmental disability – that call for ethical reflection, ultimately aimed at improving the nature and quality of practice in the whole field. Thus we hope readers will see that the issues presented and discussed are relevant to all clinical child health services.

People working in our fields are motivated by caring about, and empathy toward, young people with chronic health conditions and their families. Thus, as we began to consider the nature of a book on ethics in neurodisability, we also often came up against the reality that what a clinical audience would regard as 'ethical' practice abuts against – in fact overlaps considerably with – 'good clinical practice'. It is our impression that although we expect clinical practice to be 'ethical', and assume that we behave ethically, we rarely explicitly identify clinical or management issues as requiring an ethical discussion, let alone consult with an ethicist or ethics committee. One challenge for the authors – and perhaps for readers as well – has been to recognize these overlaps, the borderland areas, and the distinctiveness of each set of concerns. In this book, many of the issues that have an ethical dimension can also be seen to reflect effective, empathic, person- and family-centered clinical practice and advocacy. Readers can judge for themselves whether these distinctions are clear and helpful, or indeed whether they are even necessary. It has been our perception that everyday ethical issues can to some extent be contrasted to 'media hype ethics', that is, attention to the complex, highly controversial situations surfacing in clinical practice, and on which bioethics scholarship tends to focus much of its attention. Interactions with ethicists and ethics committees often involve dramatic situations associated with conflicting views and values.

After considerable discussion among the editors, and in collaboration with the Press, surveys were undertaken with members of the organisations listed in the Acknowledgments. From these surveys we were able to solicit the experiences and ideas of a large number of colleagues, whose scenarios and discussions contributed much of the material for this book. We have assembled a connected series of reflective interdisciplinary essays that address issues and challenges experienced in common practice by clinicians and clinical teams, within the perspective that we may think of colloquially as 'ethics at the coalface' or 'in the trenches'.

What do we mean by the ethical dimensions of neurodevelopmental disability?

Mac Keith Press focuses its academic attention on the broad area of neurodevelopmental medicine. For this reason, the material presented in this book has been solicited from health professionals who work in this area of child health. It is important, therefore, to offer a brief contextual background.

There are a number of implications of the contemporary concepts about children and neurodevelopmental disability, described in Chapter 2, that have ethical dimensions that we have explored in this book. We believe that these fundamental shifts in how childhood disability is thought about, assessed and managed should lead to major changes in the field of childhood neurodisability. These changes include, among many, the language of 'disability', the importance of child and family development, the roles and engagement of families as partners with professionals in the Internet age, and the formal recognition of the rights of children and the rights of people with impairments. Among the challenges for the field are how to work ethically within the constraints and regulations of existing systems; how the services and activities of health professionals should be delivered; and what is implied by changes to the organization and provision of services regarding what we do and how we do it. Into this mix fall the ethical dimensions to which this book turns its attention.

Even apparently ordinary interactions and navigation of relationships between professionals and families of children with chronic health conditions (or with the young people themselves) require a thoughtful understanding that potentially everything we do, or do not do, can/does have an ethical dimension. This may be a statement of the obvious, insofar as ethical frameworks should inform all human interaction. Professionals have responsibilities at multiple levels in these relationships, and an awareness of special aspects of vulnerability specifically related to the inherent asymmetry of such relationships. In addition, what we have in mind here are some of the particular complexities of clinical practice when such activities involve populations who have traditionally been marginalized, whose voices have been muted, and whose value to the broader community has been questioned.

Furthermore, in a book meant to be useful to readers around the world, we have been pleased to secure contributions from a wide range of colleagues addressing clinical and ethical matters in ways we believe will be enlightening for everyone. To address these issues in the full light of contemporary thinking requires that these issues be discussed openly – a goal of this book.

The purposes of this book

Given this background about the changing climate of childhood disability and the recognition that ethical dilemmas potentially inhabit every corner of the field, our goal with this book is to explore the interface between good clinical practice and ethical practice, and bring to life some of the ethical issues professionals experience in the field. To do so we have tried to articulate how we see the ethical dimensions of all aspects of clinical practice, and equally to reflect on how ethical principles should inform the further development, structure, concepts and content of the field. We hope to encourage people to consider issues of daily clinical life in the context of the perspectives that our authors have contributed to the continuing development and refinement of the world of neurodisability and the care of children with chronic health conditions. As an outcome of the book, we hope to promote a shared (or at the very least enriched) vision of how we can identify and address ethical issues – including how we can potentially prevent them from doing harm or creating problems – by developing partnerships with families and young people with impairments, and with colleagues, and of course with ethicists!

It is the hope of the editors and publishers of this book that in addition to its exploration of 'everyday' ethical issues and dilemmas in our field, the book will provide material for use as an educational resource. We imagine chapters of the book becoming the focus of discussion in book or journal clubs, and in programs for inter-professional education and collaboration, as a way to bring to light (and to formal consciousness) the kinds of issues our authors have identified and discussed. In fact, these discussions could broaden the ethical arena to include alternative approaches for both the analysis and any potential resolution of dilemmas.

To this end, we have identified three or four 'Themes for Discussion' at the end of most chapter. These issues are in no way meant to be anything more than examples of the kinds of topics we believe should provide continuing opportunities for dialog and discussion. In this way the book may provide educational material and become the kick-off point for conversations among professionals at every stage of their experience, and hopefully also between professionals and program managers, funders and policy-makers. If this happens, the book will have served one of its key purposes.

As with so many of the issues and questions identified in this essay, and in this book, there is rarely a clear answer. There is also usually more than a single ethical aspect to a clinical scenario. The reader will recognize that there is an apparent overlap in some of the clinical scenarios (e.g. those that unfold in the ICU or in rehabilitation settings). However, the subsequent discussions emphasize different ethical aspects. We believe that it is worth asking rhetorically whether, by framing these common clinical challenges within an ethical as well as a service delivery context, we might provoke more, and more serious, discussion of the need to bring these issues forward and resolve them more effectively than is often done.

Chapter 1

A parent's perspective on everyday ethics

Jennifer Johannesen

Prologue

Healthcare providers encounter ethical dilemmas all the time, even if those dilemmas do not make the evening news. This book is a testament to the myriad of these daily challenges. In some cases, dilemmas arise due to difficult decision-making in the face of uncertainty. Other dilemmas surface because, as often happens, reasonable people can disagree, or because someone – a practitioner or family member – has questioned or challenged the status quo. As a parent of a child with severe impairments, I am heartened by this inquiry and the authors' desire to illuminate these 'everyday' challenges faced by healthcare providers. Not only might readers recognize themselves or their patients in the scenarios but they may also discover a wealth of creative approaches to address these dilemmas. Raising awareness of ethical issues in everyday clinical encounters can only serve to benefit the relationships between providers, patients and caregivers, and to improve outcomes for patients and their families.

However, the approach to compiling this book – inviting healthcare providers to recount and analyze their own ethical dilemmas – is not without some risk. For example, we might erroneously consider these self-identified dilemmas to be comprehensive or complete; or we might misunderstand a particular creative solution to be the *right* solution, or the *only* solution; or we might miss other ethical dilemmas that cannot be seen when launching this inquiry from the perspective of the healthcare provider or institution. Although we might be tempted to assume that a well-considered ethical analysis is inherently bias-free (or, rather, includes all known and relevant perspectives), we might also consider that ethical questions raised by the family, or by the patient, might invite entirely different questions.

For example, an institution's concerns about resource allocation may raise questions about ventilator use, while a parent's concerns regarding resource allocation may raise questions about how to divide her time between her children (with and without impairments). A clinician may judge that a particular treatment is not worth the risk, while a parent wants to show her child she is doing everything she can to help them; in this case, their notions of beneficence are quite different. We might also consider a growing debate in the literature about use of the 'best interests' standard (e.g. Rhodes & Holzman 2014; Veatch 1995), which cannot be determined without a value judgment of what 'best' means, or even of what 'interests' mean. In other words, we ought to consider that an expression of interest in ethical inquiry must also be assumed to be an expression of bias. Perhaps this is unavoidable: the inquiry must be launched from *somewhere*.

Many of the scenarios described in this book are recognizable to me as the primary decision-maker in my young son's years-long, intensive journey through pediatric medicine, neurology, neurosurgery, developmental services and therapy. Although I experienced them from the other side – the patient's side – the scenes feel familiar. At the time, I could sometimes see that there was a dilemma *of some kind* going on, but I would not have known the specific concerns as identified by the healthcare provider. As a parent, I was contemplating issues of a different sort.

In this chapter, I will suggest some areas for ethical consideration that may not be immediately obvious to healthcare providers when self-identifying ethical issues. I will also be referencing personal anecdotes to illustrate these issues, and so must start with a brief background of our family.

Family background

My son Owen, my first child, was born in 1998. He had already had a complicated journey – he had hydrops fetalis, requiring chest and abdominal shunts (inserted *in utero*) to relieve accumulating fluid. His birth was preterm (at 32 wks) and he stayed in the neonatal intensive-care unit (NICU) for three months.

Owen did not develop typically. He missed milestone after milestone, never gaining functional control of his trunk, head or extremities. He required full assistance for all aspects of daily living: he was non-ambulatory, incontinent and deaf; he had virtually no functional use of his hands; he received a percutaneous gastrostomy tube (or g-tube) around 4 years of age and an intrathecal baclofen pump when he was 9 years of age (the pump malfunctioned and was later removed); and he had fully supportive assistive equipment, including a stander, neck-and-head support and a custom wheelchair. His health was surprisingly robust, with the exception of frequent aspiration pneumonias. (His respiratory health improved significantly after he got his g-tube.)

Owen had a brother, Angus, who was 2 years younger. Angus was Owen's chief companion and advocate, proudly holding his hand or pushing his wheelchair, shrugging off stares from other kids and criticizing adults for talking to Owen 'like a baby'. My partner Michael was an active father and deeply accepting of who Owen was. I was in charge of Owen's routines and therapies, and ensured he received exemplary care, services and treatment. Michael and I separated in 2007, but quickly established a friendly and consistent routine of sharing care of the boys, with Owen's caregivers working with him wherever he happened to be.

Owen died in 2010, at the age of 12. His death took us all by surprise, as he had been in good general health for the previous year or two and did not appear frail. He died sometime in the night, while the household slept. His official cause of death was sudden unexpected death from epilepsy (SUDEP) (see Chapter 27), which according to the coroner was admittedly a diagnosis of elimination. (Owen had not had a seizure since he was an infant.)

We were not disappointed by the lack of diagnosis. Throughout his life, Owen's constellation of symptoms was never diagnosed as anything other than cerebral palsy, yet there was no evidence of brain injury, congenital anomaly or other clues that might lead us to an underlying cause for his impairments. We were used to not knowing.

I think most of our healthcare providers would agree: I appeared to be a confident, capable decision-maker and caregiver. I was decisive, generally unsentimental, and open to being wrong if provided with facts. We were, in many ways, an ideal 'patient family' – we were engaged and cooperative, with few social, cultural or financial barriers to pursue treatments or therapies. My decisions were never questioned because I seemed so knowledgeable and *reasonable*.

In this context, my parental decision-making autonomy appeared to be complete. However, as illustrated by the following anecdotes, I was perhaps not as informed as I thought I was.

Policy nudges

When Owen was diagnosed with profound hearing loss

Owen 'failed' his auditory evoked potentials while still in the NICU. His profound hearing loss was confirmed when he was around 2 years old. I remember how the audiologist sat us down to deliver the news. 'I'm sorry', she said, eyes downcast. She let us know that someone would be in touch soon, to discuss next steps. After all we'd been through with Owen, the audiologist's apology seemed unnecessarily grim – we were pleased to have Owen home with us and generally healthy. We did not think of the diagnosis as a 'problem'.

Two weeks later I received an excited call from the hearing clinic at the hospital. We were asked to come in for an information session, now that we were on the list. I paused before responding: 'What list?'

The hospital clinic automatically placed children with profound hearing loss on the cochlear implant waiting list. They were keen to get new children assessed and 'processed' quickly. When we attended the information session, we found out why: the clinic had received funding to do a certain number of implants in a certain amount of time. The allotted time was coming to an end, and the surgeon wanted to move through the waiting list before the deadline. His presentation during the information session was focused on this funding.

Later, I asked our assigned social worker why Owen was placed on the cochlear implant list when it had never been discussed. She seemed surprised at the question, and reminded us that the cochlear implant is what the hospital provides as treatment for profound hearing loss. According to the hospital, the cochlear implant was simply 'the next step'.

A parent's perspective

After this experience, I became wary of process and protocol. I wondered how many other times I had been subtly guided toward 'decisions' without even noticing. What is most noteworthy here is that I only noticed the 'nudge' because I did not think Owen's hearing loss was a problem. I had *reason* to second-guess the default assumption that I would want to pursue the cochlear implant. Other families who did pursue the cochlear implant may *not* have had reason to question this treatment, and possibly many were satisfied and would not have decided otherwise. However, the ethical problem remains: informed decision-making and patient autonomy are compromised when an in-built process assumes that a particular treatment will follow, which can easily be perceived (and adopted by the parent) as a *decision*.

It is plausible that healthcare providers may be unaware that these policy nudges are in place. It is also plausible that policies like these are developed to aid efficiency: could it be that at one point a patient had been overlooked, necessitating automatic referral to the waiting list for everyone after that?

Policies and procedures may have unintended consequences, and it is worthwhile to query the effects of 'due process' at all stages. Healthcare providers could investigate the path of referral, both into and out of the clinic, to discover if there are hidden nudges or influences that may compromise parent or patient informed consent. Additionally, healthcare providers may inquire of parents and families as to how they arrived at their decisions, allowing providers to evaluate the integrity (and consequences) of institutional policy as it relates to shared decision-making.

Broken communication

The DBS consultation

Owen's dystonia and spasticity were compounded problems – one made the other worse. He had already had an intrathecal baclofen pump, which had malfunctioned and had been removed. His spasticity, then, was untreated and his dystonia made his discomfort worse. His unpredictable movements also made carrying and caring for him difficult. His neurologist suggested we learn more about deep brain stimulation (DBS). We were referred to a neurosurgical specialist.

When we arrived, the specialist checked Owen over. She weighed him, moved his limbs, inquired about his movements, asked about his general health and medical history. When she was finished, she made her announcement: 'Yes, he would be a good candidate'. The surgery might have a positive effect on his movements. She went on to tell us about the supporting data, research and statistics. Then she stopped and simply looked at us, waiting for a response.

Her 'yes' had come so quickly that Michael and I felt a little stunned. I also felt sad about the prospect of another surgery, particularly one I perceived to be risky. We began to discuss next steps when I realized how quickly I had gotten ahead of myself. I reminded myself that we were there to find out if DBS was a good option for Owen, not if Owen was going to be a good candidate for DBS – a subtle but important difference. The specialist, on the other hand, was doing an assessment. I was asking if we should, and she was answering if we can.

How quickly I heard the 'yes' to mean that she was recommending the surgery specifically for Owen!

A parent's perspective
As healthcare produces more and more subspecialties, parents must learn to navigate an ever-growing myriad of appointments, facilities and approaches. In some ways, this is the easy part of having a child with complex needs; we become very skilled at managing busy schedules. Despite this efficiency, parents can remain fairly naïve or inexperienced at evaluating the *merits* of consultations, the *quality* of interactions and the *intentions* of the parties involved (to name just a few aspects worth assessing). Parents would do

well to ask themselves, What is the purpose of this meeting? Is it necessary for me or my child? What do I need to know? Am I expected to make a decision during the meeting? Am I prepared to make a decision?

At the appointment described above, the specialist and I were essentially talking past one another. She was answering a different question than the one I had in mind, yet neither of us realized it at first. We were using the same terms, referring to the same child and discussing the same procedure, yet we had different motivations, and therefore were seeking different answers.

Parents of a child like Owen often function as a link between specialists, risking a 'broken telephone' effect of miscommunication and misunderstanding. Had I not caught my own misassumptions, I may very well have told our neurologist that the neurosurgeon strongly recommended the surgery. Thus a 'new' truth would have been born, attached to words the neurosurgeon had never said.

Admittedly, this is tricky territory. This is more than a matter of parental understanding or comprehension, which may be rather easier to parse out. Instead, this may be a matter of differing motivations, resulting in a kind of information distortion. Although we might be assured that all parties are aligned to a single vision of supporting the child, parents may not be especially attuned to noticing when they are unconsciously trying to match what they *hear* to what they *want*. In these moments, it is essential that healthcare providers are rigorous in their attention to transparency about their own roles, interests and motivations. By doing so, the healthcare provider helps to support and preserve a parent's ability to make informed decisions.

Autonomy without guidance

Owen's struggles with feeding

By the time Owen was 4 years old, he was exceptionally thin. Feeding continued to be extremely difficult: he aspirated liquids and solids alike, could not chew effectively, and had razor-sharp teeth (due to acid wear from reflux) that cut through his lips and inner cheeks. If he was sick, it was almost impossible to get him to ingest antibiotics, pain relievers or any other medications; because of his reflux, he often vomited whatever food we could get into him. Yet, I was determined to persist in feeding him by mouth. Not once in our frequent feeding clinic appointments was a g-tube mentioned. Instead, after every swallow study, I was given careful instructions for thickening his liquids, pureeing his solids, timing his swallows, positioning his head and neck, and encouraging chewing. I was praised for 'sticking with it'.

On one (final) occasion, I was given instructions that, if followed, required that I feed Owen for over 6 hours every day! I confided in a friend (who was also a nurse) – she encouraged me to ask about getting a g-tube. I was resistant at first, insisting that because it was never suggested, he didn't need it. Eventually I gave in. After an assessment (at my request), we arranged for the procedure to be done in the coming weeks. With the g-tube, Owen gained weight, his sleep improved and his aspiration pneumonias became much less frequent.

A parent's perspective

Even though I appeared to be 'doing fine' with feeding, Owen was not fully thriving. He was underweight and sickly, he was not getting all of his medications orally, and we were exhausted from feeding difficulties. Furthermore, the doctor who recommended our feeding plan failed to notice how much time would be required to feed Owen according to his prescribed schedule. I believe that because I was a confident, determined parent, and because I didn't complain, an appropriate alternative to feeding was never suggested. I interpreted the silence to mean that he didn't need a g-tube, and therefore did not ask about it until I was desperate.

In this situation, it could never be suggested that I did not have full autonomy – it was indeed my choice to feed Owen orally, and my choice to request a g-tube. However, we might also see that I was in need of honest counsel (to see our reality) and supportive encouragement (to explore other options), neither of which I received from our feeding specialists.

By providing autonomy *alone*, without professional advice or guidance, healthcare providers may unintentionally be compromising the ability of parents to provide optimal care for their child. In my opinion, parents (particularly those with children with complex needs) need professional guidance and advice – *sometimes, even when unsolicited* – in order to make informed decisions. This may include 'giving parents permission' to consider alternatives that they might either not have known existed or at times were hesitant to voice aloud.

A parent's perspective on everyday ethics

The anecdotes described above only skim the surface in considering ethics. In the three vignettes, a reader may agree that things did not seem quite right – but could we consider them to be ethical dilemmas *per se*? Did any one healthcare provider act poorly, or unethically?

In truth, my interpersonal exchanges with healthcare providers, in the context of caring for my son, were generally positive, respectful and at times even enjoyable. Indeed, I am grateful for the life-saving care we received and the compassion and consideration with which it was offered. My relationships with our healthcare providers were friendly; I had no doubt that everyone on our various interdisciplinary medical teams could be trusted professionally and had my son's best (healthcare) interests at heart; I encountered no bad actors, and no mal-intent.

I believe, however, that we were primarily successful in the healthcare environment because I engaged with it *according to its own terms*. My role as 'expert parent' was carefully constructed by me to ensure that I would be heard, understood and respected. I made efforts to appear calm and organized. This was rewarded with congratulations and appreciation – recognition of a job well done, with (I imagine) not a small sigh of relief that I continued to be an 'easy' parent to counsel. Although I inserted myself actively into every clinical discussion, I was not a source of resistance or friction — I did not argue, disagree, or make demands. Instead, I *negotiated* mutually acceptable terms in order to effect good outcomes for my son and my family, and this was positively received. The Family-Centred Care model was perhaps constructed with outcomes like ours in mind, where parents not only participate in decision-making, but formulate questions, educate themselves and ultimately (feel they) make satisfying, informed choices on their child's behalf (Kuo et al. 2012).

If, then, I was the ideal parent-as-advocate, what should we make of the vignettes I have just presented? To be clear, these are just three of dozens of stories I might have told. The common thread I identify throughout is that, despite my own in-the-moment positive feelings of empowerment and autonomy, I was unaware of those mechanisms that made decisions on my behalf, or that nudged me in certain directions. In other words, I was invited to make decisions only at times that were deemed appropriate by the healthcare system (and the healthcare provider), and was denied visibility into what factors informed a healthcare provider's recommendations. From a classic bioethics perspective, this easily challenges well-accepted principles of beneficence, justice and autonomy (Beauchamp & Childress 2012).

Many essays in this book present the contemplations of a healthcare provider in a clinical setting; the authors evaluate a challenging situation, consider what could occur next, and weigh options through an ethical lens or framework. In some cases, these contemplations are a direct result of parental 'friction', of the sort I mention above. It is interesting to note that many of these accounts are about families from vulnerable or disenfranchised populations. In these pages, we see dilemmas arising from encounters with families living in poverty, mothers with addiction issues, patients from different cultural backgrounds, and parents with varying levels of acceptance of evidence-based medicine. These cases certainly present personal ethical dilemmas for healthcare providers in terms of how best to manage a challenging situation, and most are handled with sensitivity and honest self-reflection. However, we should not disregard the fact that these clinician-identified ethical dilemmas are triggered by acts of 'non-compliance' by parents, notably ones who do not conform to cultural norms.

We should not accept as *coincidence* that the views of 'ideal' parents – parents who conduct themselves well – seem to be more readily accepted.[1]

A close reading of these chapters may invite the question of whether we are addressing ethical dilemmas specifically (for example, 'I am facing an ethical problem and don't know what to do') or if we are rather evaluating ethical frameworks and solutions to common challenges of living in a diverse society (for example, 'What is an ethical response to this difficult situation?'). Does this distinction matter? Perhaps not, if we are primarily concerned with supporting problem-solving for the healthcare provider. I suggest, however, that addressing clinical challenges with ethical approaches is not enough; we should not absolve ourselves from the perhaps more daunting task of remedying – indeed, working to prevent – ethical problems in the wider healthcare system in which these challenges occur, and which compromise parents' ability to care for their child.

Epilogue

When considering clinical encounters through an ethics lens, healthcare providers usually make an effort to include the family or parents' perspective. This helps to provide a more robust ethical analysis, which will hopefully lead to optimal or improved decisions or outcomes. However, the healthcare providers' *interpretation* of the parents' perspective may not be the same as the parents' perspective *itself*.

In this chapter, I have highlighted moments in which healthcare providers may find opportunities to support a parent's informed decision-making and autonomy. The three issues I identified – policy nudges, broken communication and autonomy without guidance – are just the tip of the iceberg; further exploration of parent and family perspectives will surely yield more, as will close examination of ethics as enacted (or not) by the wider healthcare system.

The project of this book is to explore everyday clinical situations, cases and scenarios through an ethical lens or framework, to discover ways in which healthcare providers can improve relationships with parents, outcomes for their patients, and their own

---

1   Despite my positive relationships with healthcare providers generally, I could easily have been the subject of one of the chapters in this book, as a parent whose decisions did not align with our healthcare providers' recommendations. In Owen's later years, I chose to withdraw him from many therapeutic programs and interventions, pursuing only those therapies that addressed specific medical problems. This was due in large part to my growing dissatisfaction with therapies aimed at normalizing Owen, rather than supporting him in his differences. I wrote about this extensively in *No Ordinary Boy* (Johannesen 2011). I believe I was not challenged on these decisions because, as mentioned earlier, I was considered an ideal parent. (Nonetheless, some of these decisions on my part may have been interpreted differently by our healthcare providers.)

self-reflexive skills (to name just a few of the possible benefits). Certainly this is a laudable task. However, we must be careful to not allow 'ethics' to become merely a problem-solving tool, or a blunt instrument by which to earn trust from parents. I think parents can sense these efforts, which may lead to or reinforce skepticism and distrust. For ethics to be meaningful and substantive, it should rather be part of an overarching *ethos* of transparency and respect that infuses all interactions, processes and systems – even if there is no dilemma at hand.

References

Beauchamp TL, Childress, JF (2012) *Principles of biomedical ethics* 7th edn. New York, NY: Oxford University Press.

Johannesen, J (2011) *No ordinary boy*. Toronto: Low to the Ground.

Kuo DZ, Houtrow AJ, Arango P, Kuhlthau KA, Simmons JM, Neff JM. (2012) Family-centered care: Current applications and future directions in pediatric health care. *Matern Child Health J* 16: 297–305.

Rhodes R, Holzman IR (2014) Is the best interest standard good for pediatrics? *Pediatrics* 134(Suppl 2): S121–S129.

Veatch RM (1995) Abandoning informed consent. *The Hastings Center Report* 25: 5–12.

Chapter 2

Present-day health and neurodevelopmental disability

Peter L. Rosenbaum and Gabriel M. Ronen
with contributions by Barbara J. Cunningham

Prologue

The neurodevelopment conditions of childhood are often accompanied by enormous challenges and a sense of hopelessness, frustration and failure for persons with impairments, their families, healthcare providers, the community and society at large (Young Bradshaw 2015). The past quarter century has seen a number of significant developments in the field of neurodevelopmental disability. These include broad conceptual shifts about health, functioning, quality of life and legal rights for persons with disabilities, as well as developments relating specifically to children or to the idea of 'disability'. Many of these ideas have emerged gradually and imperceptibly, while others have appeared to be more dramatic and potentially transformative. In this book, we wish to highlight a number of the less apparent changes and developments in the field that have informed our thinking.

Trends and concepts about health, disability and 'evidence'
- Our concept of 'health' has evolved beyond the WHO's 1946 definition – health as 'a state of complete physical, mental and social wellbeing'[1] – toward a conceptualization as a continuous scale of 'the ability of persons to function in

1 Preamble to the Constitution of the World Health Organization as adopted by the International Health Conference, New York, 19–22 June 1946; signed on 22 July 1946 by the representatives of 61 States (Official Records of the World Health Organization, no. 2, p. 100) and entered into force on 7 April 1948.

a manner acceptable to themselves, in ways that include their expectations and opportunities, even in the presence of impairments' (Huber et al. 2011).

- We value a focus on the approaches proposed by the WHO's International Classification of Functioning, Disability and Health (ICF and ICF-CY; WHO 2001, 2007, respectively), including ICF-related concepts such as taking a strengths-based approach to people with impairments and their families, recognizing the importance of functioning and participation.

- Acknowledging the social determinants of health, there is now an explicit interest in the contextual role of 'environment' – in fact the many environments and socio-ecological factors (human, structural, physical and sociopolitical) that influence the lives of people, including those with impairments and their families. This focus includes an imperative to try to change and improve the environment as well as (indeed sometimes instead of) the person or the impairment (Baumeister & Leary 1995; Harris 1995; Parker et al. 1995).

- The 'disability paradox', a term coined by Albrecht and Devlieger (1999), is another related concept. Those authors and others showed that there is an increasing body of evidence that indicates that it is difficult to attribute better or poorer health and quality of life solely to the biological aspects of a disease and its medical treatment. In fact, many individuals with impairments, including children, consider their life to be as satisfactory and fulfilling as that of individuals from the general population (Mezgebe et al. 2015).

- There has been recognition of the moral responsibility that people with impairments and disabilities must not be undervalued, and that their legal rights must be respected. These developments have been illustrated by major international organizations, while important civil and criminal lawsuits in North America provide evidence of the ethical imperative that now must inform all our actions. These concepts recognize the personhood and autonomy of children, including those with impairments. They include the UN Convention on the Rights of the Child (United Nations 1989) and the UN Convention on the Rights of Persons with Disabilities (United Nations 2006). The European Parliament and many individual countries around the world have endorsed these conventions (Jennings 2013).

- The introduction of evidence-based medicine, including the development of valid child- and parent-reported outcome measures and carefully designed studies, as well as the development of approaches and frameworks in medical ethics, are opening opportunities for novel empirical research such as enabling narratives, capturing the perspectives and experiences of stakeholders, and involving interdisciplinary deliberations (Hanisch 2013). However, in this era where evidence often evolves or changes constantly, we need to recognize that these shifting sands create clinical and ethical caution where the 'best available evidence' is only present 'for a fleeting moment in time' (Noritz 2015).

How do we think and talk about childhood disability?
- Although there is still a long way to go, modern thinking increasingly recognizes children with impairments as valued members of society, with identification of their vulnerability, the challenges they face regarding disease and disability, and the responsibilities of professionals as well as the 'community' and policy-makers to support these young people and empower them to emerge successfully from their journey through childhood able to take their rightful place as adults in their communities (Turnbull et al. 2001).

- Children are now increasingly being recognized as autonomous participants in their own care, for which informed consent, assent and dissent can be obtained, and informed choices are given within shared and participatory clinical approaches (Leikin 1983; De Lourdes Levy et al. 2003).

The role of the family and quality of life
- We recognize the importance – indeed the primacy – of the family across all areas of child health, with the expectation that the services we offer should be 'family-centered'. Among the implications of this change in practice are the challenges posed to professionals, traditionally empowered to be 'experts', who now are being expected to be 'partners' with the people who 'have it' – because we now seek, and hopefully listen to, those voices. We also recognize the need to invite families to participate in decision-making by them and about them (Hoffmann et al. 2014).

- In healthcare generally, and notably in the field of childhood disability, there is an increasing focus on 'quality of life' and subjective well-being (Renwick 2013; Ryff & Keyes 1995), and especially individuals' self-reported valuation of their own lives (Lohr & Zebrack 2009). This is happening in the face of impairments and functional challenges that traditionally were viewed with a combination of pity and negative judgments about the (lesser) 'value' of the people who experience these impairments. This development has major implications for what health professionals say and do, and how we value fellow humans with both visible and invisible functional challenges.

The nature of services for children and youth with developmental disabilities
- All our work in childhood neurodisability is done within settings that value – in fact demand – interdisciplinary perspectives, teamwork and collaboration, empathy, and of course privacy and confidentiality.

- We are no longer simply trying to 'fix' impairments (usually an impossible and naïve idea) or to promote 'normal' or 'complete' function; rather, we strive to optimize functional capacity and performance, motivate young people to enhance their capability, promote good quality of life and enhance societal participation.

- With increasing attention to screening for neurodevelopmental impairments (often performed prenatally as well as in early postnatal life) and early intervention, there is at times a considerable element of uncertainty about whether a child in fact has a problem, whether and how to describe and label the situation, and what to do in the face of the often-imperfect diagnostics and interventions currently available or offered.

The ethical dimensions of neurodevelopmental disability: a child and family's journey into childhood 'disability'

One logical way to consider opportunities to identify ethical issues in clinical practice in developmental disability is to reflect on the journey that a child and family often follow from the time of first concern or suspicion of a fetus or child's impairment to their full engagement with programs and services, often over several years. This set of ideas is scarcely exhaustive, but is offered to encourage people to recognize what other healthcare professionals have identified as the 'ethics in childhood neurodisability'. These are issues we frequently encounter and for which we may search for an appropriate ethical framework to assist us to analyze and resolve such situations successfully. We have tried to provide a few examples of the myriad ways in which clinical practice in developmental disability raises issues we believe have an important ethical dimension.

How does a family's journey into 'developmental disability' begin?
Initial encounters between a family and the 'system' happen when a family is referred to services because of concerns about a child's impaired development, worrisome symptoms or tests (usually based on the parents' own observations), and a family seeks answers. Their entry into the system may happen quickly and smoothly, but more often than not in many parts of the world there are long waiting lists for initial or specialist assessments, let alone intervention. Needless to say, for a family with worries about their child's health or developmental status, the waiting is likely to add tremendously to the existing uncertainties and emotional turmoil. Furthermore, in young children suspected of having disorders that threaten their developmental progress, time is certainly of the essence. Delays to access appropriate diagnostic and intervention services can be deleterious for the child and their family and can be unethical. (It is helpful to recall the classic maxim 'Primum non nocere' (first do no harm), one of the principal precepts of medical ethics on which all healthcare students and presumably other practitioners in training, are raised from early in our education. Thus it is fair to ask: do waiting lists do 'harm'?)

Of course, long waiting lists are usually a systems issue rather than the sole responsibility of individual practitioners. One might ask, however, about the opportunity for front-line

practitioners to help to identify, advocate, address and remedy this concerning and developmentally inappropriate reality. To the extent that these early encounters may be formative for a child and family, there is an argument for at least considering this issue as an ethical dilemma regarding resource allocation. There is no doubt that accelerating services at the front end may create challenges elsewhere in the system, but we believe that developing (and of course then evaluating) alternative models of service delivery that 'front-load' the engagement of child and family with the health and therapy systems may be beneficial, even if this happens at the 'expense' of later visits (the nature and frequency of which could and should be the focus of other discussions).

The processes of assessment and communication
When the family and child are first seen, a host of assessments are traditionally planned and carried out. Assessments may be needed for diagnostic purposes (e.g. What exactly are we dealing with?). They may enable us to understand the extent of the issues (e.g. How serious is it?). They can allow us to obtain a comprehensive understanding of the ways in which this condition is affecting this child and family. Other assessments, particularly in relation to chronic conditions, are useful to describe the levels of function, though these too often focus on describing the ways in which function is impaired rather than using a strengths-based assessment to describe what is 'working' for that person.

Thus, a traditional approach to assessment in childhood neurodisability has been to identify – often in considerable detail – the problems/challenges/deficits that children (and indeed sometimes their families) are found to have. Many people may still feel that this approach is a necessary starting point for treatment and management. One might, however, ask whether knowing what is 'wrong' will help practitioners to know what is 'right', what 'works' and what strengths the child and family demonstrate, as well as what goals and interventions are valued by parents. Reconsidering the processes by which assessments are done – emphasizing child and family strengths rather than focusing on problems – can also provide opportunities for the discussion of ethically appropriate alternative ways to communicate with families and to build trust.

This leads to the following question: Is it appropriate – is it ethical – to focus pre-dominantly on problems (which are, of course, the parents' prime concerns and why they are referred to our services)? The ethical challenge might be framed as the extent to which we are able and willing to create a 'balanced scorecard'. Such an approach to assessment and the formulation of a 'case' would begin with an account of child and family strengths and the love they have for each other. It would also identify parents' values and concerns, and it would propose intervention plans with the family using these details as building blocks. In other words, there is an opportunity for both individual practitioners and service programs to consider the basic assumptions we make about our work, and about how we wish to think about 'childhood disability': whether to continue taking a deficit approach, or to change to an approach that considers differences and opportunities to exploit best abilities, even in the face of impairments.

Another potential ethical issue in investigation and assessment includes questions about whose needs are being served, especially when investigations are undertaken that may be 'interesting' for the clinician but less important to the family (Mac Keith 1967). Some of the questions posed at assessment may be of greater importance to the clinician or researcher than they are relevant to child and family (e.g. What are the biomedical or psychological underpinnings of this condition?). These considerations can become particularly acute when costs in terms of money or risk are involved. There is also a potential to uncover findings (too easily assumed to be 'abnormalities') of uncertain meaning (as can happen, for example, with genetic panels, whole exome sequencing or imaging studies), possibly leading to a need for further explorations to define these unanticipated findings. What are our responsibilities to the child and family when these unanticipated findings appear. Do we communicate the fact and possible meaning of these findings (often while facing uncertainty), and if so, how (Gupta et al. 2010)?

Diagnosis, formulation and prognostication
In a clinical field fraught with imprecision and uncertainty due to the complexity of the conditions under consideration, there are often challenges associated with making a clear and precise biomedical diagnosis. Many of the conditions with which we have experience (e.g. cerebral palsy, epilepsy, autism spectrum disorder or intellectual impairment) are typically described or labeled phenomenologically as syndromes, and are discussed in terms of impaired function or certain features rather than being characterized with the kind of biomedical precision possible in some areas of medicine (e.g. by identifying specific biological mechanisms). This has implications when it comes to counseling families about 'treatment', because, sadly, there are still huge gaps in our knowledge of what approaches work best, for whom, at what age and stage of their development, and for what goals. Equally challenging are the limitations in our ability to address the prognosis for many of the disabling impairments of childhood where in the absence of systematic evidence-informed data, especially across the life span, we rely on experience, perhaps skewed toward the more complex end of the spectrum based on our work in specialty centers.

With respect to the outcome stage of the assessment phase of the family's journey, what are our ethical responsibilities regarding prognostication? Describing an expected biomedical or developmental prognosis might be ethically challenging in the absence of an understanding of the 'person' in whom the 'condition' is found (Jan & Girvin 2002). How comfortable are we with delivering uncertainty, ambiguity and 'bad news'? What are our responsibilities to families when we know clearly what the situation is (based on a definitive diagnosis) compared to when the clinical story is unclear? These rhetorical questions are raised to identify opportunities for training ourselves, and each other, in the ethical conduct of these practical but challenging aspects of work in neurodisability, where uncertainty is such a common companion on the family's, and our, journey. Whether they want to or not, today's families easily become medical experts of their child's condition and thus expect to be full partners in the medical team's decisions.

Discussing the future
Predicting future trajectories is thus another everyday ethical issue that warrants discussion. There is a school of thought that argues that we owe it to families to honestly lay out the 'realities' or 'truth' of their child's situation, perhaps rather starkly, and not give 'false hope'. An alternative mode of thought recommends an approach called 'prognostication' on an individualized basis, talking (for example) about 'this child with these manifestations of CP' and not about 'CP' in general (Siegler 1975). Furthermore, before discussing prognosis it is essential to understand the family's long-term expectations and goals as nested within their values and culture. The literature on 'truth disclosure' (discussed in detail in this book) is consistent in identifying this essential part of the family's experience as a process rather than an event.

It is our belief that this process of communicating well with families is a very important part of how we treat people, and sets a tone for a family's levels of trust and respect for – or, sadly, their distrust and suspicion of – the professionals with whom they subsequently come into contact. We believe that this is fundamentally an issue of empathic care and an ethical issue regarding the behavior and attitudes of both professionals and the systems in which we work. Experts have written extensively on this topic, recommending that professionals communicate with warmth and compassion, talking with both parents together, in private, at a pace they can handle, reporting our current level of knowledge or lack thereof – though not necessarily telling every detail we know at a first visit – using plain non-jargonized language and providing enough time and opportunities for questions and clarification of the issues being presented (Levetown et al. 2008). A follow-up appointment within a few days – with the grandparents and other people important to the family present whenever possible – can be an incredibly helpful opportunity for further 'telling' and clarifying the issues.

While communication with families is critical, communication between colleagues is another ethical issue that needs to be considered (Clarke et al. 2007). When a professional new to the child and family undertakes new evaluations, and especially when they repeat what has already been done in prior settings, parents often ask us 'Don't you people talk to one another?'. When we fail to communicate effectively with our co-professionals, and to trust the findings uncovered by capable colleagues, we can convey a lack of faith in others and also raise concerns that there must be more to be learned before people are ready and able to act. On the other hand, how much concrete information do we need in order to develop and implement a management plan that addresses functional issues regarding, for example, enhancing independence, communication or self-help skills? How many (really how few) of our interventions to promote these functioning goals are condition-specific? Parents have often said they want less assessment and more treatment. What then is an ethically defensible balance between assessment and management? Might the use of electronic medical records contribute to better communication – assuming people do their homework before a child is assessed?

Organization and delivery of services
There are important implications in the way that hospital-based or community services are organized and made available to children with neurodisabilities and their families. All programs and services have to deal with waiting lists, and make a host of decisions about the best approaches to cope with them. These decisions include, as but a few examples, inclusion and exclusion criteria for a program; defining the catchment area from which children and families will/will not be seen; whether to give priority to children with certain diagnoses, or age groups, or those who qualify for the clinical services of the region. The list is long and challenging.

The structure, nature and quality of the services should all have an ethical foundation. Does the service provide only assessment and consultation back to the referral source? What follow-up services are/should be provided, and for what length of time after assessment? Do the specialty services create a dependency for children and families? What are the professional pressures we face as service providers – on the one hand, long waiting lists, and on the other a need to know what happens to the children and families we see when they are starting their journey into the world of neurodisability and later on in life? There are also major issues associated with the way services are funded and paid for in different communities, where the availability of services may be significantly impacted by policies concerning these issues.

A structural challenge: assessment only or assessment and follow-up?
Some programs undertake assessment as a prelude to ongoing management and follow-up in which they expect to retain some involvement. There are, however, 'assessment centers' in which a detailed assessment is carried out and findings are reported to the referring person, followed by discharge of the family to that referral source for continuing management and care. Whether a program undertakes both assessment and follow-up, or provides only a detailed specialty assessment, there are complex ethical issues to be considered. For this reason, decisions about which strategy to employ in one's practice or community can be (should be) framed and examined through an ethical lens.

Assessment and ongoing management require human resources, which take time and energy that could otherwise be directed to the needs of the next family on the waiting list. Decisions about taking this approach to service provision should be made with the clear recognition that an active ethically informed choice to provide assessment and management has been made regarding how this program will contribute its resources to the fabric of the community's services for children with impairments and their families.

On the other hand, a single assessment process followed by discharge to others in the community can be equally challenging for everyone concerned. However excellent the clinical assessors and their processes have been, their evaluation of a situation provides essentially a point-in-time snapshot of the child's and family's issues, done outside their own environment. There are several reasons for at least one or two follow-up appointments after an initial evaluation visit. Such a process allows the professionals to review with the family whatever disclosures took place at the first visit, and enables the family to ask the questions that may have emerged following the first visit. This is also an opportunity for the family to clarify the nature of the condition and the plans for management, to consider their long-term goals pertaining to the medical plans, and to review whatever questions they may have about short- and long-term prognosis, potentially when alternative medical treatment methods are also being considered. Equally importantly, the professionals can ask the family to recount what they heard at the initial assessment, what they have learned about their child's situation from friends, family and the Internet, and what additional issues they now want to discuss.

Another dimension of the process of follow-up concerns the opportunity for the professionals to experience and learn about the progression of the child and family on their journey into the world of childhood neurodisability. Are the initial formulations about the clinical situation in fact accurate, or are there new developments that might amplify or indeed change what was originally seen and considered? How well can the management plans be implemented in the family's home community, and are they having the expected effects on functioning and comfort, or should the strategy be modified in some way? How is a family adjusting to the reality of their child's impairments? There is a long list of important questions, issues and learning possibilities, and these issues can only (or certainly best) be addressed with follow-up visits with the disclosing professionals.

It is therefore worth considering the ethical question of whether 'assessment' alone serves families best, or whether at times it creates more challenges than it resolves.

A framework for decision-making in planning treatment and management
In childhood neurodisability we have traditionally applied the classical clinical paradigm that leads us directly from making an accurate diagnosis to recommending a relative specific intervention, with much less success. First, 'diagnosis' in many areas of

developmental impairment may at best provide descriptive names of conditions rather than being able to specify precise biomedical entities that afford a direct connection to biomedically-based treatments.

Consider two of many examples. 'Cerebral palsy' and 'autism' describe phenomenological patterns of impaired function, but do not themselves identify a specific entity, biomedical substratum or management approach clearly based on biological processes. The same can also be said for many of the epilepsies. Diagnoses like Duchenne dystrophy, fragile-X syndrome, neurofibromatosis type 1, or Down syndrome are associated with a more precise and specific biological 'explanation' of the developmental and functional limitations. However, even in these latter conditions with an identifiable biomedical underpinning, the name tells us very little about the individual child's functional needs or strengths, or the family's needs and wishes for information or short- and long-term management in relation to the family's expectations and hopes.

At times in clinical practice there is a strong relationship between the effectiveness of interventions for an identified problem and the degree of certainty with which practitioners can recommend that treatment. The other side of that reality is that when the evidence of efficacy is limited, or the applicability of 'this' treatment to 'that' condition is not clear, it is less easy to be definitive about our decision-making process when recommending interventions. In these circumstances professionals might experience discomfort with knowing how best – under conditions of uncertainty – to be helpful to families of children with impairments. This imprecision might lead, in turn, to challenges in planning management and potentially over-treating, with the risk of doing harm, and perhaps even creating a feeling of distress (Duffy 2009).

A related challenge in clinical management in childhood neurodisability is the extent to which our best ideas are supported by sound evidence. In an era of 'evidence-based medicine', the field of childhood disability can seem to be a 'poor cousin' compared to some areas of pediatric medicine like oncology care, which are practiced on a far firmer evidence-based scientific grounding than is usually true in our branch of child health. In reality we often have more, and more solid, evidence regarding what does not work than what does. Thankfully, in a few areas like the management of infantile spasms, studies are beginning to provide more robust evidence for optimal treatment.

In the face of this reality, what are our ethical responsibilities toward recommending management and treatment strategies? Are we justified in being highly critical of so-called complementary and alternative therapies of uncertain value (and sometimes great costs in time and money) when our orthodox beliefs are often not well supported either? How well do we communicate with families regarding the levels of evidence about the interventions we recommend? What are our ethical responsibilities in these discussions? How do we balance being honest and fully transparent about uncertainty while communicating some level of confidence that the advice we offer is well intentioned, is unlikely to cause harm, and is directed at specific and measurable (usually short-term) goals (Bell et al. 2012)?

Ongoing management and follow-up: where does 'compliance' fit?
There are, once again, many issues that raise concerns for service providers, of which only a few are touched on here. A traditional idea about 'clients' has been our (professionals') expectation that people should take our advice – they should 'comply' with our recommendations! We can too easily be upset by 'non-compliance', as if people who fail to implement our treatment ideas are somehow delinquent, and are perhaps wasting our time. An alternative interpretation is that unless we have clearly built trust, guided and negotiated both the family's (and if possible the child's) goals and made recommendations consistent with both their goals and the resources of time, energy and technical abilities to meet those goals, we may be misinterpreting our failure of transparent communication as a family's 'bad' behavior. This misinterpretation may lead us to be angry or frustrated, and perhaps even to discontinue treatment, when in fact a different understanding of the issues might lead to a very different resolution of the problem. Do we think of these issues as 'ethical' challenges?

A related theme concerns so-called 'hard-to-serve' families, about which others have written in this book (see Chapter 17). As with 'non-compliance', there is a sense that people who miss appointments or are hard to locate constitute a challenge to our systems. An alternative interpretation might well include a consideration of other realities for a family. Their child's impairments might be but one of many challenges they face – and might, to them, be lower on their priority list than we expect them to be (recognizing that we often know only that aspect of a family's issues with which we are professionally involved). There may be social, economic, language, cultural, distance or other barriers to their ability to access even the best of services. Is it therefore ethical to mandate a specific number of attendances, and use failure to meet this criterion number as a basis for discharging children and families? Might an alternative approach be to consider the policies of our programs and to balance considerations of service demands and resources with sensitive, flexible and humane policies that acknowledge the complexities of the lives of many of the families we serve?

In an era that prizes 'Family-Centered Services' (FCS) there is an ethical imperative to balance our best professional experiences and perspectives with the values, goals and wishes of families. There is a belief in some quarters that FCS means that service providers become the handmaidens of families, responsible for doing everything the family requests. This is a naïve and frankly a cynical view of reality. FCS involves professionals and families negotiating shared goals and defined outcomes, with agreed-upon processes to try to achieve those goals. This means that, unlike the 'old days', when professionals made the decisions and 'ordered' the treatments, we have a responsibility to engage in and navigate relationships with families on their terms to address their issues framed within their values and priorities (King et al. 2004; Rodriguez-Osorio & Dominguez-Cherit 2008).

Of course, such an approach still requires professionals to act within the bounds of evidence, to engage in ethically sound behavior and to follow the guidelines of our professional associations (address these various guidelines). When families' goals and wishes are considered to be in some way inappropriate or outside our scope of practice, good clinical and ethical practice requires that we work together to find common ground, mutually agreed-upon goals and accepted guidance. If that becomes impossible, there should be a shared agreement to part ways or even to agree to disagree on a single point (like immunization) without general judgments or recriminations on either side. After all, some of these families may want to stay or re-enter our systems later on. In fact, healthcare providers need to respect the patients' and parents' autonomy, even among those with potential limitations of cognitive and informational constraints, or limited willpower (Ronen & Dan 2013).

Ongoing management means ongoing recalibration of child and family development, resynchronization with ever-changing family values, evaluating goal achievement, setting new goals and re-evaluation of the whole situation. In the field of neurodisability, few if any children are 'cured', and unfortunately patients with severe neurological impairment often deteriorate in important aspects of their health and function throughout life. This means that there may always be differences between these young people's capacities and whatever is considered typical or age-appropriate. At times, the calibration of services has to move toward the palliative spectrum of management to support comfort for the child. The more important question concerns the extent to which the child, youth and family have achieved their goals, and whether there is a need for ongoing 'active therapy'. The ethical dilemmas here include the importance of being clear whose needs and goals are being addressed (the family's, the young person's or the professionals'). Among the many rocky shoals of this issue is the potential for differences of opinions among these many protagonists – issues that are identified and addressed in some of the stories that are told in this book.

When do child services stop?

One additional area of both clinical and ethical complexity concerns the reality that children with impairments grow into adults with these conditions. They rarely die (unless their impairments are profound) or get 'better'. In fact, based on simple population demographics in the western world, there should be about three times as many adults with all these 'children's conditions' as there are children and adolescents.

Sadly, when they age out of child and youth services, these emerging adults 'fall off the cliff' (a metaphor used by parents in many countries) and essentially risk becoming invisible. The clinical and ethical challenges now beginning to be addressed in many centers concern the responsibilities of child and youth disability programs either to continue to provide effective 'transition' services or to work with adult-oriented colleagues and community resources to ensure that the emotional, physical, social and other gains that these former 'children' have achieved are not lost through the changed nature and limited availability of adult health and social services. These adults with childhood-onset conditions may have different and at times difficult trajectories of health, impairment or disability. They may develop 'new' adult onset symptoms or impairments, causing new disabilities and discomfort, with little professional knowledge, understanding and empathy.

Advocacy and health promotion
Advocacy is another major component of our ethical responsibility toward both our own patients and the population of children and families that they represent. This obligation stretches far beyond our professional duty of good clinical practice (Gruen et al. 2004). The act of advocacy includes taking part in guaranteeing equal rights for individuals with neurodevelopmental conditions in our own communities but also worldwide (United Nations 2006). Advocacy also involves us in engaging in health promotion, which implies enabling individuals and groups to increase control over and to improve their own health and well-being by helping to change their environments, including policies, programs and practices, and to help these people achieve their needs and aspiration (Morris & Shilling 2013; WHO 1986). This may also include helping them facilitate their rights as human beings in building romantic and sexual relationships and experiences (Wiegerink & Roebroeck 2013). In other words, ethical principles and practices can be considered to extend well beyond the clinic and the individual, and to encompass the world of 'disability'.

References

Albrecht GL, Devlieger PJ (1999) The disability paradox: High quality of life against all odds. *Soc Sci Med* 48: 977–988.

Baumeister RL, Leary MR (1995) The need to belong: Desire for interpersonal attachments as a fundamental human motivation. *Psychol Bull* 117: 497–529.

Bell E, Wallace T, Chouinard I, Shevell M, Racine E (2012) Responding to requests of families for unproven interventions in neurodevelopmental disorders: Hyperbaric oxygen 'treatment' and stem cell 'therapy' in cerebral palsy. *Dev Disabil Res Rev* 17: 19–26.

Clarke PG, Cott C, Drinka TJ (2007) Theory and practice in interprofessional ethics: A framework for understanding ethical issues in health care teams. *J Interprof Care* 21: 591–603.

De Lourdes Levy M, Larcher V, Kurz R, Ethics Working Group of the Confederation of European Specialists in Paediatrics (CESP) (2003) Informed consent/assent in children. Statement of the Ethics Working Group of the Confederation of European Specialists in Paediatrics (CESP). *Eur J Pediatr* 162: 629–633.

Duffy LV (2009) The nurse's role in treatment decisions for the child with neurological impairment. *J Neurosci Nurs* 41: 270–276.

Gruen RL, Pearson SD, Brennan TA (2004) Physician–citizens–public role and professional obligations. *JAMA* 291: 94–98.

Gupta S, Kanamalla U, Gupta V (2010) Are incidental finding on brain magnetic resonance images merely incidental? *J Child Neurol* 25: 1511–1516.

Hanisch H (2013) Politics of love: Narrative structure, intertextuality and social agency in the narratives of parents with disabled children. *Social Health Ill* 35: 1149–1163.

Hoffmann TC, Légaré F, Simmons MB et al. (2014) Shared decision making: What do clinicians need to know and why should they bother? *Med J Aust* 201: 35–39.

Harris JR (1995) Where is the child's environment? A group socialization theory of development. *Psychol Rev* 102: 458–489.

Huber M, Knottnerus JA, Green L et al. (2011) How should we define health? *BMJ* 343: d4163.

Jan M, Girvin JP (2002) The communication of neurological bad news to parents. *Can J Neurol Sci* 29: 78–82.

Jennings S (2013) Advances the rights of children with neurodevelopmental conditions. In: Ronen GM, Rosenbaum PL, editors. *Life quality outcomes in children and young people with neurological and developmental conditions*, pp. 166–190. London: Mac Keith Press.

King S, Teplicky R, King G, Rosenbaum P (2004) Family-centred service for children with cerebral palsy and their families: A review of the literature. *Semin Pediatr Neurol* 11: 78–86.

Leikin SL (1983) Minors' assent or dissent to medical treatment. *J Pediatr* 102: 169–176.

Levetown M, American Academy of Pediatrics Committee on Bioethics (2008) Communication with children and families: From everyday interactions to skill in conveying distressing information. *Pediatrics* 121: e1441–e1460.

Lohr KN, Zebrack BJ (2009) Using patient-reported outcomes in clinical practice: Challenges and opportunities. *Qual Life Res* 18: 99–107.

Mac Keith R (1967) The tyranny of the idea of cure. *Dev Med Child Neurol* 9: 269–270.

Mezgebe M, Akhtar-Danesh G, Streiner DL, Fayed N, Rosenbaum PL, Ronen GM (2015) Quality of life in children with epilepsy: How does it compare to typical children and children with cerebral palsy? *Epilepsy Behav* 52(Pt A): 239–243.

Morris C, Shilling V (2013) The role of parent and community organizations in child health promotion. In: Ronen G, Rosenbaum PL, editors. *Life quality outcomes in children and young people with neurological and developmental conditions*, pp. 357–368. London: Mac Keith Press.

Noritz G (2015) How can we practice ethical medicine when the evidence is always changing? *J Child Neurol* 30: 1549–1550.

Parker JG, Rubin KH, Price JM, deRosier ME (1995) Peer relationships child developmental and adjustment: A developmental psychopathological perspective. In: Cicchetti D, Cohen D, editors. *Developmental psychopathology, Vol. 2. Risk disorders and adaptation*, pp. 96–161. New York, NY: Wiley.

Renwick R (2013) Quality of life for young people with neurological and developmental conditions: Issues and challenges. In: Ronen G, Rosenbaum PL, editors. *Life quality outcomes in children and young people with neurological and developmental conditions*, pp. 22–35. London: Mac Keith Press.

Rodriguez-Osorio C, Dominguez-Cherit G (2008) Medical decision making: Paternalism versus patient-centered (autonomous) care. *Curr Opin Crit Care* 14: 708–713.

Ronen GM, Dan B (2013) Ethical considerations in pediatric neurology. *Handbook Clin Neurol* 111: 107–114.

Ryff CD, Keyes CL (1995) The structure of wellbeing revisited. *J Pers Soc Psychol* 69: 719–727.

Siegler M (1975) Pascal's wager and the hanging of crepe. *N Engl J Med* 293: 853–857.

Turnbull RH III, Beegle G, Stowe MJ (2001) The core concepts of disability policy affecting families who have children with disabilities. *J Disabil Stud* 12: 133–143.

United Nations (2006) *United Nations Convention on the Rights of Persons with Disabilities;* http://www.un.org/disabilities/convention/conventionfull.shtml (accessed July 2014).

United Nations (1989) *Convention on the Rights of the Child*, adopted and opened for signature, ratification and accession by General Assembly resolution 44/25 of 20 November 1989, entry into force 2 September 1990, in accordance with article 49.

Wiegerink D, Roebroeck M (2013) Romantic relationships and sexual experiences in young people with neurodevelopmental conditions. In: Ronen G, Rosenbaum PL, editors. *Life quality outcomes in children and young people with neurological and developmental conditions*, pp. 107–119. London: Mac Keith Press.

WHO (1986) *The Ottawa Charter for Health Promotion*. Geneva: World Health Organization Press; http://www.who.int/healthpromotion/conferences/previous/ottawa/en/index.html.

WHO (2001) *International Classification of Functioning, Disability and Health*. Geneva: World Health Organization Press.

WHO (2007) *International Classification of Functioning, Disability and Health – Children and Youth Version*. Geneva: World Health Organization Press.

Young Bradshaw D (2015) Reflections: Neurology and the humanities. Wastebasket patient. *Neurology* 84: 2002–2004.

Chapter 3

Can moral problems of everyday clinical practice ever be resolved? A proposal for integrative pragmatist approaches

Eric Racine

Clinicians who care for children with neurodevelopmental impairments are likely to face situations that raise ethical questions.[1] Such situations may take various forms and engage a range of decisions or aspects of clinical care. Announcing a diagnosis to parents who fear a condition with a poor prognosis for their child; discussing options with well-intentioned parents who plan to use complementary and alternative medicine; engaging a teenager in a confidential conversation about sexual practices; determining if the access criteria for a specialized program are unfair to a specific child or family – these are all examples of situations (some of which are discussed in this book) where conflicts can surface between different 'good' or 'right' behaviors or decisions. Depending on the nature of the situation, the 'right' or 'best' thing to do may not be obvious to those concerned, including the clinician, the family members, the child or the community. In a situation requiring the involvement of ethical thinking and problem-solving, the guidance offered by 'common wisdom', 'common sense' or 'common morality'

---

1   In this chapter, the term 'moral' will be used chiefly to allude to *behavior* and *situations*, that is, morality, while 'ethics' captures the *discipline concerned with moral questions* and its attempt to provide a reasonable process of problem resolution to moral problems, that is, ethical responses that mobilize more resources than common morality. *Ethics takes morality as its object.*

fails to offer any definitive or convincing path to follow. Alternatively, this 'common wisdom' may simply not be shared by different individuals. Thus, different views compete on what is the right or best thing to do. When conflicts occur between two (usually) mutually exclusive options the ethical question is said to take the form of a 'dilemma'.

Ethics, as a disciplined and thorough investigation of matters of morality, was introduced by ancient Greek culture as a conscious effort to scrutinize such questions and dilemmas through reason and deliberation. It was based on the conviction that the application of reason[2] can help human beings find some common agreement on how to resolve problems of individual and public morality. However, ethical questions can be daunting, in particular because they can challenge us on our principles and our most profoundly held moral beliefs about ourselves and others. Some people are pessimistic that these questions can ever find any satisfactory resolution and that all options are equal (relativism) or that any preference is as worthy as someone else's because no objectivity can be achieved (subjectivism).

At the same time, a deliberate and articulated attempt to deal with moral questions using reason (e.g. arguments, evidence) can collide with beliefs based on personal convictions or by some custom (e.g. tradition, community, religion). Indeed, when individuals have to argue and justify their stance on a question of morality, they draw on their own convictions and sense of what they consider to be a good life, excellent professional conduct, or beliefs about what constitutes physical or psychological health and well-being. It is therefore no surprise that clinicians and parents sometimes struggle with decisions involving moral issues. To fully consider these issues, one needs humility, as well as open-mindedness and a propensity to reflect on one's own beliefs and actions. Engaging in ethical deliberation can be a challenge for clinicians, but can be even more challenging for parents (and other caregivers) who lack the knowledge and experience of clinical situations held by the clinician. How can they each be made to feel more comfortable in their moral perspective? How does one start a conversation to pave the way toward a reasoned solution regarding the tension at hand? More generally, can moral problems[3] of everyday clinical practice ever be resolved?

This chapter presents a cursory background on bioethics as an interdisciplinary field dedicated to moral problem-solving in the fields of health and biomedical sciences. First, some explanations on common perspectives in bioethics are offered. Second, inspired

---

2   In the sense of Ancient 'reasonableness' such as finding the 'golden mean' or the equilibrium between two extreme attitudes. Finding the golden mean is not equivalent to the arithmetic mean (simple halfway mark between two extremes) (Aristotle 2011).

3   The term 'problem is used to avoid an intellectualist reduction of such situations to 'questions' or 'issues', which can be 'answered'. When alluding to the resolution of a moral problem, the term 'response' is used as much as possible in this chapter to capture the actionable and behavioral aspects at stake.

by the perspective of philosophical pragmatism,[4] and with the idea of delineating an integrative approach that captures different dimensions of moral problem-solving, I sketch common key steps involved in the resolution of moral problems. I hope that this chapter provides elements of a framework to tackle the questions discussed in other chapters (where specific cases are presented by clinicians) as well as some references for reflecting on the best path to follow to resolve these problems.

Different theoretical perspectives on what is ethics and what is considered to be ethical

Contemporary bioethics emerged in the 1960s and 1970s as a response to various trends that destabilized medicine's (and biomedical science's) sense of assuredness and faith in scientific progress (e.g. scandals in research ethics, ever-increasing specialization and depersonalization of medicine, and the emergence of individual autonomy and human rights) (Durand 1999). Modern ethics was caught off guard when asked at the time for specific guidance for crucial health policies (e.g. abortion, the contraceptive pill) and the clinical situations (e.g. brain death and organ donation) that often emerged with the availability of new technologies. A now famous American bioethicist, Daniel Callahan, wrote in these early days about the methodologies and the disciplinary status of bioethics that 'there was nothing whatever in my philosophical training which had prepared me to make a flat, clear-cut ethical decision at a given hour on a given afternoon' (Callahan 1973 p. 68). The situation called for the development of an interdisciplinary dialog between biomedical sciences and the humanities and took the form of 'bioethics', which aimed to be more applied than philosophical ethics, more secular than theological and religious ethics, and more interdisciplinary than traditional medical or nursing ethics. All those fields (and others) would eventually be summoned in order to define the changing contours of this interdisciplinary and practically oriented field. To give a sense of existing theoretical and methodological approaches, I will describe two concrete theoretical strands that have taken shape in bioethics and that are often alluded to in ethical debates.

One strand resides in the principles of biomedical ethics. The 'four principles of biomedical ethics' (principles of autonomy, beneficence, non-maleficence, justice) were first generated as a result of the extensive work of the National Commission for the

---

4   Pragmatism here designates a school of American philosophical thinking that stressed, in the domain of ethics, that the model of scientific thinking (its structure) could be a useful model for ethical inquiries. Too multifaceted to review even briefly, philosophical pragmatism implied the recourse to interdisciplinary scholarship; a commitment to take into account experiential knowledge (perspectives) and the impact of context on moral agents; engagement in open-ended (democratic) deliberation about moral matters; and so on. The common equation between pragmatism and a simple, practically oriented outlook in ethics is a most unfortunate event, and far removed from the meaning of the original intellectual movement (Gouinlock 1994).

Protection of Human Subjects of Biomedical and Behavioral Research in the 1970s. The result of this American commission, which investigated different abuses in biomedical and psychological research (e.g. Tuskegee experiments, psychosurgeries), culminated in the famous Belmont Report, which established three principles as the basis for thinking in research ethics (The National Commission for the Protection of Human Subjects of Biomedical and Behavioral Research 1979).[5] These famous principles were then analyzed in greater depth by a philosopher, Tom Beauchamp, and a philosopher-theologian, James Childress, to generate a practical approach to resolve ethical dilemmas in clinical care and beyond, based on four principles, with the first edition in 1979.

The use of the four principles of biomedical ethics has how become commonplace in the clinical sciences and, of course, in bioethics. Yet, in spite of its popularity, the approach is often applied simplistically. First, the principles themselves are not 'specified', as Beauchamp and Childress recommend. Many users of the method do not take the time to determine what the principles mean or entail in a concrete situation, which is this formal process of specification. However, this should be at the basis of applying the method. For example, whose 'autonomy' are we talking about (e.g. of the parents or of the developing child)?[6] And how does a certain choice or option really favor autonomy? What are we capturing concretely under the principle of beneficence and what is the factual evidence substantiating the claims of benefits of a specific intervention? Such questions should be part of a due process of principle specification.

Second, the principles are often wielded in a way that does not respect their normative equivalence. They are *equally* important, although respect for autonomy is often used as a bioethics trump card. Moreover, the principles need to be situated in a constructive dialog. Beauchamp and Childress – relying on the method of 'reflective equilibrium' proposed by John Rawls (Rawls 1971/1999) – recommend that we find the solution that is most coherent with our moral beliefs to resolve the conflict between competing principles. This exercise starts from our 'considered judgments', that is, 'the moral convictions in which we have the highest confidence and believe to have the lowest level of bias' (e.g. judgments about the wrongness of racial discrimination)

---

5   The Belmont Report uses 'respect for persons' to capture both the principle of autonomy and the principle of non-maleficence. These two principles are now usually discussed separately.

6   There is often confusion in pediatrics ethics literature with respect to this question. Although respect for autonomy is relevant in dealing with youth and even younger children, it remains that the parents' autonomy, strictly speaking, does not have its customary relevance in defining what is the best decision for the child. Parents have a primordial say in proposing what is in the best interests of the children, but this is not based on the respect for their own autonomy as parents but rather on their privileged position to define and enact what is in the child's best interests (Committee on Bioethics 1995). Accordingly, the decision-making authority of parents can be revoked if their decisions are counter to the child's best interests even if their decisions could be considered autonomous. This being said, parents may have a right to be informed by clinicians in order to best decide what is in their child's best interests (not their own) and plan according to such information.

(Beauchamp & Childress 2009 p. 382). It attempts to seek coherence between beliefs and principles by seeking to analyze them in light of the highest or most generalizable principles. When some equilibrium is achieved, it never reaches complete stability because the 'pruning and adjusting occur continually in view of the perpetual goal of reflective equilibrium' (Beauchamp & Childress 2009 p. 382). Most often, the balancing and weighing of principles is not explicitly carried out following a due process of reflective equilibrium as recommended by this approach.

It is important to keep these basic caveats about specification and reflective equilibrium in mind to ensure that the approach does rely on a defendable methodology and a clear effort to bring 'method to the madness' of ethics. This being said, there are legitimate criticisms of the approach, and these often constitute the starting point of other approaches in bioethics (e.g. narrative ethics, feminist ethics, casuistry or 'clinical ethics') (Doucet 1996).

A second methodological and theoretical strand, often pitted against the principles of biomedical ethics, has emphasized the contextual and practical dimensions of ethics under the name of 'clinical ethics'. In the early 1980s, some clinicians and other scholars felt that 'principlism' (a term used to criticize this common approach) offered[7] an impractical way of dealing with morally problematic situations. It was found to be too theoretical, too focused on the principles, and not sensitive enough to the clinical features of a case or a clinician's judgments. This led to the development of 'clinical ethics' both as a specialized field of bioethics as well as a specific case-orientation to health ethics (Siegler et al. 1990). The triumvirate of a historian-theologian (Jonsen), physician (Siegler) and lawyer (Winslade) wrote a book titled *Clinical Ethics: A Practical Approach to Ethical Decisions in Clinical Medicine*, first published in 1982 (Jonsen et al. 2010), which relied heavily on the renewal of case-based ethical analysis or 'casuistry', a term used by the Jansenist Blaise Pascal to denounce its historical abuse by Jesuits (Jonsen 1991; Jonsen & Toulmin 1988). Following this approach, four 'topics' (medical indications, quality of life, patient preferences, contextual features) provide the 'essential structure of a case in clinical medicine' and are to be duly considered (Table 3.1). Based on a first examination of the topics, relevant ethical principles (essentially the same as those of Beauchamp and Childress) are then considered to determine which are most important and guiding in the clinical situation (Jonsen et al. 2010). Through this analysis, the clinician is able to decide which decision would be ethically optimal by comparing what is good ethical practice in this case versus other cases, and decisions made in similar and different cases are compared. This is analogous to case law in jurisprudence applied to ethical reasoning.

Nowadays, the term 'clinical ethics' has come to designate a broader field of inquiry, often described as a subfield of bioethics, with loose connections to the original framework

---

7   It is also true that the version offered by Beauchamp and Childress at that time did not reflect the more comprehensive theory featured in the subsequent editions of their book.

Table 3.1 The four topics relevant to ethical decision making in medicine

Medical indications	Patient preferences
The principles of beneficence and non-maleficence	The principle of respect for autonomy
(1) What is the patient's medical problem? Is the problem acute? Chronic? Critical? Reversible? Emergent? Terminal?	(1) Has the patient been informed of benefits and risks, understood the information, and given consent?
(2) What are the goals of treatment?	(2) Is the patient mentally capable and legally competent, and is there evidence of incapacity?
(3) In what circumstances are medical treatments not indicated?	(3) If mentally capable, what preferences about treatments is the patient stating?
(4) What are the probabilities of success of various treatment options?	(4) If incapacitated, has the patient expressed prior preferences?
(5) In sum, how can this patient be benefited by medical and nursing care, and how can harm be avoided?	(5) Who is the appropriate surrogate to make decisions for the incapacitated patient?
	(6) Is the patient unwilling or unable to cooperate with medical treatment? If so, why?
Quality of life	**Contextual features**
The principles of beneficence and non-maleficence and respect for autonomy	The principle of justice and fairness
(1) What are the prospects, with or without treatment, for a return to normal life, and what physical, mental and social deficits might the patient experience even if treatment succeeds?	(1) Are there professional, interprofessional or business interests that might create conflicts of interests in the clinical treatment of patients?
(2) On what grounds can anyone judge that some quality of life would be undesirable for a patient who cannot make or express such a judgment?	(2) Are there parties other than clinicians and patients, such as family members, who have an interest in clinical decisions?
(3) Are there biases that might prejudice the provider's evaluation of the patient's quality of life?	(3) What are the limits imposed on patient confidentiality by the legitimate interests of third parties?
(4) What ethical issues arise concerning improving or enhancing a patient's quality of life?	(4) Are there financial factors that create conflicts of interest in clinical decisions?
(5) Do quality-of-life assessments raise any questions regarding changes in treatment plans, such as forgoing life-sustaining treatment?	(5) Are there problems of allocation of scarce health resources that might affect clinical decisions?
(6) What are plans and rationale to forgo life-sustaining treatment?	(6) Are there religious issues that might influence clinical decisions?
(7) What is the legal and ethical status of suicide?	(7) What are the legal issues that might affect clinical decisions?
	(8) Are there considerations of clinical research and education that might affect clinical decisions?
	(9) Are there issues of public health and safety that affect clinical decisions?
	(10) Are there conflicts of interest within institutions and organizations (e.g. hospitals that may affect clinical decisions and patient welfare?

Source: Reproduced from Jonsen et al. 2010.

described by Jonsen, Siegler and Winslade. Yet, there are common features in this literature that stress the importance of clinical cases, although clinical ethics now often captures the patient's or family's points of view and reflects greater sensitivity to the pluralism encountered in contemporary clinical practice.

Beyond these two important approaches, many others have emerged in modern bioethics and reflect, to some extent, the different philosophies of the healthcare professions and different understandings of how moral issues should be considered. Feminism and feminist theory have yielded several distinct proposals including explicit considerations about gender rather than sex and how power structures have disempowered patients and families, notably women and the roles that have traditionally been attributed to them. A good example of a feminist case analysis method is presented by DeRenzo and Strauss, which proposes different types of questions to (1) identify the salient features of the case; (2) frame the questions; and (3) negotiate the charted course (DeRenzo & Strauss 1997). Within this second set of questions, particular attention is dedicated to the examination of hierarchical relationships and issues of imbalance in power. Care ethics, inspired by the moral psychology of Gilligan (Gilligan 2001) yielded another feminist approach motivated by a commitment to reinforce the role of the healthcare professions in *caring* (but which are often focused on *curing* as some authors of this book rightfully point out). In some versions of care ethics, gender, and especially the role that nurses have played (and critical analysis about the roles they have not been fully able to play), are front and center stage (Fry et al. 1996; Wyness 1989). Other like-minded proposals describe a general commitment of the 'healing professions' to restore the fundamental role of beneficence in health professions (Pellegrino & Thomasma 1988). Finally, narrative ethics has called for a generous understanding of the 'framing' of cases beyond the point of view that a clinician brings to the discussion (Charon & Montello 1999).

A proposal for an integrative approach

There is much diversity and richness in modern bioethics that can support in-depth analyses and discussions. Even if some of the exchanges between different approaches are framed as 'debates' taking place along inescapable fault lines, there are also views that try to integrate this rich theoretical and methodological diversity within more integrative approaches based on pragmatist and feminist theory (Mahowald 1994; Miller et al. 1996; Sherwin 1999). Relying on yet another philosophical tradition, pragmatism (James 1907/1995), I sketch for readers (Fig 3.1) a way in which some of these approaches can be mobilized to help clinicians and their patients and families engage in the resolution of ethical dilemmas following a series of simple steps. Many of these steps are embedded in existing methodologies and scholarship, and what I propose follows other similar proposals based on integrative models, philosophical pragmatism or a combination of both (Andre 2002; Doucet et al. 2001; McGee 2003; Rest 1986; van der Scheer & Widdershoven 2004). It is important to note that, in daily activities, common sense, or 'common morality', very often suffices to deal with questions that involve moral

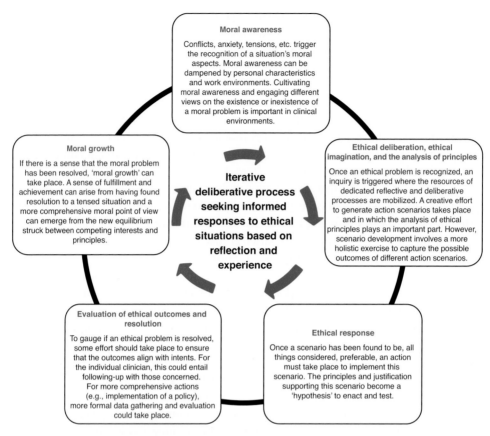

Figure 3.1 Summary of an integrative pragmatist approach to moral problem solving.
Source: Adapted from Racine 2013.

issues. In fact, these aspects are almost omnipresent in clinical decisions. However, it is when common morality falls short of providing guidance that a process of moral problem resolution (which involves ethical analysis and deliberation but also concrete responses) is required.

Moral awareness

For clinicians facing a morally problematic situation[8] one of the very first steps is to understand the nature of the challenge at hand. Of course, the recognition of the existence of the moral dimensions of a situation relies on the existence of an individual's moral sensitivity

8   The term 'a morally problematic situation' is used instead of the narrower 'ethical question' to capture that the cognitive dimension of the problem faced goes much beyond the cognitive, explicit and single stakeholder perspective. We also refrain from using the term 'case', which is shorthand for a clinically defined situation, that is, not a term capturing the perspective of other stakeholders such as the child or parents.

to the existence of a problem. The moral aspect of a situation is based on the perspective and experience of those involved, hence the actual recognition of this moral dimension (e.g. through the existence of a feeling of uncertainty or disquiet, an awareness of tension among protagonists) is instrumental in bringing the dilemma or situation to light.

However, many factors can hinder the recognition of a situation's moral aspects. The negative impact of the training of clinicians has been notoriously faulted for diminishing moral awareness and sensitivity, that is, the 'hidden curriculum' (Hojat et al. 2009; Ward et al. 2012). This is thought to result in an important decline of empathy in third-year medicine students. The reasons 'explaining' this trend remain debated (e.g. desensitization provoked by the absence of role models in mentors; emotional detachment and cynicism induced by intensive training); however, it remains a valid point that the years that clinicians spend in training blunt their overall moral sensitivity. Another factor is the experiential asymmetry between, for example, parents and clinicians. What may seem an obvious situation for a clinician (e.g. discourage the use of non-evidence-based complementary and alternative medicine) may be more complex from the standpoint of parents because they are in parental relationship with their child and have obligations and sentiments for the child's welfare that the clinician may simply not recognize and understand. In contrast, the clinician may have seen many similar cases, have scientific knowledge to inform their reasoning, and be more distant from the actual stakes. Another possible factor that can hinder the recognition of a situation's moral aspects is a lack of humility on the part of the clinician, who entertains a sense of certainty about his or her moral judgments similar to the certainty exhibited in clinical practice. This self-assuredness can easily become an obstacle to the recognition of the moral stakes in a clinical case, as well as come across as resistance and arrogance and contribute to a defensive attitude to admitting uncertainty to parents or others (including themselves).

Certainly, many other factors can obfuscate the recognition that a situation raises ethical stakes and issues. Given the existence of these many impeding factors, a clinician must be aware of what triggers his or her own moral sense and reflect on the reasons why others would approach things differently. Because clinicians have fiduciary obligations to their patients, they must cultivate a generous understanding of what a moral situation can be to ensure that the well-being and best interests of their patients are not obfuscated by biases induced by differences of culture, language or socio-economic status. Of course, cultivating a moral sensitivity is no simple feat, and no one has 360 degrees of moral awareness. At the same time, clinicians must be attuned to cues that signal angst, conflict and tensions of a moral nature within clinical situations. Narrative approaches that call for active listening and generous comprehension of others' points of view can be useful sources to consult and read about to refine one's moral sensitivity (Charon 2001; Charon & Montello 1999). They also offer examples of clinicians who have put the values and interests of patients at the centre of clinical practice.

Empirical research in bioethics sometimes based on narrative approaches has also generated much research on the perspectives of different stakeholders (clinicians, children, parents, society) that can also help refine one's understanding of the stakes in a given situation including in neurodevelopmental disability. For example, previous research has shown how disrespectful and belittling attitudes in everyday clinical practice can impact the self-esteem of individuals with cerebral palsy (or persons with other neurodevelopmental impairments) and therefore cause disability as conceptualized by the World Health Organization (2001, 2007). In addition, this attitude discourages their participation in decision-making (Larivière-Bastien et al. 2011). Research on the perspective and experience of stakeholders is consistent with a consultative and collaborative approach to first understanding the nature of a moral situation. Of course, nobody's understanding and awareness will ever be perfect or complete, and these will probably keep evolving as new facts are brought to light. However, a bracketing of one's initial judgment can help one engage in a meaningful exercise to better understand the moral aspects of a situation in a comprehensive way beyond its description as a 'case', following clinical terminology and perspectives, or through the four principles, which can betray someone's initial understanding of a moral problem (Fiester 2015).

Ethical deliberation, ethical imagination and the analysis of principles

Once a situation is recognized as being morally problematic, a deliberate effort can take place to analyze more objectively the different principles at stake or the actions at hand. Unfortunately, this part of moral problem resolution is often boiled down to an analysis of ethical principles. In the best cases, the principles will be *specified* based on a generous understanding of the situation. That being said, the effort may nevertheless remain an intellectual exercise disconnected from action. An interesting strategy for inserting traditional ethical analysis into action-oriented thinking consists in framing ethical analysis as an effort to identify and/or generate different action scenarios and compare the merits of scenarios, not only from the standpoint of ethical principles, but also for their feasibility. The philosopher John Dewey envisioned that moral deliberation was a form of dramatic rehearsal of different action scenarios (Caspary 1991; Dewey 1922). Dewey writes that 'deliberation is a dramatic rehearsal (in imagination) of various competing possible lines of action. It starts from the blocking of efficient overt action, due to that conflict of prior habit and newly released impulse to which reference has been made. Then each habit, each impulse, involved in the temporary suspense of overt action takes its turn in being tried out. Deliberation is an experiment in finding out what the various lines of possible actions are really like'.

In this process, imagination and prospective thinking play a key role in helping clinicians and those involved in a problematic moral situation to brainstorm and envision creative solutions. Closer to home, the Canadian bioethicist Hubert Doucet has structured this process into a comparative exercise where those involved in a morally problematic situation identify at least three distinct scenarios (to avoid the dichotomy induced by a decisional dyad). Each scenario is then fleshed out in terms of its implications and factual aspects (e.g. likely outcomes) and then for each scenario the ethical principles favored, and those also neglected, are identified (Dion-Labrie 2009).[9] Doucet has argued that clinical teams involved in such an exercise are engaged because the ethical deliberation is tied to the actual actions that a team could undertake instead of trying to strike some ideal equilibrium between ethical principles. Accordingly, deliberation is a process by which the initial problematic moral situation finds a response in an actionable scenario.

Deliberation can occur in oneself, but its basic meaning stems from actual human group deliberation. Accordingly, many case analysis methods in bioethics suggest that groups be involved in open discussion to benefit from a richer set of moral perspectives and also, practically speaking, to engage different stakeholders in the ensuing decision because, in the end, scenarios will have to be debated for their merits and one of them selected as the preferred action scenario. In my own work with colleagues, we have attempted to support such activities through working group deliberations (Racine et al. 2014), but they can take many shapes, provided that some basic procedural features ensure a fair process (Moreno 1990).

Ethical responses

Unfortunately, academic ethics often stops once principles are analyzed: once a 'question' is 'answered', the case is closed. This falls short of the needs of clinical practice where 'problematic moral situations' need actual 'responses'. In fact, clinical ethics remains only half-useful if it does not lead to some actionable scenario. Indeed, there is much to be said about medicine's contribution in prompting the redevelopment of practical forms of ethics (Toulmin 1982).

Responses to a moral situation can be manifold (e.g. a change in attitude, a change in treatment plan, a referral to another clinician or health service resource) and may even include the *status quo* as the most desirable action once different action scenarios have been duly considered. Individual clinicians may have less of an issue in enacting a response because they, as professionals, have leeway and some independence in the exercise of their professions. However, preparing a response can also involve other members of a clinical team, parents, the child, health services or specific programs. In such cases, the implementation of the response will call for collaborations, communication and negotiations with others involved, much like any other form of change

---

9   This method is one of the few that also include the implementation of the scenario and its evaluation.

that affects work environments. Clinical ethicists, that is, those who have specialized training in dealing with clinical cases as well as familiarity with healthcare settings, can be a resource here. They are a resource regarding 'process' that hopefully precipitates a 'reasonable' response, rather than being the people who 'make the decision' for clinicians. As with any situation, change done to solve a moral problem will face resistance based on a host of factors (e.g. 'local' clinical culture, compensation or remuneration scheme of clinicians). It is not unreasonable to think that a well-intended action scenario with little attention to implementation can easily become disastrous and counterproductive. This is rather common wisdom, as those involved in a clinical ethics situation will probably foresee. However, this aspect has been poorly integrated into ethics scholarship thus far, perhaps because it falls outside of academic work proper, or because it is beyond the traditional boundaries of philosophical ethics, which, in general, privileges cognition and reasoning skills and not really action and behavior. Another factor is that it is unlikely that a scenario will be 'perfect' in the same way that an idea could be perfect, and thus it represents a lesser intellectual interest for those who view ethics as essentially an academic exercise. However, it is likely that implementation science, health management and administration and other disciplines could in the future be useful contributors to further our understanding of the common and specific approaches that can be used to facilitate ethical change in a clinical environment.

Evaluation of ethical outcomes and resolution

From the perspective of philosophical pragmatism, the scenario generated as a result of moral deliberation – and implemented – constitutes a 'hypothesis' to be put to the test of reality. As with any hypothesis, observations and experience will be key in assessing the actual value of this hypothesis. However, once a solution has been conceived and implemented, how do we know that a right or good thing has been done? The answer to this question is of paramount importance but very complex to settle in a simple yet rigorous way. For the practicing clinician, the feeling that the initial tension has diminished or the conflict resolved may be an experiential way of understanding that the problem has been resolved. This being said, a sense of satisfaction is not the only guidepost, as one could be satisfied with what ends up being a suboptimal response but one that might support one's personal views. A satisfactory response should be one where all stakeholders also find a sense of resolution or progression.

At this point in time, the evaluation of outcomes from an ethical standpoint is another rather unexplored terrain in bioethics. Some research, for example, has assessed whether clinical ethics consultations have been successful, and proposals have been made to develop metrics (Batten 2013; Scheirton 1993; Svantesson et al. 2014), but more remains to be done. Likewise, few studies have evaluated or assessed in some way whether implemented ethically oriented changes have had good outcomes and consequences (and for whom), and whether the ethical integrity of the individuals involved has been preserved or fostered. Such metrics (e.g. increasing good outcomes, ensuring professional conduct and integrity) actually allude to the components of general ethical theories (e.g. utilitarianism/consequentialism, deontology, virtue theory) (Dubljević & Racine 2014). However, these theories are often pitted again each other because they focus on distinctive aspects of a moral situation (Dewey 1966). Therefore the normative criteria according to which an ethical dilemma is found to be 'resolved' remain hard to articulate, even if required to close the loop, so to speak. From the standpoint of clinicians, some validation with patients, families and colleagues can help ensure that one's 'resolution' is also found by others to be satisfactory. From the standpoint of academic bioethics, different methods could be deployed (e.g. qualitative research, patient-reported outcomes measures) to help progress in this area, provided that there is a fairly generous and practical appreciation of what a 'resolution' can constitute, because perfection in action (in contrast to perfection in thought) will not be achieved. For institutions and professional societies, ensuring that any new practice or guidance is made public may be an additional criterion to ensure that there is accountability for the reasons supporting an option or policy.

Moral growth

One final note, and perhaps even less explored, is the prospect that the exercise of resolving moral problems stands to make a positive contribution to the life of those involved in it. The philosopher John Dewey went as far as to propose that a sense of growth and fulfillment could be generated by the resolution of a moral problem and thus make significant contributions to the meaningfulness of one's life. As a clinician, a parent or another stakeholder surmounts such a problem, he or she grows and develops the capacities of engaging with others and of living well with limitations associated with the actual health condition of the child. They nurture an ability to deal with difficult and profoundly challenging questions, and they cultivate the arts of deliberation and dialog to pursue collaborative problem resolution. This is similar to what the Ancients described as 'wisdom' (*phronesis*) and the sense of well-being, happiness and accomplishment that Aristotle captured in the concept of *eudaimonia* that can be generated from the exercise of this wisdom. Although these concepts were generated in ancient times, they capture a fundamental truth about the profound worth of ethical action and ethical persons. This is even more relevant in our modern times, as ever increasing societal and technological complexity reveals how profoundly important ethical inquiry is to our individual and collective lives.

To conclude this chapter, it is important to stress some of the limitations of the thoughts shared with readers. First, as can be easily imagined, any moral problem resolution represents a dynamic equilibrium, satisfactory but somewhat unstable and temporary and sometimes idiosyncratic to specific situations. Stated another way, everyday moral problems in clinical practice can be resolved with humility but certainly not definitively. If medical practice or societal norms evolve, for example, a previously struck equilibrium can be disrupted, creating a potential need to revisit existing approaches. Second, those interested in learning more about specific ethical theories will find an abundance of scholarship on any of the given authors and theories mentioned briefly here. Third, the pragmatist framework described, and inspired by the writings of John Dewey and others, is presented in general terms and in a way that connects to my own experience of helping individuals or groups dealing with moral problems. There is clearly a need for further thought on the integration of the knowledge and wisdom generated through the experience of stakeholders and the structured deliberations of groups. Finally, regardless of any progress achieved, ethics, as a disciplined or structured effort, will never replace the prior existence of good will or good character. Rather, it is a tool and a resource to supplement or cultivate these moral capacities and dispositions. Hopefully, this volume, which contains powerful narratives and thought-provoking moral cases, will entice clinicians, parents, ethicists and others to work together on developing, implementing and evaluating approaches, thereby helping all of us to cultivate our moral sense and nurture our moral growth.

References

Andre J (2002) *Bioethics as a practice. Studies in social medicine no 9*. Chapel Hill/London: The University of North Carolina Press.

Aristotle (2011) *Nicomachean ethics*. London/Chicago: The University of Chicago Press.

Batten J (2013) Assessing clinical ethics consultation: Processes and outcomes. *Abbreviation is Med Law* 32: 141–152.

Beauchamp T, Childress J (2009). *Principles of biomedical ethics*. Oxford: Oxford University Press.

Callahan D (1973) Bioethics as a discipline. *Hastings Center Studies* 1: 66–73.

Caspary WR (1991) Ethical deliberation as dramatic rehearsal: John Dewey's theory. *Educ Theory* 41: 175–188.

Charon R (2001) Narrative medicine: Form, function, and ethics. *Ann Intern Med* 134: 83–87.

Charon R & Montello M (1999). Framing the case: Narrative approaches for healthcare ethics committees. *HEC Forum* 11: 6–15.

Committee on Bioethics (1995) Informed consent, parental permission, and assent in pediatric practice. *Pediatrics* 95: 314–317.

DeRenzo EG, Strauss M (1997) A feminist model for clinical ethics consultation: Increasing attention to context and narrative. *HEC Forum* 9: 212–227.

Dewey J (1922) *Human nature and conduct: An introduction to social psychology*. New York: Holt.

Dewey J (1966) Three independent factors in morals. *Educ Theory* 16: 198–209.

Dion-Labrie M (2009) *Présentation d'une grille d'analyse pour la résolution de situation éthiques problématiques en réadaptation physique*. Québec: Association des établissement de réadaptation en déficience physique du Québec.

Doucet H (1996) *Au pays de la bioéthique. L'éthique biomédicale aux États-Unis.* Geneva: Labor et Fides.

Doucet H, Larouche J-M, Melchin KR, editors (2001) *Ethical deliberation in multiprofessional health care teams.* Ottawa: University of Ottawa Press.

Dubljević V, Racine E (2014) The ADC of moral judgment: Opening the black box of moral intuitions with heuristics about agents, deeds and consequences. *AJOB Neurosci* 5: 3–20.

Durand G (1999) *Introduction générale à la bioéthique: Histoire, concepts et outils.* Montréal: Fides-Cerf.

Fiester AM (2015) Weaponizing principles: Clinical ethics consultations and the plight of the morally vulnerable. *Bioethics* 29: 309–315.

Fry ST, Killen AR, Robinson EM (1996) Care-based reasoning, caring, and the ethic of care: A need for clarity. *J Clin Ethics* 7: 41–47.

Gilligan C (2001) *In a different voice. Psychological theory and women's development.* Cambridge, MA: Harvard University Press.

Gouinlock J (1994) *The moral writings of John Dewey.* Amherst, NY: Prometheus Books.

Hojat M, Vergare MJ, Maxwell K et al. (2009) The devil is in the third year: A longitudinal study of erosion of empathy in medical school. *Acad Med* 84: 1182–1191.

James W (1907/1995). *Pragmatsim.* Mineola, NY: Dover Publications.

Jonsen AR (1991) Casuistry as methodology in clinical ethics. *Theor Med* 12: 295–307.

Jonsen AR, Siegler M, Winslade WT (2010) *Clinical ethics: A practical approach to ethical decisions in clinical medicine.* New York, NY: McGraw-Hill.

Jonsen AR, Toulmin S (1988) *The abuse of casuistry: A history of moral reasoning.* Berkeley, CA: University of California Press.

Larivière-Bastien D, Majnemer A, Shevell M, Racine E (2011) Perspectives of adolescents and young adolescents with cerebral palsy on the ethical and social challenges encountered in healthcare services. *Narrat Inq Bioeth* 1: 43–54.

Mahowald MB (1994) So many ways to think. An overview of approaches to ethical issues in geriatrics. *Clin Geriatr Med* 10: 403–417.

McGee G, editor (2003) *Pragmatic bioethics.* Cambridge, MA: MIT Press.

Miller FG, Fins JJ, Bacchetta MD (1996) Clinical pragmatism: John Dewey and clinical ethics. *J Contemp Health Law Policy* 13: 27–51.

Moreno JD (1990) What means this consensus? Ethics committees and philosophic tradition. *J Clin Ethics* 1: 38–43.

Pellegrino ED, Thomasma DC (1988) *For the patient's good: The restoration of beneficence in health care.* New York, NY: Oxford University Press.

Racine E (2013) Pragmatism and the contribution of neuroscience to ethics. *Essays Philos Humanism* 21: 13–20.

Racine E, Bell E, Yan A et al. (2014). Ethics challenges of transition from paediatric to adult health care services for young adults with neurodevelopmental disabilities. *Paediatr Child Health* 19: 65–68.

Racine E, Lariviere-Bastien D, Bell E, Majnemer A, Shevell M (2013) Respect for autonomy in the healthcare context: Observations from a qualitative study of young adults with cerebral palsy. *Child: Care Health Dev* 39: 873–879.

Rawls J (1971/1999) *A theory of justice.* Cambridge, MA: Harvard University Press.

Rest J (1986) *Moral development. Advances in research and theory.* New York, NY: Praeger.

Scheirton LS (1993) Measuring hospital ethics committee success. *Camb Q Healthcare Ethic* 2: 495–504.

Sherwin S (1999) Foundations, frameworks, lenses: The role of theories in bioethics. *Bioethics* 13: 198–205.

Siegler M, Pellegrino ED, Singer PA (1990) Clinical medical ethics. *J Clin Ethics* 1: 5–9.

Svantesson M, Karlsson J, Boitte P et al. (2014) Outcomes of moral case deliberation – the development of an evaluation instrument for clinical ethics support (the Euro-MCD). *BMC Med Ethics* 15: 30.

The National Commission for the Protection of Human Subjects of Biomedical and Behavioral Research (1979) *The Belmont Report: Ethical principles and guidelines for the protection of human subjects of research.* Washington, DC: US Department of Health, Education and Welfare.

Toulmin S (1982) How medicine saved the life of ethics. *Perspect Biol Med* 25: 736–750.

van der Scheer L, Widdershoven G (2004) Integrated empirical ethics: Loss of normativity? *Med Health Care Philos* 7: 71–79.

Ward J, Cody J, Schaal M, Hojat M (2012) The empathy enigma: An empirical study of decline in empathy among undergraduate nursing students. *J Prof Nurs* 28: 34–40.

World Health Organization (2001) *International classification of functioning, disability and health (ICF).* Geneva: World Health Organization.

World Health Organization (2007) *International classification of functioning, disability and health (ICF). Children and youth version.* Geneva: World Health Organization.

Wyness MA (1989) Caring – Is it vital to neuroscience nursing? *Axon* 9: 31–33.

Chapter 4

Prenatal consultation: ethical challenges and proposed solutions

Jennifer Cobelli Kett, Hannah M. Tully and Dan Doherty

Prologue

In the past 50 years, perinatal and neonatal care has evolved dramatically. Fetuses with congenital anomalies can now be identified prenatally through advanced ultrasound and magnetic resonance imaging (MRI) techniques. Preterm neonates who would have not have survived in previous generations can now routinely live due to advancements in thermoregulation, gentle ventilation and surfactant administration. Along with these powerful innovations have come challenging ethical questions about what we should do with the technology that is at our fingertips. Clinicians from neonatology, neurology, developmental pediatrics, radiology and many other disciplines are increasingly asked to weigh in on the difficult decisions faced by families and medical teams in circumstances similar to the above cases.

Intense debates regarding the ethics of pregnancy termination and resuscitation at the limits of viability have been outlined extensively in the literature. In this chapter, we will accept the premise that the termination of pregnancy can be an ethically acceptable option for women carrying fetuses with major congenital anomalies. We will also accept the notion that non-resuscitation can be an ethically permissible option for infants born at the limits of viability. We will likewise accept the recommendation that such decisions should be made by caring expectant parents with the support of the medical team. We will not repeat these debates here, but will focus instead on the ethical challenges faced by the clinicians who are tasked with helping families to make these exceptionally difficult choices. The clinical scenarios that open this chapter illustrate just how challenging this can be.

Clinical scenario

Gabriella is a 35-year-old attorney in New York. She and her husband, Joseph, a financial analyst, have been trying to conceive for several years. After many cycles of IVF, they are elated to discover that Gabriella is pregnant with a baby boy, whom they plan to name Joseph Junior. However, the couple is shocked when a 20-week ultrasound reveals severe ventriculomegaly (enlargement of the fluid-filled spaces in the brain). They are concerned about what this would mean for Joseph Junior's future development. They are afraid that he will not be able to participate fully in school or social activities, and that he will require many painful medical procedures. They are also worried that their busy careers will not permit them the time and energy required to care for a child with significant developmental impairments. Although they very much wish to be parents, they are strongly considering terminating this pregnancy. They have come to the fetal diagnostic clinic for information and advice.

Joanna is a 28-year-old waitress in Texas. She and her partner, David, a truck driver, are expecting a baby girl, whom they plan to call Ella. They have two other children at home. The couple is distraught when Joanna goes into labor unexpectedly at 23 weeks. Although the obstetric team has been trying to halt Joanna's labor, they expect that she will deliver in the next several days. The couple has heard that extreme prematurity can affect a child's health and development. They are worried about what this might mean for their daughter. They are afraid that she will have a long and difficult hospital course. They are worried that they do not have enough money to raise a child with special needs and still care for their older children. They have been told that resuscitation at this early gestational age is based on parental preference. They are not sure what to do and have asked to meet again with the neonatologist on call.

What is the prenatal consultation?

Clinicians from a range of pediatric subspecialties may be asked to meet with families during pregnancy to discuss the likely diagnosis and prognosis, and options for the future. This type of consultation can generally be placed into one of two categories. In the first, clinicians are asked to meet with a woman (and her partner) who is pregnant with a fetus with suspected congenital anomalies in the outpatient setting, usually well before delivery. The goal of this type of consultation is typically to provide diagnostic and prognostic information that will assist families in decision-making about pregnancy termination (if still a legal option at the time of the consultation), fetal intervention (if available), birth planning and postnatal treatment. This is the type of consultation that would be provided to Gabriella and Joseph, in the first case. A different type of consultation would be provided to Joanna and David. This second type of consultation typically occurs when a woman is admitted to the inpatient labor and delivery unit in preterm labor. Here, the goal is generally to outline what a family might expect in the future and to assist families in decision-making about delivery-room resuscitation (for infants at the limits of viability).

Both models of prenatal consultation can be greatly beneficial to families; however, they also present several ethical challenges. For example, the nature of prenatal evaluations may limit our ability to fulfill the requirements for informed consent, including the requirement that clinicians provide material information and the requirement that decision-makers meet a threshold of competence. Other difficult issues in prenatal counseling include questions about the degree to which counseling should be directive, how best to meet other informational needs of families (i.e. for emotional or spiritual support) and to what extent it is acceptable to consider the interests of others (i.e. parents or siblings) in decision-making for a fetus or child.

Does the prenatal consultation fulfill the requirements for informed consent?

The prenatal consultation can be viewed as a type of informed consent (or informed permission) discussion, in which the clinician assists families in making a decision about a particular intervention, such as termination of pregnancy or delivery-room resuscitation. Although some prenatal consultations do not involve explicit decision-making, they almost always lay the foundation for decision-making about a future intervention such as hospitalization in the newborn infant intensive care unit or the placement of a ventriculo-peritoneal shunt.

One of the primary requirements for informed consent is the disclosure of material information by clinicians to the decision-maker (Beauchamp & Childress 2013). Unfortunately, there are inherent limitations to prenatal evaluations that may impair our ability to meet this criterion. In counseling families regarding congenital anomalies, clinicians must largely rely on genetic testing, ultrasound and MRI imaging studies for diagnosis. Although the diagnostic accuracy of these modalities has improved over time, they remain somewhat limited. For example, Limperopoulos et al. (2008) evaluated the outcome[1] of 90 fetuses with suspected posterior fossa anomalies on prenatal ultrasound. Prenatal MRI confirmed the ultrasound findings in 67% of cases, and postnatal MRI completely agreed with prenatal MRI in just 59%. This included instances of both under- and overestimation of severity (Limperopoulos et al. 2008). A similar investigation by

---

1 Editors' note: In this book we choose to use the term *prognosis* to refer to the predicted medical endpoint of a health condition, and reserve the term *outcomes* to mean the extent and impact that programs or interventions have been shown to have on its participants in real-life situations. However, there are situations where it is difficult to choose one term over the other (or to distinguish between these terms as they are often used).

Dhouib et al. (2011) that included a wider range of central nervous system (CNS) anomalies demonstrated that pre- and postnatal MRI findings were discordant 15% of the time, although an additional 32% demonstrated differences that were believed to be due to the natural course of the condition. In 9% of cases, findings evident only on postnatal MRI had a significant impact on prognosis (Dhouib et al. 2011). Even if prenatal imaging were able to detect structural abnormalities with perfect precision, systematic data on outcomes for most prenatally diagnosed neurodevelopmental conditions are limited by diverse inclusion criteria, small sample sizes, short duration of follow-up and lack of standardized outcome measures, greatly hampering our ability to provide accurate prognostic information. For example, Bolduc notes that 'despite recent advances in neuroimaging ... the neurodevelopmental and functional outcome of children with cerebellar malformations remains poorly defined. Important inconsistencies in the outcomes reported are frequent and the spectrum of disability is often broad, ranging from normal or near-normal to profound disability for a given malformation' (Bolduc & Limperopoulos 2009). A similarly wide spectrum of outcomes can be seen in other congenital CNS anomalies. For example, in a meta-analysis of 132 cases of prenatally diagnosed agenesis of the corpus callosum (ACC), a malformation that is comparatively easy to identify by MRI, 71% had a normal outcome, 14% had borderline or moderate impairments, and 15% had severe impairments. Even in those cases in which the ACC was not accompanied by additional brain abnormalities, 12% of children had severe neurological impairment on follow-up (Sotiriadis & Makrydimas 2012).

For preterm infants, there is similar prognostic uncertainty. Prior to delivery, fetal size, lung maturity and comorbidities (such as infection) are difficult to predict with precision. For example, fetal weight and gestational age assessment by ultrasound may vary by as much as 15% and 2 weeks, respectively, and even these seemingly small variations can significantly affect the prediction of outcome (ACOG 2002). In a landmark study by Tyson et al., the maximum rate of survival without profound impairment for male infants born at 23 weeks gestation was 10% for those who weighed between 401 and 500g, and nearly double (18%) for those who weighed between 501 and 600g. Similarly, male infants weighing between 501 and 600g who were born one week later (at 24 wks) had a maximal rate of survival without profound impairment of 27% (Tyson et al. 2008). These seemingly small differences in estimated weight and gestational age may translate into substantial differences in prognosis.

There are other significant challenges to interpreting neurodevelopmental outcome data for preterm infants. For example, in research studies, preterm infants may be grouped by gestational age or by birth weight. Although gestational age data are somewhat imprecise, data based on birth weight may combine older, smaller infants with younger infants who are the appropriate size for their gestational age. Because neurodevelopmental maturity is more closely tied to gestational age than size, the inclusion of more mature, growth-restricted infants in a particular group can positively skew prognostication (ACOG 2002). Additional challenges include the choice of denominator for statistics on which to develop prognoses. For example, the number of infants with neurodevelopmental impairments may be reported as a proportion of all infants whose mother went into labor at a particular gestational age, all infants who were live-born at that age, all infants who were admitted to the neonatal intensive-care unit (NICU) at that age, or as a proportion of all infants born at that age who survived to NICU discharge. The choice of denominator may dramatically affect the reported proportion who survive, or who survive without significant neurodevelopmental impairment (ACOG 2002). Additionally, clinicians may report local data (which may accurately reflect local practice, but are likely to include only a few infants who are born at the limits of viability) or national data (which include larger numbers of extremely preterm infants, but may not reflect local practice). The timing of follow-up examinations, type of follow-up performed and definition of 'impairment' may further interfere with the accuracy of outcome data.

In sum, prenatal assessment for fetuses with congenital anomalies, or those who may be delivered extremely preterm, is inherently limited. Limitations in our ability to obtain accurate data, and to provide a precise prognosis on the basis of those data, may diminish our ability to meet the informational requirement of informed consent during our prenatal consultations with families. Over time, we may be able to improve the quality of these data substantially. In the meantime, clinicians may wonder what, exactly, to say to families like Gabriella and Joseph, and Joanna and David. Explaining intricate physiology and complex outcome data is already difficult. Acknowledging the limits of these data without abandoning or overwhelming families can be exceptionally challenging for everyone.

"The requirements for decision-maker competence include the ability to understand and appreciate the decision to be made, to reason through the risks and benefits of each course of action, and to express a preference based on that assessment"

In addition to the provision of material information, appropriate informed consent also requires a competent decision-maker. The requirements for decision-maker competence include the ability to understand and appreciate the decision to be made, to reason through the risks and benefits of each course of action, and to express a preference based on that assessment (Beauchamp & Childress 2013). Unfortunately, the prenatal consultation commonly occurs in an environment that can threaten this ability. For example, during the prenatal consultation, the expectant mother is typically a patient herself. She may be undergoing tests and procedures and, in the setting of preterm labor, may be experiencing significant pain or receiving medications. The information provided during the prenatal consultation may be emotionally shocking and deeply worrisome to expectant parents. Intense emotion, shock, fear, exhaustion, distraction, pain and medication effects may temporarily impair the decision-making competence of expectant parents, as they would for any person. Although this may be true for much medical decision-making, in the context of preterm labor or pregnancies approaching the legal limit of termination, these exceptionally complex decisions must be considered under unique time pressure. It may not be possible to defer them to a time when medication effects have diminished, or emotional or physical distress has eased. Because prenatal decisions are often very complex, gravely important, irreversible and time-sensitive, decision-makers' abilities may be uniquely at risk. Being aware of this, and finding ways to support the decision-making ability of families like Gabriella and Joseph, and Joanna and David is of key importance.

Should prenatal counseling be directive?

Clinicians involved in prenatal consultation often debate to what degree the prenatal consultation should be directive: they wonder whether it is appropriate to include their own values and beliefs about the right course of action when speaking with families. However, it should be noted that it might be impossible *not* to do so. Prognostic data for infants with congenital anomalies are constantly evolving, and outcome data for preterm infants can be hugely disparate (see also Chapter 5 by Chouinard et al.). Which data we choose to include in our discussions with families already involves some degree of value judgment on the part of the clinician. However, because these numerical data appear to be completely objective, there is a serious risk that these implicit value judgments may be obscured.

With regard to explicit directiveness in prenatal counseling, past approaches have employed a paternalistic model, in which clinicians would make decisions for patients with minimal input from them, even when the decisions were deeply linked to personal values. This approach has largely fallen out of favor in the USA and was followed by the so-called 'menu' approach, in which clinicians would outline a range of treatment options without providing any guidance as to which is superior. This approach has been criticized as an abdication of the physician's responsibility. Although the concept itself is not new, much recent attention has been devoted to promoting a *shared decision-making model*, in which clinicians and families collaborate in a process that promotes respect for each party's unique experience and values (D'Aloja et al. 2010; Raju et al. 2014). In a shared decision-making model, clinicians would elicit information about the important goals of care and family values from Gabriella and Joseph or Joanna and David, and then guide the family toward the medically appropriate course of action that would best meet their needs. It should be noted, however, that individual families may prefer an alternate approach, and eliciting their preferred information preference and decision-making style in advance may be beneficial (Janvier et al. 2012; Raju et al. 2014).

What else do families want from the prenatal consultation?

A substantial component of the literature regarding prenatal consultation has focused on optimizing the transfer of information, and indeed clinicians tend to view this as a primary goal (Grobman et al. 2010; Kett et al. 2014). However, qualitative investigations involving NICU parents have demonstrated that the provision of information alone is not sufficient to meet their needs. Payot and colleagues conducted a qualitative investigation designed to understand the prenatal consultation at the limits of viability. They found that, 'For parents, scientific information, although helpful to some extent, does not suffice on its own' (Payot et al. 2007). Grobman and colleagues conducted a similar study and noted that 'Words that parents used to indicate the kind of behavior they desired [from clinicians] included: 'kind', 'soft', 'gentle', 'caring', and 'attentive'. Much of the advice centered on demonstrating compassion and empathy' (Grobman et al. 2010). Boss and colleagues likewise interviewed bereaved NICU families, who 'described religion, spirituality, hope and compassion as being the most important values they considered when making decisions regarding delivery room resuscitation' (Boss et al. 2008). In the Grobman study 'providers were specifically cautious about providing hope, perceiving it as conflicting with objective information, [although] most patients perceived no such conflict' (Grobman et al. 2010). Similarly, in the Boss study, 'Physicians who were perceived as providing more hope were not necessarily more likely to predict survival; in fact, some … predicted nearly certain death. These physicians gave parents hope because the expressed emotion and showed the parents that they were touched by the tragedy of the situation' (Boss et al. 2008). In sum, families like Gabriella and Joseph and Joanna and David are likely to want accurate information, but also to want clinicians to engage with them on an emotional level, to demonstrate compassion, to recognize their role as parents, and to provide hope wherever possible.

Whose interests matter?

Perhaps the most challenging element of prenatal counseling is determining how to consider the interests of the fetus and/or infant in the context of the interests of others. For example, Gabriella and Joseph are worried that their careers will not accommodate the time and energy that they would need to raise a child with developmental impairments. Joanna and David worry that they could not afford to do so, or that this

"Words that parents used to indicate the kind of behavior they desired [from clinicians] included: 'kind,' 'soft,' 'gentle,' 'caring,' and 'attentive.'"

type of care would limit the resources available for the care of their other children. Is it acceptable for a woman to terminate a pregnancy because she does not feel that she has the resources to care for a child with special needs? Should expectant parents be permitted to decline resuscitation for an extremely preterm infant because they are concerned about finances or the impact on their other children? One might also ask how these established, ethically permissible, actions might conflict or align with clinician obligations and duties? Owing to the complex moral status of the fetus, these questions must necessarily be treated distinctly.

Before the threshold of viability, women may seek pregnancy termination in the USA for essentially any reason. Although this is the subject of significant social controversy, it has been less controversial in medical ethics. This practice is commonly justified by an appeal to a woman's right to reproductive freedom and/or bodily integrity. Yet, the fact that termination is permissible does not obviate clinicians' obligations to provide care for the previable fetus in most cases. Chervenak and McCullough suggest that 'the pre-viable fetus is a patient solely as a function of the pregnant woman's autonomous decision to confer this moral status … When the woman withholds or withdraws the moral status of being a patient from pre-viable fetus, abortion becomes permissible in *medical* ethics, because abortion does not involve the killing of a patient' (Chervenak et al. 2007). In this framework, the status of the previable fetus is conferred exclusively by the pregnant woman. If she determines that the fetus is a patient, then clinicians have beneficence-based obligations to provide appropriate care for that patient. However, if the pregnant woman does not confer or revokes this patienthood status, clinicians' beneficence-based obligations to the previable fetus are eliminated. Although this framework has not been accepted universally, it may be useful for understanding how, prior to viability, clinicians can be obligated at times to provide termination of pregnancy and at other times to protect the health of the fetus. In this framework, it would be acceptable for Gabriella to terminate her previable pregnancy on the basis of concerns about her career.

After the threshold of viability, however, decision-making regarding fetuses may become more complex. Chervenak and McCullough state, 'The viable fetus is a patient independent of the pregnant woman's autonomy to confer this status' (Chervenak et al. 2007). In their framework, the viable fetus is always a patient (although, importantly, not yet a physically separate patient), and clinicians must weigh autonomy- and beneficence-based obligations to the pregnant woman with beneficence-based obligations to the fetus. Again, it must be acknowledged that this framework is not universally accepted. In fact, the American College of Obstetrics and Gynecology (ACOG) states that while 'most women will agree to … [fetal] treatment out of a beneficence-based obligation to their fetuses …

"parental autonomy does not permit parents to 'seriously sacrifice [one child's] … health to promote the interests of other family members'"

consent still must be based on the pregnant woman's assessment of her *own* interests. Although a parental decision may, in certain circumstances, be overridden for a child after birth, even the strongest evidence for fetal benefit would not be sufficient ethically to ever override a pregnant woman's decision to forgo fetal treatment' (ACOG 2011).

Children, on the other hand, have a clear moral status that is uncontroversial. Because they lack decision-making capacity, medical ethics has traditionally required that decision-making for them be based on an assessment of their best interests. A strict interpretation of this 'best interests standard' requires that the interests of the child are considered exclusively (Brudney & Lantos 2014). In current practice, Joanna and David would likely be asked to make a decision about the resuscitation of their preterm infant based on consideration of that child's interests alone. However, recent literature has criticized this standard as being subjective, polarizing and vague (Rhodes & Holzman 2014). Rhodes suggests that there are 'times when the interests of others may be as or more important than what is best for the patient' (Rhodes & Holzman 2014). Several authors have called for a decision-making framework that permits the consideration of individual family members, or of the family as a whole, when making decisions on behalf of children (Brudney & Lantos 2014; Rhodes & Holzman 2014; Ross 1994). Ross has suggested that a standard of 'constrained parental autonomy' may be useful (Ross 1994). She suggests that parents be given wide latitude for familial decision-making, but that their decisions be constrained by a principle of respect for persons. In other words, parents should be permitted to balance the interests of family members as they see fit, so long as they provide for the basic needs of all (Ross 1994). Importantly, although constrained parental autonomy allows parents to balance the interests of family members, it does not permit parents to 'seriously sacrifice [one child's] ... health to promote the interests of other family members' (Ross 1994). This compelling model has not been widely employed, and controversy remains in the literature regarding how much others' interests may be considered in medical decision-making for children, if at all.

Epilogue

Several ethical issues in prenatal decision-making remain unsettled. For example, there is an ongoing debate as to whether decision-making for children may include some consideration of the interests of other family members. It is likewise unclear whether decision-making for viable fetuses should be based on the interests of the pregnant woman alone, or should balance the interests of the woman and fetus. It is clear that families have requested that the prenatal consultation include not only information, but also attention to their emotional, spiritual and other needs, and a number of publications have highlighted the need for a shared decision-making model in this and other contexts. It is important to note, however, that even when the prenatal consultation is not explicitly directive, clinicians engage in implicit value judgments simply by the nature of the data they elect to share. It is also important that clinicians be aware of the ways that the nature of the prenatal consultation may impair the competence of the decision-maker and that they take steps to mitigate this when possible. Finally, it is of key importance that clinicians recognize that the nature of prenatal evaluations may limit our ability to meet the informational needs of the informed consent process. While we work to improve our data, we should be honest with patients and ourselves about its limitations.

In counseling Gabriella and Joseph, Joanna and David, and the many families like them, clinicians should consider being forthcoming about the inherent inadequacies in the data, addressing issues that may impair decision-maker competence, inquiring as to a family's preferred model of decision-making, fostering hope wherever possible and engaging with families on an emotional front. This is certainly difficult work; it can be challenging to work with families in an area in which both the science and the ethics are unsettled in important ways. It is also exciting work, which has the potential to have a lasting impact on the families in our care.

Themes for discussion

- We may have access to a variety of types of 'data' to inform our discussions with families and each other. What are these types of data, and what are the relative advantages and disadvantages associated with them?

- Situations like the ones described in this chapter put parents (and professionals) under considerable stress. Who else might – with a family's permission – be invited to participate in these discussions? How might one go about developing this idea in one's own setting?

- Given the one-at-a-time nature of clinical and ethical dilemmas such as those discussed in this chapter, what can clinicians do both to train for this kind of clinical responsibility and to evaluate 'how we did' after these kinds of events have run their course?

References

ACOG (2002) Practice bulletin number 38: Perinatal care at the threshold of viability. *Obstet Gynecol* 100: 617–624.

ACOG (2011) Committee opinion number 501: Maternal–fetal intervention and fetal care centers. *Obstet Gynecol* 118: 405–410.

Beauchamp TL, Childress J F (2013) *Principles of biomedical ethics* 7th edn. New York, NY: Oxford University Press.

Bolduc ME, Limperopoulos C (2009) Neurodevelopmental outcomes in children with cerebellar malformations: A systematic review. *Dev Med Child Neurol* 51: 256–267.

Boss RD, Hutton N, Sulpar LJ, West AM, Donohue PK (2008) Values parents apply to decision-making regarding delivery room resuscitation for high-risk newborns. *Pediatrics* 122: 583–589.

Brudney D, Lantos JD (2014) Whose interests count? *Pediatrics* 134: S78–S80.

Chervenak FA, McCullough LB, Levene MI (2007) An ethically justified, clinically comprehensive approach to peri-viability: Gynaecological, obstetric, perinatal and neonatal dimensions. *J Obstet Gynaecol* 27: 3–7.

D'Aloja E, Floris L, Muller M et al. (2010) Shared decision-making in neonatology: An utopia or an attainable goal? *J Matern Fetal Neonatal Med* 23: S56–S58.

Dhouib A, Blondiaux E, Moutard ML et al. (2011) Correlation between pre- and postnatal cerebral magnetic resonance imaging. *Ultrasound Obstet Gynecol* 38: 170–178.

Grobman WA, Kavanaugh K, Moro T, DeRegnier RA, Savage T (2010) Providing advice to parents for women at acutely high risk of periviable delivery. *Obstet Gynecol* 115: 904–909.

Janvier A, Lorenz JM, Lantos JD (2012) Antenatal counselling for parents facing an extremely preterm birth: Limitations of the medical evidence. *Acta Paediatr* 101: 800–804.

Kett JC, Woodrum DE, Diekema DS (2014) A survey of fetal care centers in the United States. *J Neonatal Perinatal Med* 7: 131–135.

Limperopoulos C, Robertson RL, Khwaja OS et al. (2008) How accurately does current fetal imaging identify posterior fossa anomalies? *Am J Roentgenol* 190: 1637–1643.

Payot A, Gendron S, Lefebvre F, Doucet H (2007) Deciding to resuscitate extremely premature babies: How do parents and neonatologists engage in the decision? *Soc Sci Med* 64: 1487–1500.

Raju TN, Mercer BM, Burchfield DJ, Joseph GF (2014) Periviable birth: Executive summary of a joint workshop by the Eunice Kennedy Shriver National Institute of Child Health and Human Development, Society for Maternal–Fetal Medicine, American Academy of Pediatrics, and American College of Obstetricians and Gynecologists. *J Perinatol* 34: 333–342.

Rhodes R, Holzman IR (2014) Is the best interest standard good for pediatrics? *Pediatrics* 134: S121–S129.

Ross LF (1994) Justice for children: The child as organ donor. *Bioethics* 8: 105–126.

Sotiriadis A, Makrydimas G (2012) Neurodevelopment after prenatal diagnosis of isolated agenesis of the corpus callosum: An integrative review. *Am J Obstet Gynecol* 206: 337.e1-5.

Tyson JE, Parikh NA, Langer J, Green C, Higgins RD (2008) Intensive care for extreme prematurity – moving beyond gestational age. *N Engl J Med* 358: 1672–1681.

Chapter 5

Evidence-based neonatal neurology: decision-making in conditions of medical uncertainty

Isabelle Chouinard, Eric Racine and Pia Wintermark

Prologue

The practice of medicine has evolved to rely upon increasingly strict rules where specific types of evidence are expected or required to support medical decisions. Evidence-based medicine (EBM) represents the most recent epitome of this evolution, although with some interesting reservations (Noritz 2015). EBM involves the application of the best available research evidence to medical decision-making (Sackett et al. 1996). Recently, however, this approach has been challenged in specialties that do not fit well within this model of practice (Upshur 2013).

Neonatal neurology is one such specialty where there is a limited pool of evidence-based guidelines, because understanding of the conditions and treatments is always evolving, and there is not always long-term follow-up on which to rely for safety. Very often, physicians face the added pressure of providing a prognosis based on 'evidence' that is unavailable given the nature of the conditions they encounter and the very experimental nature of the interventions and cutting-edge therapies used to treat their patients.

These aspects are featured in an illustrative case (of Baby Jane) that one of us (PW) faced. The case demonstrates the complexity of prognostication and engaging in end-of-life discussions for newborn infants at risk of severe neurological impairments. Specifically, it highlights the ethical dimensions of medical decision-making in the context of uncertain prognoses and the difficulties encountered in communicating these prognoses and uncertainty to families who must at times make dreadful decisions for their newborn infants.

Part 1: Evidence in neonatal neurology

Clinical Scenario: Baby Jane

I was on call that evening in the NICU as an attending neonatologist. Baby Jane had been transferred from a peripheral center where she was born, despite an uneventful pregnancy, by emergent C-section following massive vaginal hemorrhage. Baby Jane had been born unconscious, not breathing and without any heart rate. She required intensive resuscitation and eventually, at 16 minutes of life, her heart started beating. Jane's brain had suffered and clinically she met all the criteria for hypothermia treatment, which was provided along with other supportive intervention immediately upon her transfer to our NICU. Jane's father arrived a few hours later; her mother was still at the peripheral center. I had a discussion with him about the benefits and risks of hypothermia and the fact that hypothermia was the only available treatment for babies like Jane to try to prevent escalation of the brain injury. We also discussed the fact that it does not work well for all newborn infants, that some still develop persistent injuries. He listened, but he appeared extremely sad, overwhelmed and tired. He wanted to know right away if baby Jane would turn out fine and if she would respond to the hypothermia and have no brain injury. I reiterated that she was currently very sick, that it was hard at that point to predict how she was going to do and that her evolution over the next days would be the best determinant of her outcome. His wife called to get an update and he tried his best to explain what he had understood, but could not find any more courage to explain it all.

Birth asphyxia often leads to so-called neonatal encephalopathy, associated with a high risk of mortality and long-term morbidities. Birth asphyxia is considered by the World Health Organization as one of the top 20 leading causes of burden of disease in all age groups (based on disability-adjusted life years). Children who survive birth asphyxia have an increased risk of developing neurodevelopmental impairments such as cerebral palsy, intellectual disability, epilepsy, learning difficulties and visual difficulties (Oskoui & Shevell 2009).

Therapeutic hypothermia (i.e. cooling to an esophageal temperature of 33.5°C initiated within the first 6h of life and continued for 72h) is a relatively novel treatment in the NICU that has been shown in randomized controlled trials to decrease the rates of death and long-term impairments in term newborns following birth asphyxia by preventing brain injury (Shankaran et al. 2012). The advent of this therapy has changed the outcome of these newborn infants. Some asphyxiated newborns who experienced an alarming birth history, difficult resuscitation and a very abnormal initial neurological exam have improved quickly under hypothermia and have gone on to develop reasonably well. Unfortunately, this treatment is not successful in all cases and a proportion of newborn infants still develop persistent brain injury (Jacobs et al. 2013). It remains difficult for neonatologists to predict in the first hours of life which infants will respond well to hypothermia. Research has yet to elucidate why some newborn infants with similar clinical histories develop different degrees of encephalopathy, respond differently to therapeutic hypothermia and subsequently develop different types of brain injury (Tagin et al. 2012). In that regard, the practice of EBM is not well adapted to such medical situations where uncertainty prevails. Evidence gathered in the context of research such as has been done on hypothermia for neonatal encephalopathy, while helpful in prognostication, is in its infancy. As a result, prognostication in neonatal neurology is rooted in some aspects to a greater degree in clinical judgment than in evidence.

Part 2: Clinical judgment and neurological prognostication

Therapeutic hypothermia and neurological prognostication

In accordance with treatment guidelines, hypothermia was initiated within the first 6 hours of Jane's life and continued for the next 72 hours. She was hemodynamically unstable during the first days of life. Her neurological exam did not improve over the following days and she actually became less responsive. She also presented with seizures that did not respond to treatment. Overall, Jane required many significant interventions in order to keep her alive. Once Jane's mother arrived on day 3 of Jane's life, a first formal sit-down meeting was held with the parents and the health providing team. The discussion centered on communicating the very guarded prognosis and the associated risk of severe motor and cognitive impairments and on presenting the limited treatment options available, including the very real possibility of pursuing comfort measures only. I was on call again that night, which gave me an opportunity to speak with both parents. They were unable to make any decision yet, and just wanted to spend some time with Jane. At the end of the 72-hour hypothermia treatment, Baby Jane was rewarmed, but she continued to require a breathing tube and her neurological exam had not improved. A brain MRI on day 5 of life showed extensive injuries. At this time, the team once again met formally with the parents.

Neuroprognostication requires the integration of evidence from a number of sources, including patient history, clinical presentation, investigative tools and population outcome studies. Brain magnetic resonance imaging (MRI) has been adjusted for newborn infants and now makes it possible to visualize brain injuries and include them as a prognostication tool (Rutherford et al. 2010). Advanced MRI modalities assessing brain metabolism and perfusion (spectroscopy, diffusion-weighted imaging and perfusion-weighted imaging) permit even more accurate diagnosis of these brain injuries in the hours or days following the asphyxia event and play a role in informing early medical decisions and long-term prognosis (Bednarek et al. 2012; Bonifacio et al. 2012). However, up to now, studies using these new types of imaging have involved only small sample sizes, often use varied timing of imaging, and have a wide variability in length of follow-up related to neurodevelopmental outcome. In addition, proper interpretation of these new types of imaging still depends upon only a few specifically trained clinicians.

Survivors of birth asphyxia may display a wide spectrum of long-term outcomes, from no impairments, to subtle findings, to cognitive impairments, neurosensory deficits and cerebral palsy (Myers & Ment 2009). Everyday prognostication in individual newborn infants is inherently uncertain and is likely to remain so despite ongoing technological developments. Particular to neonatology, prognostic uncertainty arises from the assumed plasticity of the developing child's brain – that is, its capacity to adjust and somewhat 'regain' function – making it difficult to predict exact neurodevelopmental outcome related to a specific brain injury.

Nonetheless, early and accurate prognostication of outcome is central for discussions about long-term functional outcome and for developing treatment and management plans. This is known in the medical–ethical literature as 'the window of opportunity' (Kitzinger & Kitzinger 2013; Wilkinson 2011b). Delays in decision-making may mean that newborn infants are no longer ventilator-dependent and, consequently, may lead to the survival of infants with severe impairment, or to the need in some babies to con-template withdrawal of artificial nutrition.

In addition, there may be a lack of consistency among physicians, contributing even more to the complexity of diagnosis, prognostication and decision-making in neonatal brain injury (Bell et al. 2015). Some physicians still use the prognostication procedures that they were using before hypothermia treatment was introduced. Other physicians are more up to date with recent research and have already included new investigative procedures in their practice, even if these are still not yet considered EBM.

Prognostication of the outcome associated with neonatal brain injuries thus remains a statistical idea, or perhaps an intellectual exercise. This uncertainty complicates communi-cation and can lead to substantive ethical challenges for the families and caregiver teams.

Part 3: Parent/patient preferences

From prognostication to decision-making

Based on Baby Jane's predicted poor prognosis, the parents, along with the treating team, chose to withdraw life-sustaining interventions. On day 6 of life, the decision was made to remove her breathing tube and not to replace it should she have any new signs of respiratory failure.

The parents did not want to see their baby girl continuously suffer. She tolerated breathing on her own quite well, but she required a feeding tube. A brain MRI on day 12 of life confirmed the presence of extensive brain injuries. Her parents asked about the different possible options in this daunting situation. Upon presentation of the case to the ethics committee and considering the high risk for severe sequelae, removal of the feeding tube was presented as an option. After a few days of serious reflection, the parents opted to do this and they were moved to a unit that specialized in managing end of life care. Two days later, although Jane's parents had initially chosen to remove her feeding tube, they could not emotionally bear to continue. The feeding tube was reinserted and Jane and her parents went home.

Parents are the natural (and most often legally recognized) decision-makers for newborn infants or young children. They have to balance the best benefits for their children and consider their future, because this decision-making authority is recognized based on the understanding that parents will seek the best interests of their child (Giroux et al. 2005; Harrison & Canadian Paediatric Society 2004). For parents, the NICU environment is a transformative experience. Their expectations of holding their infants, to discover a life of joy and to share it with their close family, are shattered. They are suddenly isolated from their surrounding family in a techno-scientific environment. Their baby is placed in an isolette and hooked up to a monitoring device, with wires and tubes; she cannot be held until she becomes more stable. Alarms are ringing all around. Many features of the situation are unexpected, stressful, heartbreaking, intimidating and overwhelming. Once the initial shock settles, the parents naturally become worried and wonder about their roles as parents in this environment.

Birth asphyxia is challenging for parents to understand. They were expecting a perfect baby after a normal pregnancy until the last minute before birth, when all of a sudden something went wrong. They are now faced with the situation of their newborn infant battling for survival. In addition to getting used to being a new parent, parents of an asphyxiated or otherwise sick newborn need to adapt and adjust to this new situation. However, very often, there is a lack of time to adjust or adapt, as decisions have to be taken quickly. Clinicians can convey prognostic information to the parents, but many non-medical factors will also enter into the parents' decision-making process.

Ethical practices

Clinicians need to navigate the tension between the desire to provide objective and certain opinions (from parents, their colleagues, themselves and other healthcare professionals) and the fundamental uncertainties that shape decision-making in neonatal neurological injury. This is an ethically charged terrain where the standards of the profession, the best interests of the child and the situation of the parents all need to be factored in. The case scenario we present raises multifaceted questions for discussion. It demonstrates the complexity of making palliative care and end-of-life decisions for newborn infants with severe neurological prognosis. The case also highlights the 'type' of evidence that weighs more heavily when there is medical uncertainty.

In the following, we offer some thoughts on what can be important features of an ethical practice.

Recognizing variability and clinician biases in prognostication
Physicians have to advise about the future outcome, but also have to present the option of withdrawal from or withholding of treatment in severe cases. Large variability exists in clinicians' recommendations (Bell et al. 2015; Ganz et al. 2006; Marcin et al. 1999, 2004; Rebagliato et al. 2000; Sprung et al. 2003). Differences in knowledge, training, personal and professional experience, and religious or cultural backgrounds can all influence how a clinician will deliver a message to parents (Andrews et al. 2005; Parker & Shemie 2002). There are no standards on how to deliver a prognosis, even if some practical guideposts have been proposed (e.g. required preparation, timing of discussions and designation of the clinician to engage in discussions) (Bernat 2004; Jan & Girvin 2002; see also Chapter 8 by Novak et al.). Pitfalls in the communication of prognosis include 'inadequate time spent in discussion, use of technical jargon, biased framing of decisions, unjustified physician bias, ethnicity barriers, and surrogates' unfounded intuitions about critical illness and death' (Bernat 2004 p. 107).

Sociological studies have demonstrated the inherent social aspect of prognostication (Anspach 1987, 1993; Halpern & Anspach 1993). Prognostication can be influenced by hospital culture, patient characteristics and clinicians' backgrounds and training. According to Renee Anspach, this is even more apparent in end-of-life decision-making in neonatal intensive-care settings where prognostic uncertainty leads to factors (other than 'evidence') such as 'gut feelings' or intuition having a greater weight in the formulation of prognoses (Anspach 1987). Evidence can also be subject to different interpretations (Bell et al. 2015). Physicians working in similar environments, with similar patients, but in different countries have been found to have significantly different practice patterns. While one group used data to support discontinuing life-sustaining interventions, another used the same data to support pursuing life-sustaining management (Orfali & Gordon 2004). An ethical approach to prognostication demands a consideration of the 'social determinants' that influence the generation of these prognoses (Christakis 1999; Racine 2013). 'Recognizing social influences in prognostication is a starting point to help physicians evolve from "naive objectivity" to "social sensitivity and awareness"' (Racine 2013). The best interests of newborn infants will be best served by supporting measures to reduce this variability. Additionally, the contributions of relevant disciplines

"Recognizing social influences in prognostication is a starting point to help physicians evolve from 'naive objectivity' to 'social sensitivity and awareness'"

(e.g. anthropology of health and sociology of health) could be introduced in professional education and training to increase awareness and the identification of these
factors (Racine 2013).

A common source of moral distress for neonatologists is guilt over the long-term implications for families when neurologically profoundly impaired infants survive (Meadow
& Lantos 2009). This emotional reaction highlights how clinicians are not immune from
having their own perspective on the events surrounding their involvement in the medical
care of a child. Experiences such as those portrayed in the case of Baby Jane have an
indelible impact on clinicians, affecting their future decisions with similar patients. In
exploring their own biases, clinicians promote an approach to establishing meaningful
connections with families in caring for their severely ill child by clarifying the stance
from which they are delivering prognostic information to families.

Conveying prognosis and shared decision-making
Having discussions with a family about a child's poor prognosis is always difficult. So difficult, in fact, that physicians have historically delayed sharing information with families
in order to protect parents (and themselves) from suffering (Davis 1960). Recent studies on
the communication of prognosis to families and the associated ethical responsibilities
of clinicians have shown that families not only want to receive the information in an
honest and straightforward way, but when provided with prognostic information early
in the course of their child's illness (Lamont & Christakis 2003; Mack et al. 2006), they
can make decisions that better support their child's best interest (Mack & Joffe 2014).

Prognostication is difficult and fraught with uncertainty, but this does not preclude
clinicians from having discussions early on with families to elucidate their hopes and
fears about the care of their child even at a time where prognosis is unclear. Early communication about best- and worst-case scenarios is important not only for clinicians
to understand the family's perspective, but also because these discussions help families
reflect and consider what is important to them as they are probably living this experience
for the first time (Mack & Joffe 2014). Adapting to families' lived experiences is also
important. Advice and attitudes need to be adjusted to every parent. Some parents are
more pessimistic than their child's medical condition warrants, while others are more
optimistic and sometimes even in denial. Some parents like to receive detailed information, and others find information overwhelming. Some parents like to review the
evidence, some like to hear what the doctor would do if this were their own child, and
some like the doctors to take the decisions. A lot of parents find it difficult to imagine
the future for their child, as most of them have limited personal experience with neurologically impaired persons. Parents usually have difficulty assessing the impact of
brain injury, as the neurodevelopmental impairments are most often not yet visible in
the neonatal period. Learning about the best- and worst-case scenarios is very often
hard to place in perspective; it is dependent upon the parents' religious and cultural

background and previous personal experiences. Parents evaluate the information provided to them and make decisions from both rational and emotional standpoints (Janvier et al. 2014). When discussing a prognosis and advising about treatment plans, there is very often no one good answer, but several possible answers, and connecting with other families with similar experiences can help guide the direction of discussions. Elucidating families' hopes can provide an avenue to open the discussion and to establish what is most important to families (Feudtner 2009).

When prognosis has been established to be poor and decisions need to be taken about whether to pursue or limit life-sustaining interventions, Janvier and colleagues (Janvier et al. 2014) propose a personalized approach to communicating with families that takes into account personal biases, families' narratives, families' preferences for what information to receive and in what manner, and the emotional aspects of decision-making. Perhaps more than the content of the information that is communicated, it is the words and tone used in these delicate situations that have a lasting impact on parents. A study with parents who have lost a child to illness has shown that parents clearly recall instances in which physicians conveyed information either well or poorly (Meert et al. 2008). Parents want information to be provided in honest and comprehensive ways, despite the difficult nature of what they are facing, but they also need this information to be conveyed at a pace suitable for them in a caring and empathetic manner (Meert et al. 2008).

A shared decision-making approach, therefore, is sensitive to the nature of decision-making for children. Ethical reflection in cases like that of Baby Jane is of utmost importance and is based on the consideration of the child's expected outcome, evaluation of the harms and benefits of continued treatment, and the healthcare team's and parents' willingness to make a choice (Nelson et al. 1995). The best interest standard has been used to guide clinicians and parents in decisions that support what is most appropriate for the child. While considering the primacy of a child's interests, these interests cannot be assessed without consideration of the interests of their surrogate decision-makers (Lantos 1997; Racine & Shevell 2009; Truog et al. 2008). Open and honest communication can play a significant role in supporting clinicians and families in making decisions that are in the best interest of the child.

Guidelines that recognize the full complexity of prognostication
Uncertainty in prognosticating for newborn infants with severe neurological impairments increases the risk of making the wrong treatment decisions (Meadow & Lantos 2009; Wilkinson 2011a). The use of prognostic information in treatment decisions is a complex phenomenon that must take into account many factors. There are uncertainties in mortality and morbidity risk assessments, in the assessment of the benefits and harms of given interventions, in the social influences on the medical conclusions that have been reached, and in the many and varied extraneous factors outside the patient's condition that may in fact influence the outcome (Christakis & Iwashyna 1998). This

complexity, however, is rarely taken into account in the currently available guidelines on decision-making for critically ill newborn infants. Prognostication guidelines or algorithms are usually developed based on empirical outcome studies and do not account for factors beyond medical evidence. Furthermore, the current literature does not address the extent to which prognosis provides grounds for withholding or withdrawing life-sustaining medical treatment (American Academy of Pediatrics Committee on Bioethics 1994; Larcher et al. on behalf of the Royal College of Paediatrics and Child Health 2015). Although some studies do allude to neurological prognosis in conditions such as brain death, anencephaly and the permanent vegetative state – where there is a perception of some clarity – any conditions beyond those listed here fall within a gray zone where little guidance is available to clinicians.

There is a need for professional societies and funding bodies to support research to generate an understanding of the complexity of neurological prognostication in children experiencing birth asphyxia. The uncertainties and challenges of prognostication are not currently well captured in any resources available to clinicians. The outcomes of new procedures should be examined holistically and contextually, including their impact in end-of-life discussions and the uncertainty inherent in those decisions. In order to fully capture the complexities illustrated in the case of Baby Jane, policy-makers will need to expand their pool of research studies to incorporate qualitative research that encapsulates the voices of parents who have been through these experiences, as well as longitudinal studies that provide evidence beyond the very early childhood period.

Evolution

Jane is now 2 years 6 months old. Although she has dystonic cerebral palsy, she is continuing to make progress though at a reduced velocity. She has now started to walk using a walker, she is still partly tube-fed but has started to take some purees, she does not pronounce any clear words but communicates with signs, and she has good eye contact. I met her parents one day in the hospital when they were coming for a follow-up appointment for Jane. They mentioned that they never regretted their decision to have restarted feeding and that they were happy to see Jane's slow but continuing progresses even if it was requiring a lot of hard work on their part to stimulate her. They were still thinking sometimes about what their life would have been if Jane had been born healthy, but they love Jane as she was and she is. They also mentioned that their experience in the NICU was one experience that changed their life forever.

Epilogue

Decisions in the context of neonatal neurology, regularly including end-of-life decision situations, are not straightforward and depend on accurate prognoses. Yet variability and uncertainty in prognostication complicate this decision-making process. The case of Baby Jane illustrates a common scenario in neonatal medicine. This case speaks to the complexity of prognostication in neonatal neurology and highlights the importance of ethical behavior that includes communicating with families from early on and working toward a shared decision-making approach. The evidence available to make decisions in the case of Baby Jane was scarce and depended on newly available technology. Advances in medicine do not yet account for variability due to developing brain plasticity and probably will never account for the variability in the values of the clinicians and families of the children concerned. Evidence in neonatal neurology goes beyond medical knowledge. It merges knowledge from a variety of sources – medical, social, emotional, personal, experiential and so on. Developing medically informed guidelines and undertaking research based on outcomes for children who have experienced birth asphyxia is only part of the response. As clinicians we need to reflect on our own biases in delivering prognoses to families and need to extend this curiosity to include an understanding of the perspectives, hopes and fears of the families whose child we are supporting. Future research and practice-based guidelines can aspire to achieve the goal of guiding clinicians beyond research evidence, incorporating a wider scope of knowledge for which the need continues to be demonstrated by every case similar to that of Baby Jane's that is encountered in medicine.

Themes for discussion

- Modern medicine expects health professionals to be evidence-based and 'objective' as we consider challenging issues such as those reflected in the scenario in this chapter. However, in addition to those aspects of a clinical situation that we can assess, measure and (sometimes) influence, there is a range of social determinants that affect outcomes. How can we explicitly identify and acknowledge those personal elements so that we counsel most effectively?

- Have you experienced cases like this one, filled with uncertainty and emotion? If so, was the idea of 'ethical decision-making' ever discussed? How was that experience similar to, and different from, the story outlined in this chapter?

- In developing this book, the editors often wondered whether there were conceptual and behavioral differences between 'good clinical practice' and 'ethical practice'. What do you think?

References

American Academy of Pediatrics Committee on Bioethics (1994) Guidelines on forgoing life-sustaining medical treatment. *Pediatrics* 93: 532–536.

Andrews P, Azoulay E, Antonelli M et al. (2005) Year in review in intensive care medicine, 2004. III. Outcome, ICU organisation, scoring, quality of life, ethics, psychological problems and

communication in the ICU, immunity and hemodynamics during sepsis, pediatric and neonatal critical care, experimental studies. *Intensive Care Med* 31: 356–372.

Anspach RR (1987) Prognostic conflict in life-and-death decisions: The organization as an ecology of knowledge. *J Health Soc Behav* 28: 215–231.

Anspach RR (1993) *Deciding who lives: Fateful choices in the intensive-care nursery*. Berkeley, CA: University of California Press.

Bednarek N, Mathur A, Inder T, Wilkinson J, Neil J, Shimony J (2012) Impact of therapeutic hypothermia on MRI diffusion changes in neonatal encephalopathy. *Neurology* 78: 1420–1427.

Bell E, Rasmussen LA, Mazer B (2015) Magnetic resonance imaging (MRI) and prognostication in neonatal hypoxic-ischemic injury: A vignette-based study of Canadian specialty physicians. *J Child Neurol* 30: 174–181.

Bernat JL (2004) Ethical aspects of determining and communicating prognosis in critical care. *Neurocrit Care* 1: 107–117.

Bonifacio SL, Saporta A, Glass HC (2012) Therapeutic hypothermia for neonatal encephalopathy results in improved microstructure and metabolism in the deep gray nuclei. *Am J Neuroradiol* 33: 2050–2055.

Christakis NA (1999) Prognostication and bioethics. *Daedalus* 128: 197–214.

Christakis NA, Iwashyna TJ (1998) Attitude and self-reported practice regarding prognostication in a national sample of internists. *Arch Intern Med* 158: 2389–2395.

Davis F (1960) Uncertainty in medical prognosis: Clinical and functional. *Am J Sociol* 66: 41–47.

Feudtner C (2009) The breadth of hopes. *N Engl J Med* 361: 2306–2307.

Ganz FD, Benbenishty J, Hersch M, Fischer A, Gurman G, Sprung CL (2006) The impact of regional culture on intensive care end of life decision making: An Israeli perspective from the ETHICUS study. *J Med Ethics* 32: 196–199.

Giroux MT, Tessier R, Nadeau L (2005) *L'extrême prématurité: Les enjeux parentaux, éthiques et légaux*. Sainte-Foy Quebec: Presses de l'Université du Québec.

Halpern S, Anspach RR (1993) The study of medical institutions: Eliot Freidson's legacy. *Work Occup* 20: 279–295.

Harrison C; Canadian Paediatric Society (2004) Treatment decisions regarding infants, children and adolescents. *Paediatr Child Health* 9: 99–103.

Jacobs SE, Berg M, Hunt R, Tarnow-Mordi WO, Inder TE, Davis PG (2013) Cooling for newborns with hypoxic ischaemic encephalopathy. *Cochrane Database Syst Rev* 1: CD003311.

Jan M, Girvin JP (2002) The communication of neurological bad news to parents. *Can J Neurol Sci* 29: 78–82.

Janvier A, Barrington K, Farlow B (2014) Communication with parents concerning withholding or withdrawing of life-sustaining interventions in neonatology. *Semin Perinatol* 38: 38–46.

Kitzinger J, Kitzinger C (2013) The 'window of opportunity' for death after severe brain injury: Family experiences. *Sociol Health Illn* 35: 1095–1112.

Lamont EB, Christakis NA (2003) Complexities in prognostication in advanced cancer: 'To help them live their lives the way they want to'. *JAMA* 290: 98–104.

Lantos JD (1997) *Do we still need doctors?* New York, NY: Routledge.

Larcher V, Craig F, Bhogal K, Wilkinson D, Brierley J, on behalf of the Royal College of Paediatrics and Child Health (2015) Making decisions to limit treatment in life-limiting and life-threatening conditions in children: A framework for practice. *Arch Dis Child* 100: S1–S23.

Mack JW, Joffe S (2014) Communicating about prognosis: Ethical responsibilities of pediatricians and parents. *Pediatrics* 133(Suppl 1): S24–S30.

Mack JW, Wolfe J, Grier HE, Cleary PD, Weeks JC (2006) Communication about prognosis between parents and physicians of children with cancer: Parent preferences and the impact of prognostic information. *J Clin Oncol* 24: 5265–5270.

Marcin JP, Pollack MM, Patel KM, Sprague BM, Ruttimann UE (1999) Prognostication and certainty in the pediatric intensive care unit. *Pediatrics* 104: 868–873.

Marcin JP, Pretzlaff RK, Pollack MM, Patel KM, Ruttimann UE (2004) Certainty and mortality prediction in critically ill children. *J Med Ethics* 30: 304–307.

Meadow W, Lantos J (2009) Moral reflections on neonatal intensive care. *Pediatrics* 123: 595–597.

Meert KL, Eggly S, Pollack M et al. and the National Institute of Child Health and Human Development Collaborative Pediatric Critical Care Research Network (2008) Parents' perspectives on physician–parent communication near the time of a child's death in the pediatric intensive care unit. *Pediatr Crit Care Med* 9: 2–7.

Myers E, Ment LR (2009) Long-term outcome of preterm infants and the role of neuroimaging. *Clin Perinatol* 36: 773–789.

Nelson LJ, Rushton CH, Cranford RE, Nelson RM, Glover JJ, Truog RD (1995) Forgoing medically provided nutrition and hydration in pediatric patients. *J Law Med Ethics* 23: 33–46.

Noritz G (2015) How can we practice ethical medicine when the evidence is always changing? *J Child Neurol* 30: 1549–1550.

Orfali K, Gordon EJ (2004) Autonomy gone awry: A cross-cultural study of parents' experiences in neonatal intensive care units. *Theor Med Bioeth* 25: 329–365.

Oskoui M, Shevell MI (2009) Cerebral palsy and the transition from pediatric to adult care. *Continuum: Lifelong Learn Neurol* 15: 64–77.

Parker M, Shemie SD (2002) Pro/con ethics debate: Should mechanical ventilation be continued to allow for progression to brain death so that organs can be donated? *Crit Care* 6: 399–402.

Racine E (2013) Pragmatic neuroethics: The social aspects of ethics in disorders of consciousness. *Handb Clin Neurol* 118: 357–372.

Racine E, Shevell MI (2009) Ethics in neonatal neurology: When is enough, enough? *Pediatr Neurol* 40: 147–155.

Rebagliato M, Cuttini M, Broggin L et al. and the EURONIC Study Group (European Project on Parents' Information and Ethical Decision Making in Neonatal Intensive Care Units) (2000) Neonatal end-of-life decision making: Physicians' attitudes and relationship with self-reported practices in 10 European countries. *JAMA* 284: 2451–2459.

Rutherford M, Ramenghi LA, Edwards AD et al. (2010) Assessment of brain tissue injury after moderate hypothermia in neonates with hypoxic–ischaemic encephalopathy: A nested substudy of a randomised controlled trial. *Lancet Neurol* 9: 39–45.

Sackett DL, Rosenberg WM, Gray JA, Haynes RB, Richardson WS (1996) Evidence based medicine: What it is and what it isn't. *BMJ* 312: 71–72.

Shankaran S, Pappas A, McDonald SA et al. and the Eunice Kennedy Shriver NICHD Neonatal Research Network (2012) Childhood outcomes after hypothermia for neonatal encephalopathy. *N Engl J Med* 366: 2085–2092.

Sprung CL, Cohen SL, Sjokvist P et al. and the Ethicus Study Group (2003) End-of-life practices in European intensive care units: The Ethicus Study. *JAMA* 290: 790–797.

Tagin MA, Woolcott CG, Vincer MJ (2012) Hypothermia for neonatal hypoxic ischemic encephalopathy: An updated systematic review and meta-analysis. *Arch Pediatr Adolesc Med* 166: 558–566.

Truog RD, Campbell ML, Curtis JR et al. and the American Academy of Critical Care Medicine (2008) Recommendations for end-of-life care in the intensive care unit: a consensus statement by the American College of Critical Care Medicine. *Crit Care Med* 36: 953–963.

Upshur REG (2013) A call to integrate ethics and evidence-based medicine. *Virtual Mentor* 15: 86–89.

Wilkinson DJ (2011a) A life worth giving? The threshold for permissible withdrawal of life support from disabled newborn infants. *Am J Bioeth* 11: 20–32.

Wilkinson D (2011b) The window of opportunity for treatment withdrawal. *Arch Pediatr Adolesc Med* 165: 211–215.

Chapter 3

Chapter 6

The importance of beliefs and relationships in the decision-making process

Howard Needelman and David Sweeney

Prologue

When families and professionals encounter difficult issues, there may be differences of opinion among those involved as to what course to take. These often arise as a result of differences in the cultural or religious background of the individuals, combined with an often unclear and incomplete understanding of the facts involved at the time a decision must be reached. The final decision regarding care must be made with the patient's best interest in mind and must be ethically sound. The following scenario illustrates this situation.

Clinical scenario

In a moderate-sized Midwestern American city, at a university hospital with a 40-bed Level 3 neonatal intensive-care unit (NICU), a preterm infant is delivered at 24 weeks' gestation weighing 750g. The infant is the product of in vitro *fertilization and is now a surviving twin, the other twin having been unable to be resuscitated in the delivery room. The infant is now 1 week old and on modest ventilator support and pressors. A cranial ultrasound done at 5 days of age shows a large grade IV intraventricular hemorrhage.*

The neonatologist caring for the infant tells the parents that he wants to discontinue ventilator support. He feels strongly that if the infant survives (and he is doubtful of that), he will have 'significant cerebral palsy and be mentally retarded, never being able to speak or recognize and love other people, including his parents' (neonatologist's words).

The parents are in their early 30s and have been attempting to have children for 3 years. They are married, usually visit together, and the staff feel that they are generally in agreement over care and are supportive of each other. The father is an accountant and the mother an advertising executive, and both have master's degrees. They have healthcare insurance. Both sets of grandparents live in the city where the couple live and are a fairly good support system. The couple is active in their faith tradition and have a good relationship with the clergy. They feel that their faith tradition considers all life sacred and would have great difficulty condoning discontinuation of ventilator support under any circumstances. They are, however, concerned regarding how meaningful the life the physician describes would be.

A care conference is arranged. Present are the parents, the neonatologist, a hospital chaplain, the infant's primary nurse, a social worker and the infant's maternal grandparents. The conference begins with the neonatologist reviewing the child's course, his present status and what he feels is a dismal prognosis. Mother tears up and her husband attempts to comfort her. As this is taking place, the maternal grandmother challenges the neonatologist regarding his thoughts of the suspected prognosis, saying she believes that the child will 'be fine'. The social worker encourages conversation between the parents and physician and, with obvious tension in the room, a discussion takes place regarding the adaptive skills a child with cerebral palsy and intellectual disability might have.

The family asks to have some time and a follow-up conference is arranged for 2 days later. In the interim there is no change in the child's status.

At the follow-up conference, the same individuals are present. The father states emphatically that he and his wife appreciate the neonatologist's views regarding what he suspects will be the outcome but they want to continue ventilator support. Because the neonatologist has persisted over the last several days in pressuring to have the parents agree to discontinuation of support, they ask if it would be possible to have another neonatologist take care of the child. The father states that the disagreement over care places the family in an uncomfortable position. Unfortunately, because of subspecialty physician availability and the policy adopted by the neonatology group, this is difficult to do. The meeting ends.

At this point the neonatologist, believing that further care is probably ineffectual and that he is causing the baby undue pain, calls the administrator to ask for institutional support for the decision to remove the child from the ventilator without the parents' consent. The request has a twofold purpose. First, he would like to have the approval of the healthcare community, represented by the hospital, in proceeding against the parents' wishes. Second, the neonatology group is employed by the hospital and therefore a controversial action against the hospital's wishes could conceivably lead to termination of employment. In fact, even if the physician were not a hospital employee, the commitment of what might be conceived as ill-advised clinical care could lead to *the loss of practice privileges at the institution. The administrator says 'no'; he is afraid of bad press. Undeterred, the neonatologist then calls the hospital attorney, who also says 'no' – stating that the parents are generally considered the presumptive decision-makers in cases involving children (Ahronheim et al. 2000).*

The other neonatologists in the group, and the nursing staff, aware of the situation, suggest a meeting of the hospital ethics committee, comprising physicians, nurses, social workers, an attorney and community representatives. The result of that meeting is that it is agreed to continue support. Also, care conferences will be held at least weekly so that both the providers and family can have a chance, without the pressure of having to make momentous decisions, to share information and clarify concerns and points of view.

Discussion

This scenario presents the common issues associated with the challenges of medical uncertainty and its presentation to parents. It also illustrates differences in the desired course of treatment and the importance of understanding why those differences arise, and how conflict resolution might happen within an ethically appropriate process.

It is important to have the medical facts

It is commonly said that good ethics begins with good facts. Jonsen and colleagues state that 'every discussion of an ethical problem in clinical medicine should begin with a statement of medical indications' (Jonsen et al. 2006 p. 14). For ethical decision-making to take place, the decision-makers must have an understanding of the consequences of their actions. In this case, the likelihood of an outcome as described by the neonatologist is not insignificant. This infant's birth weight and gestational age, and the severity of the intraventricular hemorrhage in association with brain parenchymal injury, are all factors contributing to the assumption of a poor prognosis. In the Western world, the chance of survival at this gestational age is approximately 50% (Eichenwald & Stark 2008). More specific data are available that include gestational age, weight, sex, multiple status and the use of antenatal steroids to help those involved determine the probability of survival (NICHD 2012). Should the infant survive, the major sequelae likely to be seen are cerebral palsy, generally spastic diplegia or quadriplegia, intellectual impairment, epilepsy, blindness and deafness. Other sequelae could include communication difficulties, specific learning impairments, and behavioral issues such as autism and attention-deficit/hyperactivity disorder (ADHD). While the presence of a grade IV hemorrhage certainly skews the likelihood for impairment significantly, at 24 weeks' gestation the incidence of significant major morbidities for all surviving infants

"Providers must remember that it is the patient's story in which they are involved. They are not the heroes of the story, the patient is"

is probably in the 60–70% range (Eichenwald & Stark 2008). In general, the spectrum of expectations for this child ranges from an individual with severe intellectual impairment, epilepsy and autism, without communicative ability, who is wheelchair dependent, to perhaps at best an individual with cognitive limitations including learning impairment and modest behavioral issues and who needs orthotics for ambulation.

These facts must be presented in a manner that allows discussion

Is the neonatologist being inaccurate in his presentation? Does his presentation close the door to further discussion? He may be speaking from his own experience and therefore flavoring his presentation based on what he believes and has seen. He cannot separate his recommendations from at least some influence from who he is and how his religious and cultural experiences have influenced his views on death and disability (Rebagliato et al. 2000). Studies have shown that physicians rate the quality of severely impaired children's lives as poorer than the children's parents, who rate the quality as poorer than the children themselves rate their own lives (Saigal et al. 1999). Gawande (2014) speaks of physicians who are directive, those who are informative without being directive (that is, just giving the facts) and those who use the facts to help guide shared decision-making. This physician is certainly presenting data in a way to be directive. He begins with a definitive comment that he wants to discontinue care. With this as his introductory comment, he is not presenting the data in a dispassionate manner, but rather in a way that directs decision-making and, more importantly, makes it difficult for those present to propose or offer differing views. It would be far better for the neonatologist to present the facts so they could then be used in a discussion of shared decision-making. Using the metaphor adopted by Mohrmann (1988), providers must remember that it is the *patient's* story in which *they* are involved. They are not the heroes of the story, the patient is. Because so much of the rest of the infant's story will be carried out with his parents and those in his community, their opinions must carry great weight.

The medical literature is based on statistical likelihood and the potential errors associated with it (Nuzzo 2014). With the advances resulting from research in medical intervention, the curves for survival and outcomes in pediatrics are often not bell-shaped but rather become more skewed in the direction of survival and better developmental outcomes. Therefore, even with the worst prognosis, there remains the possibility of some hope both for a better prognosis than predicted and for social-emotional successes even in the face of impairments. It should be the obligation of the physician to help describe the likelihood of variable outcomes.

It is not uncommon for the healthcare provider to be in the position where her or his recommendation regarding care is dismissed by the patient or his surrogate. Although this may be due to a lack of agreement as to the medical indications for the intervention in question, it may also be due to differing cultural and religious beliefs between the surrogate and the provider. Certainly, in the latter case, the dismissal of the recommendation is understandable. In adult medicine, the patient has a history and through their voice or that of their surrogate, their desire can generally be determined. However, the issue is particularly difficult in pediatrics because it speaks to the question of who truly is the appropriate optimal decision-maker who will speak to the child's best interest. For the child approaching adulthood, decision-making is sometimes clarified by asking for the child's assent, rather than their consent. This is, of course, not true for the younger child or the child whose medical condition precludes participation in decision-making. As the attorney noted, surrogacy generally belongs to the family.

The issue at the center of these complex dilemmas is often the essential importance of effective communication. While popular culture often portrays the physician as desiring to continue treatment, in fact, the opposite scenario also often occurs. The healthcare provider recommends discontinuing treatment measures while the family desires to continue to attempt cure. Perhaps the conflict could be lessened if the discussion were about healing the patient rather than curing the disease (Flam 1994). This may allow a discussion based more on what is important for the patient as an individual with multiple needs, to enable them to accomplish a meaningful life, rather than discussing an individual who happens to have a specific condition, that is, prematurity and its sequelae. The difficulty in coming to an effective and acceptable resolution often involves a problem with effective communication.

Why, for ethical decision-making, is it important to know so much about the family?

With growing cultural, economic and ethnic diversity in many regions of the world, it is important to recognize and validate divergent views and beliefs when utilizing any bioethical principles. For example, in current North American bioethics, the principle of autonomy is founded on the view of a person as an individual. This individual is an entity complete in and of itself. Some non-Western cultures espouse a different belief in the individual. For example, to be a complete individual in a communal society, one does not exist independently of others. Fulfillment as a human person dictates participation in a community of other selves. 'A human being becomes a human being through participation in a community of other human selves' (Mkhize 2006). Therefore, the individual should be cognizant of their responsibilities and obligations regarding their family and community and should act and make decisions accordingly.

There are striking differences between, and in fact within, faith traditions regarding the ethics of some medical interventions. More orthodox traditions are often more prescriptive, while more liberal traditions may allow more latitude in decision-making. Neither must be considered good or bad. It must be remembered, however, that the child and their family will live in and be a part of the community to which they will belong for many years to come, and generally the medical environment is only a small although often important part of their life. This underscores the importance of the concept of an ethical community that facilitates moral development.

How a family understands its religious and cultural norms has its roots in the moral development of the family members, and the degree of maturity of that development helps determine what they feel are ethical decisions. The influence of religious and cultural norms will affect the neonatologist's ethical decisions, and the understanding of these norms will also be determined by the maturity of the providers' moral development. Therefore, as a group of individuals meets to determine the best plan of care for anyone who is unable to make decisions for themselves, such as an incapacitated individual or, as in this case, an infant, the degree of moral development of the key players will greatly impact the quality of the decisions. The ability of an individual to make impartial and dispassionate decisions for another person, with only the welfare of that person weighed in the balance, is directly related to an individual's moral development. Lawrence Kohlberg (1981) posited a theory, which holds that moral reasoning, the basis for all ethical behavior, has identifiable developmental stages that can be more generally grouped into levels with stages in each level. As an individual ascends to higher stages and levels, they are more able to respond in a mature ethical manner to moral dilemmas. In the scenario case, therefore, there must be an understanding of the tools available to all for ethical decision-making. Their levels of education, family support and the religious and cultural milieu in which they function will influence their ability to think and act morally.

How should the conflict be resolved?

Unfortunately, there are times when the decision-makers are unable to reach agreement.

Enlisting the aid of the hospital administrator or the hospital's legal counsel is often detrimental to the process of reaching an ethically informed decision on the best plan of care for a patient in the hospital. The duties and obligations inherent in the administrator's position create a conflict of interest, and if they are consulted in a case involving a patient at their institution, they ought to recuse themselves. They cannot simultaneously espouse the best interest of the institution and the best interest of the patient. For the attorney, at what point do ethical quandaries become captive to legal constraints? While decision-makers must be cognizant of the law, they also must remember that good law and good ethics are not necessarily the same thing. In conditions of unresolved conflict, Ethics Committees are often used to help determine community moral standards. Although their recommendations are generally not binding, their deliberations and conclusions can be helpful for decision-makers, whether they be family, medical or legal.

If, after thoughtful discussion, a provider is unable in good conscience to follow a joint plan, that party should be allowed to recuse themselves from further involvement. If, however, that individual feels that the decision being reached cannot be tolerated, it is incumbent upon them to act in a manner that aims to block it, usually leading to involvement of the judicial system. For the family, if they cannot tolerate the decision, their options are generally also limited to legal action or the request to transfer to another provider who will concur with their plan of care, usually at another institution. In this case, the transfer itself may itself pose a significant risk to the sick newborn infant.

The decision-making process

Any responsible individual may ask for an Ethics Committee review. The American Academy of Pediatrics states that these committees should be multidisciplinary and diverse in makeup (American Academy of Pediatrics 2001).

All at the table must recognize their own biases and beliefs and respect others' views. It is important in this case to have a trusted friend, confidant or clergy present to help define for all parties, including both the family and the healthcare team, not only the family's particular desires and needs but also the faith traditions or cultural beliefs that are informing the family's decisions. These advocates must, however, recognize their role and not try to become primary decision-makers and must be certain that their presentation helps set the stage for meaningful discussion.

How are judgments reached? A common framework used in the analysis of medical decision-making involves four moral principles/values: autonomy, beneficence, nonmaleficence and justice. One might ask: a framework for whom – the child or his family/community – and are these two perspectives always the same, or can they be in conflict? Should each principle have equal weight? In common clinical practice, they often do not. In this case the patient is not capable of making decisions for himself, so his parents are making decisions based on their own values and beliefs.

Ethical decision-making is not simply based on looking at these principles in isolation. Feminist ethics (Tong & Williams 2014) directs us more towards interpersonal relationships and special obligations. Care ethics focuses on care of self, care of others and the interconnection between self and others. When one is involved in ethical decision-making, it is important to keep in mind that the process will be impacted by the beliefs, values, moral imperatives and so on, of everyone involved, and for no two individuals within the process will these be identical. These differing views may seem insignificant, but when applied to bioethical principles, such as autonomy, the potential for misunderstanding and conflict is great. If the goal is to reach an ethically sound decision, it is essential to take into account multiple moral traditions, ethnic backgrounds and religious communities.

The principles of beneficence and nonmaleficence suggest we ask questions such as 'What are the goals of treatment?', 'What are the probabilities of success?', 'What physical, mental and social deficits is the patient likely to experience if treatment succeeds?', 'Are there biases that might prejudice the provider's evaluation of the patient's quality of life?' and 'Is the patient's present or future condition such that their continued life might be judged undesirable?' Issues of justice must include financial, cultural and religious considerations.

Jonsen et al. (2006) suggest that analysis be based upon medical issues, patient preferences, quality of life and contextual features. These four topics are relevant to all ethical decision-making in medicine and should be considered in the context of each particular situation.

It is difficult to respect a patient's autonomy in a case involving substitutive judgment, especially in the absence of an Advanced Directive (Jaworska 2009). It is to be hoped that the patient has shared their wishes with their primary care physician and family. Even if this has not happened, one may look at the values and decisions the patient has made in their life and use these as a guide. When the patient is an infant this process is fraught with the reality that we cannot know what the infant's preferences are and therefore the issue of autonomy becomes difficult, and we must turn to the principles of beneficence and nonmaleficence to determine what is in the child's best interest. While parents are assumed to be acting in this regard, we need to balance any decision made with the knowledge and expertise provided by the patient's physician. This may unavoidably lead to conflict. In this case the parents' religious beliefs are obviously impacting their decision to provide all treatment options, regardless of the outcome. Are parental best interest decisions unquestionable? The courts often intervene, for example in the transfusion of Jehovah's Witness children, in cases where it is felt that a standard of care is not being followed by parents.

"Perhaps the right decision lies not so much in the right answer, but rather in the right process"

In this case, a solution is formed partly by our medical knowledge and expertise, and partly by the family's belief system and their understanding of the situation. What is best for this 'precious baby'? How we view ourselves and our world, what we value, that which gives us meaning – these are the beliefs that drive our ethical decisions. This is what each of us brings to the table, and, the better we understand ourselves and the others seated with us, the more likely we are to reach an acceptable moral decision.

Given the many potential pitfalls that may be encountered during the attempt to reach a sound ethical decision, how is one to move forward in this quest? Perhaps the right decision lies not so much in the right answer, but rather in the right process. The cornerstone of working with families in difficult situations must be effective communication, communication that acknowledges the understanding and bias of all involved.

Epilogue

In this case, the hospital community, through the Ethics Committee, affirmed that the parents were acting in a way that could be considered the child's best interest and that they were acceptable surrogates. They were allowed to follow a plan of care that they felt was acceptable to their underlying beliefs. With plans for better communication in place, recognition of the changing status of patients in an intensive-care environment allows those involved to modify the plan of care in response to those changes.

Themes for discussion

- How does an 'ethical' framework for decision-making in complex situations help clinicians move beyond the basic principles of 'good clinical care'?

- In what ways might the discussions and resolutions of complex clinical dilemmas like the one presented here challenge our sense of self and our professionalism as clinical service providers?

- The views and values of the neonatologist in the case described here were clearly different from those of the family. When faced with a situation like this, what resources might be available to us to deal with the conflicts that likely arise?

References

American Academy of Pediatrics Committee on Bioethics (2001) Institutional ethics committees. *Pediatrics* 107: 205–209.

Ahronheim JC, Moreno JD, Zuckerman C (2000) *Ethics in clinical practice*. Gaithersburg, MD: Aspen.

Eichenwald EC, Stark AR (2008) Management and outcomes of very low birth weight. *N Engl J Med* 358: 1700–1711.

Gawande A (2014) *Being mortal*. London: Profile Books.

Flam N (1994) The Jewish way of healing. *Reform Judaism Mag* Summer.

Jaworska A (2009) Advance directives and substitute decision-making. In: Zalta EN, editor. *The Stanford encyclopedia of philosophy*; http://plato.stanford.edu/archives/sum2009/entries/advance-directives/.

Jonsen AR, Siegler M, Winslade WJ (2006) *Clinical ethics* 6th edn. New York, NY: McGraw Hill.

Kohlberg L (1981) *The philosphy of moral development* 1st edn. New York, NY: Harper & Row.

Mkhize N (2006) Communal personhood and the principle of autonomy. *CME: Your SA Journal of CPD: Ethics* 24: 26–29.

Mohrmann ME (1988) Stories and suffering. In: Lammers SE, Verhey A, editors. *On moral medicine* 2nd edn. Grand Rapids, MI: Eerdmans Publishing.

NICHD Neonatal Research Network (NRN) (2012) Extremely preterm birth outcome data; https://www.nichd.nih.gov/about/org/der/branches/ppb/programs/epbo/Pages/epbo_case.aspx.

Nuzzo R (2014) Scientific method: statistical errors. *Nature* 506: 150–152.

Rebagliato M, Cuttini M, Berbik I et al. (2000) Neonatal end of life decision making: Physicians' attitudes and relationship with self-reported practices in 10 European countries. *JAMA* 284: 2451–2459.

Saigal S, Stoskopf BL, Feeny D et al. (1999) Differences in preferences for neonatal outcomes among health care professionals, parents, and adolescents. *JAMA* 281: 1991–1997.

Tong R, Williams N (2014) Feminist ethics. In: Zalta EN, editor. *The Stanford encyclopedia of philosophy*; http://plato.stanford.edu/archives/fall2014/entries/feminism-ethics/.

Chapter 7

Humanism in the practice of neurodevelopmental disability: examples of challenges and opportunities

Garey Noritz

Prologue

In this chapter, we explore the concept of humanism as it relates to working with families touched by neurodevelopmental disability and illustrate this idea with a few selected vignettes. As stated by Cohen (2007), 'Humanism is a way of *being*. It comprises a set of deep-seated personal convictions about one's obligations to others, especially others in need. Humanism manifests itself by such personal attributes as altruism, duty, integrity, respect for others, and compassion.' It is this commitment to humanism that increases our expertise in caring for children with complex medical needs beyond that of skilled technicians. Just as physicians must hone their skills in taking a history, conducting a physical examination, or performing a procedure, the development and improvement of humanistic qualities takes time, experience and reflection. Through the vignettes in this chapter we present examples of issues that are common in the practice of neurodevelopmental pediatrics and which challenge the clinician to balance ethical principles while practicing compassionate, humanistic care. Three sequential main concepts are considered: breaking bad news, advising a

> "Humanism comprises a set of deep-seated personal convictions about one's obligations to others, especially others in need."

family that is making difficult decisions, and recognizing and working with families under stress.

Breaking bad news

By virtue of our work, the neurodevelopmental specialist has ample opportunity to refine their skills at delivering bad news. The most common scenario is the confirmation that the child has a particular impairment, for instance, cerebral palsy. This will be a turning point for the family. They have probably suspected that there is something 'wrong' with their child, and the clinician will now confirm it. The family will probably remember this encounter powerfully, and although their recollection of the specifics may transform over time, the attitude and humanism of the clinician (or, sadly, the absence thereof) will remain vivid in their memories.

The biggest ethical issue here is maintaining honesty and transparency. The diagnosis should be given clearly and compassionately, while avoiding the natural tendency to minimize the impact of the diagnosis. Experts in this area advise 'firing a warning shot' before disclosing the bad news; that is, let the family know bad news is coming. Once the news is delivered, there needs to be time for it to be digested. The experienced specialist knows how to use silence and is comfortable doing so.

Delivering the name of the condition (e.g. 'cerebral palsy') is only part of the task. Next, the family needs to hear, to the greatest extent possible, what impact the diagnosis will have on this specific child and the family. This should not merely be a listing of the ways in which the child will be 'abnormal'. Modern ethical practice demands that the person with impairment be seen as a valued member of society. As such, a list of impairments is less helpful than a discussion of the child's strengths – and there are always strengths.

In those situations where data are available to guide the discussion, information must be presented honestly; for example, a 10-year-old with cerebral palsy who does not have head control is not going to walk, regardless of any intervention (Rosenbaum et al. 2002). However, we rarely have the specifics that families want, and this reality also needs to be presented honestly. At best, we can often only prognosticate generally; for example, most people with Down syndrome continue to require some assistance throughout their lives.

Beginning with this first 'bad news' visit (event), the neurodevelopmental specialist can help the family begin to understand the challenges that they and their child face. It is likely that the family does not have much direct experience with people with disabilities and thus have only negative expectations. An important task after naming the disorder is to explore the known treatment and prognostic information, including a reframing of expectations. (Additional deliberations on delivering 'bad news' are discussed in Chapter 8 by Novak et al.)

Decision-making for children with neurodevelopmental disability

Clinical scenario

A 4-month-old term girl (Laura) with a chromosomal abnormality and hydrocephalus presents to our neurodevelopmental clinic for a first visit. She was just released from the neonatal intensive-care unit (NICU) and the team there asked us to take over her primary care. The NICU team presented a very grim picture of Laura's prognosis and the palliative care team worked with Laura's mother (Dinah) to explore her goals and wishes for her daughter. Dinah is a single, teenaged woman, estranged from her own family; Laura's father has been involved intermittently. Dinah decided that she did not want Laura to undergo painful procedures to prolong her life. A ventricular-peritoneal shunt and gastrostomy tube were offered by the surgeons, but with the support of both NICU and palliative care teams, these interventions were declined. Laura was discharged with home-based palliative care services and a nasogastric tube for supplemental feeding.

This case scenario is a typical presentation for the kinds of patients seen in a neuro-developmental clinic. These clinics tend to be situated in large children's hospitals and provide neurodevelopmental assessments and medical care for an array of patients with varied neurological impairments. Commonly, these patients are seen because of cerebral palsy, autism, myelomeningocele, genetic disorders and neuromuscular diseases. Although many of these conditions are considered 'static' or 'non-progressive', all the children are evolving naturally (development happens in children with impairments and in their parents). In addition, there can be an evolution of symptoms or impairments, which require ongoing medical management. As part of their complex medical issues, these children often have impairments in multiple domains, with significant cognitive and behavioral issues. Some such clinics will see both adults and children; some will provide primary care in addition to subspecialty services. Most will have vital resources available – such as social workers, dieticians, psychologists and chaplains – to assist in the biopsychosocial aspects of care.

Serious conditions such as these often beget ethical dilemmas. Most families are unprepared to handle the physical and emotional burdens of having a child with limited function and potentially a limited life expectancy. There is little evidence available to guide clinicians and families through the critical choices that must be made in the care of such patients; without a clear path to guide medical decision-making, ethical tensions become prominent, as we must balance the core principles of beneficence and non-maleficence, autonomy and justice.

Issue 1: pain of unclear etiology

Dinah reports that having Laura at home has been very stressful. Laura cries frequently and is difficult to console. Neither the infant nor her mother sleeps much. The baby is eating poorly.

Dinah worries that her daughter is in pain and also that she has made the wrong decision to place limits on medical care.

When we examine Laura, she is irritable and afebrile. Her head is large and the anterior fontanelle is bulging. She has dysmorphic facial features and emerging spasticity. There are no corneal abrasions, hair tourniquets, bony abnormalities, ear infections, abdominal tenderness, diaper rash or other obvious sources of pain.

Irritability is a common complaint raised by families of children with neurological impairments. Pain is frequently postulated as a generator of irritability, although this can be difficult to establish in the preverbal or non-verbal patient. A reasonable rule (promulgated by this author) is that pain is present if the family believes it is.

The ethical principle of *justice* demands that pain in a person with impairment should be treated as aggressively as it would be in any other person, but there is the added challenge of elucidating the cause of pain (for causal treatment) and monitoring the response to treatment. In these patients there are a myriad of possible pain generators, which can be caused by the underlying disease (e.g. hip dislocation in spastic cerebral palsy) or by a treatment of the disease (e.g. pancreatitis as a result of valproate therapy for seizure control), or indeed it can be completely unrelated to the condition (e.g. otitis media or constipation, as in any child).

The use of strong pain medicines, such as opioids, is often avoided by clinicians and families because of the worry of 'doing harm' by introducing dependency or respiratory depression. When used cautiously and appropriately, however, there is little actual risk of either (Friedrichsdorf & Kang 2007).

Irritability unrelated to pain is also common in patients with neurological impairment and can be caused by a number of factors. These might include frustration from poor communication, unrecognized seizures, psychiatric symptoms such as depression and anxiety, poor sleep, overstimulation or hunger. Irritability is a common side effect of several antiseizure medications. There is also an ill-described (but commonly cited) syndrome of 'neuroirritability' (Schwantes & Wells O'Brien 2014).

Issue 2: clinical uncertainty in diagnoses

Based on Laura's symptoms and exam, we believe that the most likely cause of her irritability is headache from untreated hydrocephalus. As this is our first time working with this family, we begin to explore Dinah's decisions using an ethical framework. She was able to articulate (tearfully) how she had considered whether to allow for ventricular shunting; she understood that Laura might live longer with a shunt, but there would also be pain and potential complications from brain surgery. She understood that while shunting might fix her hydrocephalus, it would not improve her chromosomal abnormality. Without using the terms beneficence and non-maleficence, she effectively discussed this tension.

Issue 3: uncertainty of prognoses

Following this discussion, we validate her desire to promote Laura's comfort and present two treatment options: her headache could be treated with pain medications alone, or by placement of a ventricular shunt. We attempt to be clear in our uncertainty as to what is the preferred approach.

Children with neurological impairment and life-limiting conditions, even when aggregated, are rare. To a large extent, each situation is unique. As such, it is usually difficult to prognosticate outcomes of a particular course of therapy in a specific child. This uncertainty is central to the ethical dilemmas in the care of patients with these impairments, as neither benefits (principle of beneficence) nor harms (principle of non-maleficence) can be accurately predicted before the therapy is undertaken.

Dinah decides to have Laura undergo placement of a ventriculoperitoneal shunt, which is performed successfully. Laura seems better, with less irritability and improved oral feeding. She is discharged but returns to our office with recurrence of irritability and vomiting. We order magnetic resonance imaging (MRI) and call the neurosurgeon, who reevaluates her and believes the shunt to be draining well. Our team, the neurosurgeon and Dinah have to decide what to do next, realizing that the shunt may not have alleviated the cause of the irritability.

The care of patients with neurodevelopmental impairments is fraught with second-guessing. As procedures and treatments are more often temporizing than curative, families and clinicians have ample time to agonize and re-agonize about these decisions. When the players in these debates are not on the same page, there can also be an undercurrent of blame, such as when one parent wants to choose an aggressive treatment and the other is ambivalent, or when the family feels pressured by the clinical team to do (or not do) something. Clinical team members not involved in the original decision may criticize choices down the road, sometimes years later. At issue here is the protection of the family's *autonomy* to act in the child's best interests; despite disagreement by other interested parties, it is imperative that the neurodevelopmental specialist advocates for the family and child (Noritz 2015). The exception would be if the clinician thinks that the family autonomy is straying into maleficence, or doing harm.

Laura is admitted to the hospital for evaluation, which includes phlebotomy, bladder catheterization and tapping the shunt for cerebrospinal fluid (CSF) examination. None of these assessments is revealing and despite continued irritability, she is discharged. She is readmitted 24 hours later with the same symptoms and is similarly re-evaluated, with similar results. Although he believes the shunt to be functioning normally, the neurosurgeon suggests exploring the shunt in the operating room. Dinah consents to surgery and the shunt is indeed found to be working well. However, following the surgery, Laura cannot be extubated. Several more attempts to extubate her fail over the next week, and continued mechanical ventilation via tracheostomy is offered.

There is often a common tension between chronic care providers and acute care providers, and this needs to be recognized and appreciated in order to serve the patient well. The acute care provider, such as the intensivist, is expert in life-sustaining procedures such as mechanical ventilation. They have probably seen many patients with severe impairments and supported them through grave situations. However, the particulars of each situation are new and specific to this child and family. Because of the previous work and relationship with the family, the neurodevelopmental specialist's assistance can be vital in helping the family and intensivist through the next decision-making process.

The palliative care team is again consulted and works with Dinah, exploring the option of ventilation and tracheostomy. Dinah reiterates her desire to make sure Laura is comfortable, and does not want her to 'live on machines'. Dinah tells the pediatric intensive care unit (PICU) staff that she will not consent to tracheostomy. One member of the PICU staff is uncomfortable with this course of action and requests a consult from the ethics committee to explore whether the failure to offer life-sustaining therapy constitutes discrimination against a person with a 'disability'. The committee judges that this is within the realm of ethical practice – that Dinah, using substituted judgment, is acting for Laura's best interests.

Laura is extubated with symptoms of dyspnea managed by opioids and benzodiazepines; she dies comfortably in her mother's arms later that night.

Parents under stress and their responses: an ethical analysis

No training exists to help parents understand the 'rules' for interacting with a healthcare team. Parents must learn to be effective advocates for their children, while avoiding the insulting labels too often assigned (very inappropriately) by professionals, of parents being 'difficult', often meant as 'overbearing', 'demanding', 'in denial' or 'crazy'. Because of the uncertainties surrounding the care of children with impairments, parents in the neurodevelopmental clinic are particularly prone to being tagged with this kind of pejorative label. However these terms are applied, justice demands that the children of every type of parent receive our best efforts. It needs to be remembered that we often don't see parents at their best – they need us most when they are tired, stressed, anxious or scared.

> *"It needs to be remembered that we often don't see parents at their best – they need us most when they are tired, stressed, anxious or scared"*

There are several common identifiable parental 'phenotypes' (perhaps unfairly caricatured), each with its own ethical challenges. Several are described below to elucidate the ethical points, along with strategies for working with such parents. It should be noted that these descriptions are not mutually exclusive. It should also be noted that these are not meant to be derogatory, but rather are presented as archetypes for illustrative purposes. These behaviors can be regarded as coping mechanisms gone awry. By recognizing what we may feel is problematic coping, we can approach parents 'where they are at' and attempt to improve care for the child and the family (Grossberg 2008).

The parent with boundless optimism

Alex is an 8-year-old male with dystonic cerebral palsy; he has a cochlear implant and gastrostomy tube. He is dependent for all of his activities of daily living and has no means of self-mobility. Alex's parents are determined that he will live a 'completely typical life'. Despite the many hours that his hands-on care consumes, they have declined nursing help at home. He goes to a mainstream school and participates in adaptive recreational activities. He has an older brother and a younger sister, both of whom are having trouble in school and are difficult to redirect at home. In the office, the parents excitedly tell you all of the things that Alex is doing, and deflect any conversation with any negative connotation.

Parents who present this perspective may outwardly deny that the impairment affects their family at all, or even that the child has any impairment. They may believe that to say anything about the impairment (even if it is constructive) is to say something negative about *the child*. This is often a response to difficulties the family has experienced in the integration of the individual in society. The parent may not feel that there is a safe place to discuss the difficulties of parenting a child with an impairment.

While *boundless optimism* in a family may make for pleasant interactions, there are times when this armor of denial must be chipped away in order to facilitate more transparent communication. A parent exhibiting these characteristics may have difficulty recognizing functional decline or suffering, and over time, they may have trouble recognizing their own infirmities, mental health challenges or advancing inability to provide care. Although it is easy to collude with the parent and pretend that everything is fine, it would not be *beneficent* to perpetuate a fiction. If the clinician detects stress within the family, it should be named. If there is decline, the clinician must insist on investigation. In the case above, it is clear that there are familial difficulties related to the child's care, and the clinician could help by exploring sibling dynamics; each child in this family needs the attention of the parent to achieve optimal functioning. (See also Chapter 19 by Blasco.)

The parent with a tendency to be pessimistic

Sam is a 16-year-old boy with severe autism, insomnia and behavioral problems that include self-injurious behavior. He communicates occasionally with pointing and grunting; even this is inconsistent. He has seen many developmental specialists, psychologists and psychiatrists, both in our town and at national referral centers. He has been on many psychotropic drugs, none of which has worked and most were stopped for apparent side effects. At your visits, Sam's parents have a long list of complaints, including his behavior, but also his bowel habits, abdominal pain, insomnia, headaches, sinus problems and acne – and all of your proposed solutions are declined, as they 'didn't work before'. In your estimation, the parents are depressed and very fatigued.

The pessimistic parent has a very negative outlook on life. Complaints are many, centered on both the plight of the child and past interactions with the medical system. Proposed solutions are quickly dismissed as unworkable. When the clinician offers therapies believed to be *beneficent*, the parent will assume *maleficence*, often leading to treatment inertia.

Pessimism can be infectious. Despite starting from an optimistic place, staff working with the family begin to succumb to negativity. The parent may or may not have an underlying affective disorder; they assuredly have residual grief from the loss of the 'normal' child. Parents of children with serious impairments commonly report a significant lack of sleep for both child and caregiver (Tietze et al. 2014). No-one is at their best when sleep-deprived, and the psychomotor effects of sleep deprivation may be easily confused with depression (Green 2007). This can only be sorted out by honestly discussing what is observed in the office, for example, anhedonia, irritability, hopelessness and so on. Our psychosocial partners in psychology, social work or chaplaincy are instrumental in caring for these families. (See Chapter 20 by Reddihough and Davis.)

Often, the child is the only one in this case scenario not beaten down by gloom. The individual with an impairment may, within their frame of reference, make significant achievements, and the parent may have difficulty recognizing these. Here, the clinician may have to advocate for the child's *autonomy* and *value* in the face of a parent who has difficulty recognizing it.

This is a situation that can be improved by attention to family dynamics. Respite can be helpful, as can individual or family therapy for the parents.

The 'nurse' parent

This is the parent who delivers intensive-care unit (ICU)-level care in their home. They keep voluminous medical records, vital signs, stooling charts and frequently speak in medical jargon.

George is a 12-year-old boy with severe spastic cerebral palsy, frequent respiratory infections and epilepsy, who is monitored for heart rate and oxygen saturation 24/7. His parent finds that the heart rate is elevated above his baseline for an evening. Otherwise, he seems to be acting well. The parent calls and requests that you order a chest X-ray, blood count and urine culture by catheterization, to be done at an outpatient lab close to their home, rather than bring him to you (or any other doctor) for evaluation. The parent states that they know something is wrong based on past instances when elevated heart rate heralded an infection, which resulted in a 'terrible' hospitalization. They want to figure out what is wrong and get appropriate antibiotics started before there is a need for an ER visit or hospitalization.

This is a very experienced and savvy parent, who holds the (usually correct) belief that their child is still alive because of their care and advocacy. This parent is the expert in the child's medical care and can often sense when something is seriously wrong. If the child is admitted to the hospital, this parent is often very critical of members of the nursing staff, who do not care for their child the way they are cared for at home. (This includes both the mechanical aspects of nursing care, as well as the emotional and empathic dimensions of care.)

A common problem for this type of parent is 'losing the forest for the trees'; they become focused on biomedical details rather than the life experience of the child. Often, this is a coping mechanism on the parent's part – they channel the stress and helplessness of raising a child with neurological impairment into a 'take charge' kind of attitude. In this author's experience, this is notably common among parents who are also professionals in their community, such as physicians, executives and engineers.

The ethical issue here is that this parent needs limits set on their *autonomy*. While sending the patient to the outpatient lab without a clinical evaluation might be more convenient for the family and clinician, it flirts with the unlicensed practice of medicine and an abdication of professional responsibility. Note that in the vignette above, it is the parent who 'wants to figure out what is wrong', and the physician is merely a clerk for ordering tests, rather than a healthcare provider.

The parents' hard work and expertise should be validated, but there are cases where limits need to be set and mutual expectations discussed. Although George may have many doctors and nurses, he will only have one or two parents. It may be helpful to help them develop their parental roles beyond medical caregiving.

The 'naturalistic' parent, distrustful of conventional medicine

This is the parent who scours the Internet for alternative treatments for their child's medical problems.

Mary is a 10-year-old girl with spinal muscular atrophy type II. She uses bilevel positive airway pressure (BiPAP) at night and when not feeling well; she is fed mostly by gastrostomy. Her parents give her a dozen or so dietary supplements that they believe are improving her muscular function. These include turmeric for preventing contractures, creatine to boost muscle strength, human breast milk (from a milk bank) to boost immunity and a home-blended, low fat, low protein diet to improve digestion. They have declined all vaccinations, including influenza. Mary regularly receives chiropractic treatments. Her parents tell you they are planning to start giving Mary marijuana oil, as they have heard that it may reduce fasciculations, which are interfering with sleep.

This is the parent who wants to do things as 'naturally' as possible. They are suspicious of mainstream medicine and frequently ask about alternative healing methods, generally termed 'complementary and alternative medicine' (CAM) (see also Chapters 12 and 13). They are always ready with a story about how a suggested medication caused a terrible side effect, often in a report from the Internet. They are frequently a proponent of the latest naturalistic fad – currently medical marijuana, previously antioxidants or mega-dose vitamins.

The ethical issues with this type of parent involve respecting both parental and clinician autonomy as regards unproven treatments. It is a rare circumstance where a parent should be mandated to allow a treatment that they think harmful, such as blood transfusions for the child of Jehovah's witnesses. The clinician's autonomy needs to be respected as well, and they should not be expected to prescribe treatments they consider unwarranted or dangerous, such as hyperbaric oxygen for the treatment of cerebral palsy. This leads to tension between the clinician and family in defining beneficience and *non-maleficence*, balancing the unknowns of 'natural' treatments versus the known problems of 'traditional' medications.

The clinician must have an honest discussion of the knowns and unknowns regarding the treatment of neurodevelopmental impairments. It is clear that CAM treatments are common in the chronic incurable diseases that we treat (Hurvitz et al. 2003); we must help the family recognize that 'natural' does not necessarily mean safe and that the Internet is full of scams and unvalidated testimonials, without reports of possible failures and harm that has been done.

When CAM is requested, the clinician and family should discuss whatever CAM has the best evidence behind it and choose that which is least likely to cause harm and financial burden. The clinician must attempt to maintain trust and collaboration, whatever is chosen. Rarely, reports to protective services are warranted in the face of dangerous treatments. In the case above, the clinician needs to be aware of local laws that govern the use of medical marijuana, as well as uncertainties regarding which formulations the family might obtain, as well as dosing. The increase in public acceptance of marijuana used for 'medical' purposes does not mean that there is scientific evidence of benefit (Ammerman et al. 2015).

Epilogue

The care of individuals with impairments is an inherently humanistic endeavor, and ethical issues are commonly encountered. As parents are the experts in their children and (usually) their best advocates, great deference must be given to their autonomy to act in the best interest of their child, using substituted judgment. This does not mean that professional responsibility is abdicated, nor is the moral responsibility to help families understand the consequences of their decisions lessened. Providing services using a compassionate family-centered, collaborative approach to decision-making is likely to help everyone prevent at least some of the ethical dilemmas that easily arise in this complex branch of child health. The neurodevelopmental specialist, who often has a relationship with the family spanning years, is well suited to the complex medical and psychosocial care needed by families of children and adults with impairments.

Themes for discussion

- There is a tendency, described in this chapter by Noritz, for health professionals to categorize parent 'types' in caricatures. What can we do both to avoid this and to identify and discuss it in our teams when we hear this happening?

- In an effort to express empathy, many of us may say to a family 'I know what you are going through'. This can elicit anger and distress among parents who challenge this statement. Without appearing to sound trite, how else can we indicate to families that we 'feel their pain'?

- Perhaps the most important resources we have as developmental service providers working with families like those discussed in this book are compassion and time – yet time in particular is prized by the 'systems' in which we work as the resource we must use 'efficiently'. How do we reconcile what appear to be competing demands on the resource of time?

References

Ammerman S, Ryan S, Adelman WP, The Committee on Substance Abuse TCOA (2015) The impact of marijuana policies on youth: Clinical, research, and legal update. *Pediatrics* 135: 769–785.

Cohen JJ (2007) Viewpoint. Linking professionalism to humanism: What it means, why it matters. *Acad Med* 82: 1029–1032.

Friedrichsdorf SJ, Kang TI (2007) The management of pain in children with life-limiting illnesses. *Pediatr Clin North Am* 54: 645–672.

Green SE (2007) 'We're tired, not sad': Benefits and burdens of mothering a child with a disability. *Soc Sci Med* 64: 150–163.

Grossberg RI (2008) Psychoanalytic contributions to the care of medically fragile children. *J Psychiatr Pract* 14: 307–311.

Hurvitz EA, Leonard C, Ayyangar R, Nelson VS (2003) Complementary and alternative medicine use in families of children with cerebral palsy. *Dev Med Child Neurol* 45: 364–370.

Noritz G (2015) How can we practice ethical medicine when the evidence is always changing? *J Child Neurol* 30: 1549–1550.

Rosenbaum P, Walter S, Hanna S et al. (2002) Prognosis for gross motor function in children with cerebral palsy: Creation of motor development curves. *JAMA* 288: 1357–1363.

Schwantes S, Wells O'Brien H (2014) Pediatric palliative care for children with complex chronic medical conditions. *Pediatr Clin North Am* 61: 797–821.

Tietze AL, Zernikow B, Michel E, Blankenburg M (2014) Sleep disturbances in children, adolescents, and young adults with severe psychomotor impairment: Impact on parental quality of life and sleep. *Dev Med Child Neurol* 56: 1187–1193.

Chapter 8

Truth with hope: ethical challenges in disclosing 'bad' diagnostic, prognostic and intervention information

Iona Novak, Marelle Thornton, Cathy Morgan, Petra Karlsson, Hayley Smithers-Sheedy and Nadia Badawi

Prologue

Clinical scenario

From the very beginning, it was clear to me that something was very wrong with my baby. For the 9 months of my campaign to find answers, the health professionals and specialist doctors we consulted either dismissed our concerns or told us that our daughter was 'a slow starter' and a 'lazy baby'. Only one doctor suggested that significant spasticity was evident. Without much further explanation or words that comforted, he simply referred us to a specialist cerebral palsy service organization. At our initial visit, after lots of prodding and poking and testing reflexes and the like, a staff doctor there turned to me and declared, 'Yes, she's one of ours!' The clinical 'baldness' of the pronouncement was probably the most impactful. There had to be a better way to break this news ... perhaps a message that firstly affirmed my instincts as a mother and secondly, a positive message that help was at hand. Had this happened, I think I would have felt more in control of not just my emotions, but of the overall situation. (Personal communication Marelle Thornton, AM, DipTeach)

Over 85% of the time, parents know that their child has cerebral palsy before the diagnosis is given (Baird et al. 2000; Klein et al. 2011). Despite this, receiving the diagnosis can be both traumatizing and socially stigmatizing (Green 2002), and discrimination can be experienced even within the health system (Larivière-Bastien et al. 2011). The set-up and way in which parents are told their child has an impairment affect their emotions and beliefs, attitudes to their child and future, and impressions of the health system (Jan & Girvin 2002). Thornton's 'clinically bald' experience of receiving her daughter's diagnosis of cerebral palsy is a poignant example of what not to do, and implores us to learn better ways of breaking bad news.

Informing a parent that their child will have a life-long impairment is likely to cause shock, disappointment, anxiety, loss, grief, guilt and challenge:

"The diagnosis itself, even if expected, is experienced as a unique and powerful form of interpersonal loss."

The diagnosis itself, even if expected, is experienced as a unique and powerful form of interpersonal loss. It is the loss of an imagined reality … The diagnosis of a disability violates [pre-planned] narratives in dramatic and intense ways … It's a death, because it's not the child you think of … (Green 2002 pp. 21–22)

Assessing the family's perception of where they are at, in their process, is important. Over time, parents' feelings of denial and loss are replaced by an intense desire to do everything that might help their child (Piggot et al. 2002). As a result, parents want to be told both the good and bad news about their child's diagnosis and prognosis, and to be given information about how to help. Most of the time, health professionals underestimate just how much information parents want (Girgis et al. 1998; Green 2002; Tattersall et al. 1994). Giving knowledge and information to the family helps parents make decisions and regain a sense of control about the future, and affects their satisfaction (Pain 1999).

What does it mean to be an ethical source of support? An important first step is to establish shared decision-making between families and professionals, underpinned by the belief that families know their child best and want to help (Dunst 2002; Rosenbaum et al. 1998). Even though a diagnosis can cause stigma, diagnostic labels can also open doors to intervention services, which most parents understandably want as soon their child is diagnosed. This chapter will outline the major types of diagnostic and prognostic news, as well as evidence-based intervention decision-making that typically needs to be communicated to parents of children with cerebral palsy over the lifespan. It outlines an ethical and evidence-based framework for communicating this often difficult and complex information in a way that facilitates family coping, taking into consideration unique family characteristics.

The ethics of sharing news

Ethics attempts to answer questions about which professional standards and behavior we should accept and why (Beauchamp & Childress 2001), and is therefore integral to sharing news.

> Present information in a manner, language and volume which that are appropriate for the parents and in a way that gives focus to the positive qualities of the child, not just a commentary which focuses upon his/her atypical symptoms. As parents we often ask inappropriate, irrelevant and irrational questions about our child or about the nature of the disability or program. Please don't be too harsh with your answers, or discount the question as worthless. Parents' concerns are very real to them. (Personal communication Marelle Thornton, AM, DipTeach)

The principles of informed consent and respect for autonomy have created an ethical and legal obligation to provide families with as much information as they want about their child's impairment and treatment (Baile et al. 2000) and invite them to shared decision-making. Codes of ethical conduct seek to protect children and families from therapeutic harm, neglect and mistreatment, and these codes encompass sharing bad news in a way that does not cause harm. A vital aspect of ethical practice is therefore good communication, tailored to the child and family (Chauhan & Long 2000), addressing the family's emotions with empathic responses. The four major ethical principles and their relationship to sharing news are now described (Beauchamp & Childress 2001).

Non-maleficence

Truth telling is fundamental to ethics, and yet some believe that withholding the truth might protect parents and thus *do no harm* (i.e. non-maleficence). Truth, however, is a subjective concept (Chauhan & Long 2000). Truth telling by definition involves communicating information comprehensively, accurately and objectively, while fostering understanding, and as such, respects parental autonomy (Beauchamp & Childress 2001).

> Information about the nature of the disability, problem or disorder is most valuable to parents. Parents need to be encouraged to be as well informed as possible about their child, treatment programs, alternative methodologies and progress being made by the child. (Personal communication Marelle Thornton, AM, DipTeach)

It is not uncommon to fear that telling the truth, when the news is bad, will cause unwelcome emotional reactions with long-term harmful consequences. And it is true that when news is withheld or delivered in an abrupt manner, parents' mental health can worsen (Baird et al. 2000; Girgis & Sanson-Fisher 1998). Even if negative emotions occur initially, in the longer term families tend to reframe their experience to gratitude, peace of mind, a positive attitude, and acceptance (Girgis & Sanson-Fisher 1998; Schuengel et al. 2009). A mother of a child with cerebral palsy reflected:

> I can't say that I would have chosen this complicated path for my life. I most assuredly would not have chosen [it] for my daughter ... I can say that the experience has changed who I am and the way in which I view the world ... It has also broadened my image of what it means to live a good and worthwhile life. (Green 2002 pp. 30–31)

Families indicate that compassionate delivery of news is as important as the content of the news itself: 'The truth must always be told but with empathy, compassion and hope. Provide information on what can be done to help' (Personal communication Marelle Thornton, AM, DipTeach). In other words, a hopeful framework can make a positive difference to how families perceive the healthcare received.

What is hope and its relationship to truth telling in healthcare? Hope is an emotional attitude encompassing desiring an event; believing the event is congruent with personal values; imagining the event is possible; and acting in a way that corroborates hope (Simpson 2004). Is it possible to deliver bad news in a compassionate way so as to convey hope? Parents suggests yes, and comment that

> Giving realistic, positive and hopeful messages to parents about their child is the start of providing good support to people with disabilities through their whole lives. (Harnett et al. 2009 p. 37)

Furthermore, if hope is thought of as a series of small collective expectations, rather than one single entity that might be dashed, it is easier to deliver bad news compassionately (Feudtner 2009). You can say that you wish the news were different. Then as the parent begins to understand the news, you can move to explaining the hope that remains (Feudtner 2009). For example: 'Given what you are now up against, what are you hoping for?' (Feudtner 2009 p. 2307).

"if hope is thought of as a series of small collective expectations, rather than one single entity that might be dashed, it is easier to deliver bad news compassionately"

Autonomy

Respect for autonomy means respecting parents' freedom and choice to make decisions based on their own values, providing they act in the best interests of the child, even when professionals' viewpoints differ (Chauhan & Long 2000). As children grow up and find ways to communicate their preferences, it may become apparent that children and parents do not always agree. Children are not an extension of their parents

(Racine et al. 2014). A balance needs to be struck between respecting child self-determination and parents consenting on behalf of the child, especially when it may not be possible for a child to understand or experience immediate treatment benefits (e.g. preventative dental treatment). However, for families to be as autonomous as possible in the face of good and bad news, families need be given the truth and the necessary information to be free to choose their course of action (Chauhan & Long 2000). For families of a child with an impairment, multiple installments of 'bad' news are likely. The news might begin with the threat of a miscarriage or preterm birth, and progress to complex decisions about life-saving care in the neonatal intensive care unit, followed by discussion around risk of impairments.

> When they told me that my best option was to actually let my son go, [I wondered] what type of parent would I be by bringing a child into this world that will need constant 100% care ... What quality of life am I giving him because he will have cerebral palsy? Every day I'd look and think, especially for the first two months, am I doing the right thing? ... I don't feel selfish for what I've done ... I loved that I chose this for my life, [and] that he's got all the help he's needed. (Personal communications with a mother of child with cerebral palsy, who had a history of multiple miscarriages)

More questions than answers exist about how best to care for an infant in the neonatal intensive-care unit (NICU) who might die or survive with life-long impairment (Liben et al. 2008). The challenge of supporting parents to make decisions about active care in the NICU versus allowing a natural death for infants with life-threatening illness or a probable long-term severe disability is filled with complex ethical dilemmas. In these sorrowful circumstances, information-giving must be a process not an emergency event (Alderson et al. 2006). Parents value understanding the facts about the infant's current and future quality of life; the chance of getting better; and current pain and discomfort levels (Meyer et al. 2002). It is important to explore sensitively a good quality of life for the child and parent versus a good death for the child (Liben et al. 2008). Parents must be given real choices, information about the least harmful decision, time to reflect and the right to refuse (Alderson et al. 2006). It is important to affirm and support parental decision-making and to remain physically present through the process of death if this is the chosen path (Brosig et al. 2007; Sullivan et al. 2013).

Beneficence
The ethical principle of beneficence involves providing information about the treatment's potential benefits as well as balanced communication about the potential risks or harms (Beauchamp & Childress 2001). When striving to adhere to the ethical principles of 'do good' and 'do not harm', ethical consideration must be given to the timing and evidence-based content of messages.

Challenges of starting school

By the time our daughter was ready to start school, it was fairly plain to us that she would probably never walk independently, but that first conversation about a wheelchair was very confronting. A wheelchair seemed to be the symbol that all hope was lost and this was as good as it was going to get for her. And so too was the announcement by the speech pathologist that a symbol board was being prepared for her. In hindsight, why couldn't these messages have been delivered in a way that promoted discussion and brought us to an understanding of the freedom and benefits that mobility aids and communication devices would give our daughter, rather than what seemed presented as a full stop in a sentence about the future? (Personal communications Marelle Thornton, AM, DipTeach)

The severity of cerebral palsy cannot always be prognosticated early, and the early years often include a series of disappointments, as milestones such as walking are not met. Parents have the challenge of choosing from a variety of rehabilitation and medical intervention options, including some that they may not personally want (e.g. a wheelchair). Parents often continue to prioritize walking over wheeled mobility well into the school years (Chiarello et al. 2010; Pollock & Stewart 1998), even when it might not be realistic for the child, as they experience feelings of guilt when tapering walking interventions (Gibson et al. 2012). A number of tools exist to discuss likely prognosis, including neuroimaging for prognostication, the Gross Motor Function Classification System (GMFCS) (Palisano et al. 1997; Rosenbaum et al. 2008) and the Manual Ability Classification System (MACS) (Eliasson et al. 2006). The gross motor curves (Hanna et al. 2009; Rosenbaum et al. 2002) provide more specific information about the likelihood of walking. Classifying a child's functional mobility as GMFCS Level IV or V early, and describing what this probably means for the future, is therefore a meaningful discussion with implications for current intervention plans (e.g. use of wheeled mobility) and long-term expectations. Professionals need to communicate clearly the meaning of mobility, why independent mobility is important for overall development, and the advantages of early powered mobility, such as how it might empower self-initiated conversation (Jones et al. 2012). The health professional must assess whether there is some risk of harm to the parent in sharing this information; or whether this prognostic information belongs to the child and parent, and thus whether there is some harm to the child by not discussing it.

Justice

The ethical principle of justice means that professionals must also ensure fair and equitable treatment throughout the life cycle from referral to diagnosis and intervention. Because young children and adolescents with intellectual disability cannot independently consent to treatment without their parents, professionals must also advocate for what is in the best and fairest interest of the child by explaining all of the available treatment options and the likely consequences of acting and not acting (Stewart et al. 2006; Zeigler 2003).

For example, many intervention options for cerebral palsy are advertised, described and even filmed on the Internet. Parents search out what they can do to help their child but can easily be overwhelmed by the volume of often-conflicting information, and sometimes feel compelled to try all of it. Studies show that parents forego leisure opportunities, family holidays and health services for themselves in order to purchase a wide range of services to help their child (Bourke-Taylor 2015). It is therefore important for professionals to guide and assist parents to navigate the complex web of modern intervention options using an evidence-based framework while respecting the autonomy of parents to choose what they believe is best for their child. For example, should a child lose their playtime and holidays in pursuit of better functional outcomes from more intense therapy? Or would playtime and family holidays give the child a better quality of life?

An evidence-based process for sharing news

It is becoming increasingly clear that the way in which medical and prognostic information is shared has a long-lasting impact on the ongoing relationships of families and people with impairments with the health system. It is likely that there will be more than one occasion where difficult news will need to be delivered to families of children with impairments. Certainly, giving the diagnosis is a key moment, but as the child grows there are likely to be other instances that might feel to families like 'more bad news'.

> It is particularly important that 'bad news' moments over time are acknowledged and that professionals are reminded and equipped with a way to deal with these moments in an ethical way and with as much sensitivity as the 'original bad news' – diagnosis. In fact the delivery of these 'other' pieces of bad news can also have lasting impact on families and their interrelationships. (Personal communications Marelle Thornton, AM, DipTeach)

In the interests of a trusting and effectual partnership, it is imperative that better methods of communication are put in place. In order to address all four ethical principles effectively, as previously outlined, within the difficult context of sharing bad news, some degree of standardization of language grounded on evidence-based guidelines is appropriate. There are several areas of medicine that have made notable gains and we suggest that these could be adapted for this use.

Best available evidence from randomized control trials on sharing 'bad' news originates chiefly from the cancer field, but nevertheless offers the disability field important lessons, including that families are more hopeful when (1) the diagnosis is disclosed face to face with a high degree of individuality, intimacy and privacy, (2) the diagnosis is given by someone with a connection to the family, (3) the presence of supportive accompaniment is an option at the time of diagnosis, (4) available medical information is given with realism and hope, (5) the diagnostician describes anecdotes of actual families who have overcome similar problems, (6) information is given about support groups, (7) families perceive they are encouraged to take control of their own care and that the care is the best medical science has to offer, and (8) professionals are emotionally supportive and will not abandon them as a consequence of the diagnosis (Sardell & Trierweiler 1993; Walsh et al. 1998).

The process of disclosing bad news can be viewed as an attempt to achieve four essential goals: (1) information-gathering so as to determine the family's knowledge, expectations, and readiness for news; (2) provision of clear information matched to the family's needs; (3) reduction of the emotional impact and isolation experienced from hearing bad news; and (4) development of a treatment plan based on the family's input (Baile et al. 2000). The SPIKES protocol is the most widely cited evidence-based framework for communicating bad news effectively (Baile et al. 2000). Below, we outline the SPIKES protocol devised in the oncology field, and apply the cerebral palsy evidence base to this framework as a suggested way forward for the disability field. The SPIKES framework can be adapted at various points in the family's journey to ensure best practice communication strategies are used.

The six steps of the SPIKES protocol

Step 1: S – SETTING UP the interview

Breaking 'bad' news is never easy, but it is important it is done well (Novak & Msall 2014), so preparation on the part of the professional is required. Mental rehearsal is a good preparation technique that professionals can use to help manage the stress and planning to handle difficult questions well (Baile et al. 2000). Ninety-two percent of parents think that it is important for professionals to plan to give positive information about the child in the midst of giving a diagnosis and realistic prognoses, so as to foster their hope about the child as a person (Harnett et al. 2009). Setting up the physical space for delivering the news is also important (Baile et al. 2000). Parents also recommend using a quiet, private office (Ahmann 1998; Rahi et al. 2004); scheduling at least two face-to-face diagnostic information sharing sessions (Calam et al. 1999; Hallberg et al. 2010), because coming to terms with diagnosis is a process rather than a one-off event; and ensuring both parents and the infant are present for the diagnostic meetings (Ahmann 1998; Huang et al. 2010) to ensure the discussion

"it is important for professionals to plan to give positive information about the child in the midst of giving a diagnosis and realistic prognoses, so as to foster their hope about the child as a person"

is about the real child, and to promote recall and foster emotional support. Planning the interview probably should always include a plan to audio-record the discussion so that family and friends can have a permanent record to which they can listen as many times as necessary, revisiting issues where there may be uncertainty about exactly what was said, and how it was said.

Step 2: P – Assessing the family's PERCEPTION

Next, *before you tell, ask* (Baile et al. 2000). The use of open-ended questions assists the professional to gain an accurate picture of how the family perceives and understands the situation (Baile et al. 2000): for example, 'What have you been told so far?' 'What is your understanding of why we did the MRI?' Based on the answers given, the professional then can reframe any misunderstandings and tailor information to suit the individual family (Ahmann 1998; Baile et al. 2000; Hallberg et al. 2010). Parents recommend providing honest, transparent and specific information about future prognosis (Reid et al. 2011): for example, 'It sounds like you are asking me if your child will walk? Have you heard of the Gross Motor Function Classification System? It is a tool we use to help parents understand the likelihood of their child walking. Let's have a look at the tool together and you can identify which level you think your child is functioning at. Then we can discuss what this usually means. Does that sound okay?'

Step 3: I – Obtaining the family's INVITATION

When the family explicitly requests and invites more information, the invitation lessens whatever anxiety the professional might be feeling (Baile et al. 2000). To set up the invitation, questions might be formulated, such as 'How would you like me to give you the results?' Parents also recommend inviting their questions (Reid et al. 2011): for example, 'Most parents have lots of questions. What are your questions?' It is important for professionals to communicate explicitly that they are willing to hear the family's questions both in the present moment and at a later appointment (Baile et al. 2000).

Step 4: K – Giving KNOWLEDGE and information to the family

Warning the family that there is 'bad' news ahead can lessen the shock and facilitate information processing (Baile et al. 2000). Given this pre-framing, the medical facts can then be provided clearly and not overly bluntly, regularly confirming understanding and communicating that intervention help is available (Baile et al. 2000). Parents recommend using simple, direct, jargon-free language (Ahmann 1998; Reid et al. 2011), using a hopeful, empathic and supportive tone (Ahmann 1998), providing written information to allow later absorption (Jedlicka-Köhler et al. 1996; Klein et al. 2011) and providing information about the child's strengths as well as limitations, to promote developing an optimistic outlook (Ahmann 1998): for example, 'I have some bad news I need to share with you today. I wish that the news were different. The assessments ...

are indicating that your child has a condition called cerebral palsy. Cerebral palsy is a physical disability, resulting from damage to the part of the brain controlling movement … For 80% the cause is unknown – so this is not your fault. Cerebral palsy is permanent and life-long, but life expectancy is almost always normal. Two in three children with cerebral palsy will walk and three in four will talk … The good news is, all children with cerebral palsy can learn and progress. We know how to help. Is that something you'd like to talk more about?' (Novak & Msall 2014).

> Supply parents with appropriate literature or steer them towards other sources of information, so that they can digest the content in their own time and at their own pace. This will assist thought … and provide some confidence in talking to others. (Personal communications Marelle Thornton, AM, DipTeach)

Step 5: E – Addressing the family's EMOTIONS with empathic responses
Responding to emotions is one of the most difficult challenges of breaking bad news (Baile et al. 2000). Acting empathically involves observing the emotions, naming the emotions, identifying the reasons for the emotions, and allowing the family to express their feelings (Baile et al. 2000). Parents recommend inviting discussion about feelings, because it promotes trust and confidence in the parents' ability to cope and increases satisfaction with the disclosure process (Ahmann 1998) – for example, 'Understandably you look very sad. It's very normal to feel sad and stressed with this type of bad news. Would you like to tell me more about what you are thinking and feeling?'

Step 6: S – STRATEGY and SUMMARY
Before discussing a treatment plan, it is important to check with the family to see if they are ready for such a discussion. Families given the opportunity to formulate a clear plan for the future, and ideas about how to help their child, feel less anxious and uncertain (Baile et al. 2000). Parents also recommend arranging both parent-to-parent and family support, as parents indicate this to be a key strategy for long-term coping (Reid et al. 2011); appointing a key worker for debriefing plus helping parents to gather information and navigate service entry (Rahi et al. 2004); and arranging follow-up early intervention, preferably initially at higher intensity to help parents to come to terms with what is required of them (Piggot et al. 2002): for example, 'Who do you have in your life that supports you? Is there someone you can call or visit to discuss today's difficult news? Many parents tell me they also like to talk to another parent who has been through this before. Is that something you'd like me to arrange?'

Epilogue

Ethical dilemmas abound in the disability field. Dilemmas arise during information sharing and treatment decision-making that require professionals to share the truth, seek informed consent, respect autonomy and communicate treatment beneficence without maleficence. Uptake of evidence, including the use of the SPIKES framework and parental advice in delivering the bad diagnostic and prognostic news, may change parents' experiences for the better. Truth telling with hope is important, and professionals should work with families to explain the evidence for or against an intervention and work with the family to find an effective alternative.

Themes for discussion

- Telling the 'truth' is a complex and challenging task, and elicits a wide range of emotions. What are your experiences of this process? Why does it cause professionals so much difficulty?

- What processes can professionals use to acquire and practice the skills needed to be an effective communicator of 'bad news'?

- How can professionals evaluate the quality and impact of their communication skills? Are such processes and resources available in your setting, and if not, can they be developed?

References

Ahmann E (1998) Review and commentary: two studies regarding giving 'bad news'. *Pediatr Nurs* 24(6): 554–556.

Alderson P, Hawthorne J, Killen M (2006) Parents' experiences of sharing neonatal information and decisions: Consent, cost and risk. *Soc Sci & Med* 62(6): 1319–1329.

Baile WF, Buckman R, Lenzi R, Glober G, Beale EA, Kudelka AP (2000) SPIKES – A six-step protocol for delivering bad news: application to the patient with cancer. *Oncologist* 5(4): 302–311.

Baird G, McConachie H, Scrutton D (2000) Parents' perceptions of disclosure of the diagnosis of cerebral palsy. *Arch Dis Child* 83: 475–480.

Beauchamp TL, Childress JF (2001) Beneficence. In: Beauchamp TL, Childress JF, editors. *Principles of biomedical ethics* 5th edn. New York, NY: Oxford University Press.

Bourke-Taylor H, Cotter C, Stephan R (2015) Complementary, alternative and mainstream service use among families with young children with multiple disabilities: family costs to access choices. *Phys Occup Ther Pediatr* 35(3): 311–325.

Brosig CL, Pierucci RL, Kupst MJ, Leuthner, SR (2007) Infant end-of-life care: the parents' perspective. *J Perinatol* 27(8): 510–516.

Calam R, Lambrenos K, Cox A, Weindling A (1999) Maternal appraisal of information given around the time of preterm delivery. *J Reprod Infant Psyc* 17(3): 267–280.

Chauhan G, Long A (2000) Communication is the essence of nursing care. 2: Ethical foundations. *Br J Nurs* 9(15): 979–984.

Chiarello LA, Palisano RJ, Maggs JM et al. (2010) Family priorities for activity and participation of children and youth with cerebral palsy. *Phys Ther* 90(9): 1254–1264.

Dunst CJ, Boyd K, Trivette CM et al. (2002) Family-oriented program models and professional helpgiving practices. *Fam Relations* 51(3): 221–229.

Eliasson AC, Krumlinde Sundholm L, Rösblad B et al. (2006) The Manual Ability Classification System (MACS) for children with cerebral palsy: Scale development and evidence of validity and reliability. *Dev Med Child Neurol* 48: 549–554.

Feudtner C (2009) The breadth of hopes. *N Engl J Med* 361(24): 2306–2307.

Gibson BE, Teachman G, Wright V, Fehlings D, Young NL, McKeever P (2012) Children's and parents' beliefs regarding the value of walking: Rehabilitation implications for children with cerebral palsy. *Child Care Health Dev* 38(1): 61–69.

Girgis A, Sanson-Fisher RW (1998) Breaking bad news. 1: Current best advice for clinicians. *Behav Med* 24(2): 53–59.

Green SE (2002) Mothering Amanda: Musings on the experience of raising a child with cerebral palsy. *J Loss Trauma* 7(1): 21–34.

Hallberg U, Oskarsdottir S, Klingberg G (2010) 22q11 deletion syndrome – the meaning of a diagnosis. A qualitative study on parental perspectives. *Child Care Health Dev* 36(5): 719–725.

Hanna S, Rosenbaum P, Bartlett D et al. (2009) Stability and decline in gross motor function among children and youth with cerebral palsy aged 2 to 21 years. *Dev Med Child Neurol* 51(4): 295–302.

Harnett A, Tierney E, Guerin S (2009) Convention of hope-communicating positive realistic messages to families at the time of a child's diagnosis with disabilities. *Br J Learn Disabil* 37(4): 257–264.

Huang YP, Kellet UM, St John W (2010) Cerebral palsy: Experiences of mothers after learning their child's diagnosis. *J Adv Nurs* 66(6): 1213–1221.

Jan M, Girvin JP (2002) The communication of neurological bad news to parents. *Can J Neuro Sci* 29(1): 78–82.

Jedlicka-Köhler I, Gotz M, Eichler I (1996) Parents' recollection of the initial communication of the diagnosis of cystic fibrosis. *Pediatrics* 97(2): 204–209.

Jones MA, McEwen IR, Neas BR (2012) Effects of power wheelchairs on the development and function of young children with severe motor impairments. *Pediatr Phys Ther* 24(2): 131–140.

Klein S, Wynn K, Ray L et al. (2011) Information sharing during diagnostic assessments: What is relevant for parents? *Phys Occup Ther Pediatr* 31(2): 120–132.

Larivière-Bastien D, Majnemer A, Shevell M, Racine E (2011) Perspectives of adolescents and young adults with cerebral palsy on the ethical and social challenges encountered in healthcare services. *Narrative Inquiry Bioethics* 1(1): 43–54.

Liben S, Papadatou D, Wolfe J (2008) Paediatric palliative care: Challenges and emerging ideas. *The Lancet* 371(9615): 852–864.

Meyer EC, Burns JP, Griffith JL, Truog RD (2002) Parental perspectives on end-of-life care in the pediatric intensive care unit. *Crit Care Med* 30(1): 226–231.

Novak I, Msall M (2014) Cerebral palsy. In: Malcom WF, editor. *Beyond the NICU: Comprehensive care of the high-risk infant.* New York, NY: McGraw Hill Professional.

Palisano R, Rosenbaum P, Walter S, Russel D, Wood E, Galuppi B (1997) Development and reliability of a system to classify gross motor function in children with cerebral palsy. *Dev Med Child Neurol* 39(4): 214–223.

Pain H (1999) Coping with a child with disabilities from the parents' perspective: The function of information. *Child Care Health Dev* 24(4): 299–312.

Piggot J, Paterson J, Hocking C (2002) Participation in home therapy programs for children with cerebral palsy: A compelling challenge. *Qual Health Res* 12(8): 1112–1129.

Pollock N, Stewart D (1998) Occupational performance needs of school-aged children with physical disabilities in the community. *Phys Occup Ther Pediatr* 18(1): 55–68.

Racine E, Bell E, Shevell M (2014) Ethics in neurodevelopmental disability. In: Bernat JL, Beresford R, editors. *Handbook of clinical neurology: Ethical and legal issues in neurology Series 3*, Chapter 21. Edinburgh: Elsevier.

Rahi JS, Manaras I, Tuomainen H, Hundt GL (2004) Meeting the needs of parents around the time of diagnosis of disability among their children: Evaluation of a novel program for information, support, and liaison by key workers. *Pediatrics* 114(4): e477–e482.

Reid A, Imrie H, Brouwer E et al. (2011) 'If I knew then what I know now': Parents' reflection on raising a child with cerebral palsy. *Phys Occup Ther Pediatr* 31(2): 169–183.

Rosenbaum P, King S, Law M, King G, Evans J (1998) Family-centred service: A conceptual framework and research review. *Phys Occup Ther Pediatr* 18(1): 1–20.

Rosenbaum P, Palisano R, Burlett D, Galuppi B, Russel D (2008) Development of the gross motor function classification system for cerebral palsy. *Dev Med Child Neurol* 50: 249–253.

Rosenbaum PL, Walter SD, Hanna SE et al. (2002) Prognosis for gross motor function in cerebral palsy: Creation of Motor Development Curves. *JAMA* 288(11): 1357–1363.

Sardell AN, Trierweiler S (1993) Disclosing the cancer diagnosis procedures that influence patient hopefulness. *Cancer* 72: 3355–3365.

Schuengel C, Rentinck IC, Stolk J et al. (2009) Parents' reactions to the diagnosis of cerebral palsy: Associations between resolution, age and severity of disability. *Child Care Health Dev* 35(5): 673–680.

Simpson C (2004) When hope makes us vulnerable: A discussion of patient-healthcare provider interactions in the context of hope. *Bioethics* 18(5): 428–447.

Stewart D, Stavness C, King G, Antle B, Law M (2006) A critical appraisal of literature reviews about the transition to adulthood for youth with disabilities. *Phys Occup Ther Pediatr* 26(4); 5–23.

Sullivan J, Monagle P, Gillam L (2013). What parents want from doctors in end-of-life decision-making for children. *Arch Dis Child* 99: 216–220.

Tattersall MHN, Butow PN, Griffin AM, Dunn SM (1994) The take home message: Patients prefer consultation audiotapes to summary letters. *J Clin Oncol* 12(6): 1305–1311.

Walsh RA, Girgis A, Sanson-Fisher RW (1998) Breaking bad news 2: What evidence is available to guide clinicians? *Behav Med* 24(2): 61–72.

Zeigler VL (2003) Ethical principles and parental choice: treatment options for neonates with hypoplastic left heart syndrome. *Pediatr Nurs* 29(1): 65–74.

Chapter 9

Different perspectives, different priorities: using a strengths-based approach to gain trust and find common ground

Dinah S. Reddihough and Jane Tracy

Prologue

Every child and family we see in our clinic challenges us to do better. Every child offers opportunities to deepen our understanding of the needs of families, every family brings a set of unique and special circumstances, and every child and family with complex needs presents ethical challenges for those involved in their care. This case scenario highlights six areas of practice in which ethical dilemmas arose for us when the beliefs and perspectives of clinician and family differed in the following areas:

- Giving/obtaining an accurate history

- Appropriate medication use

- Building the best possible life for this child

- Investigations and interventions required

- The child's right to communicate

- Priorities for intervention

Each of these words describing elements of care carries with it a subjective, value-based judgment. When values are not shared between clinicians and the family, significant tensions can arise, and these in turn can create ethical challenges. As clinicians, we try to build and maintain constructive relationships with family members while at the same time navigating a path between our responsibility to do what we perceive as being in the best interests of the child and respecting the autonomy and integrity of the family. It is not always a clear or easy path to follow.

Clinical scenario

I am a pediatrician and work with a multidisciplinary assessment team. On the outpatient list today, I note the name of a child not previously seen in this clinic. She is 14 years of age and according to the referral letter, has a diagnosis of cerebral palsy although the cause is not documented. She has recently moved with her family from the countryside to suburban Melbourne.

Obtaining an accurate history

It is the end of a busy clinic. Molly enters the room in a dilapidated wheelchair accompanied by her parents, who both seem stressed. Molly's sitting posture is poor and her clothes are disheveled. I ask why they have come to the clinic today. They respond by explaining that they require some assistance with bathing Molly as she is maturing and the father feels he can no longer assist with this aspect of her care. I get the feeling the parents are defensive and evasive as I ask more about Molly's past history. The parents tell me that Molly was dropped when she was eight months old and was taken to a hospital. They say they were never told whether this caused or contributed to her impairment, and that they don't think any tests were done to understand the cause of Molly's impairment. Molly's parents appear reluctant to answer further questions, including those I ask about obstetric and family history. I am not clear whether they are apprehensive about disclosing details about Molly and their family, whether they are overwhelmed by being in the clinic, or annoyed that they have had to come to the clinic today. Perhaps they cannot fully comprehend the reason for all of my questions and believe the only issue of relevance is the management of her personal care. It is the end of the day, the team is tired and I notice one of the therapists glancing at her watch.

When families bring a child who is not able to speak for herself to health professionals, what right does the family have to withhold information from health professionals that may influence care? As a doctor I have been trained to want to know more and to take a thorough history. I feel frustrated and impatient with their answers when I sense their reticence is hindering an honest and trusting relationship that needs to be built and is blocking my access to the information that I require. I feel the tension between their right to privacy and my need for knowledge in order to do the best for the child.

'Appropriate' medication use

Molly's mother reports that Molly has seizures most days although it is difficult to gain a clear understanding of when these started and the nature and duration of these episodes. The family doctor has prescribed anti-seizure medication. The parents were advised to give this medication twice a day but they only administer it every second day, as 'she gets too tired otherwise'.

What are the best interests of the child in this situation? Taking medication intermittently is less likely to be effective. However, the parents believe that they are doing what is best for their daughter. I feel very concerned for Molly. Her parents are playing a mediating role between the doctor and their daughter, but do they understand the implications? Are they capable of making informed decisions about the appropriate use and dose of anti-seizure medication? Should I be making a judgment about this when I only met these parents 30 minutes ago? Have they been adequately informed in the past about the importance of regular dosing to maintain blood levels and therefore effective treatment? Is this the right time to embark on a conversation about the need for regular administration when they may interpret my comments as criticism and they are already defensive? What are the safety and ethical implications of leaving Molly on a subtherapeutic dose? These questions race through my mind as I continue with the history.

Building the best possible life for this child: community inclusion

Molly's parents report that she spends her days at home, cared for by her mother and other family members. She has never been to school. The parents tell me that she could not possibly learn as she has no speech and that they would worry about her safety if they were not with her. The parents do not receive any funded assistance with Molly's personal care and she does not participate in any community or social activities apart from family functions.

What are the child's rights here? Does she have the right to attend school and participate in her community when her parents have an alternative view of what is best for her? Her parents do not believe she could benefit from going to school and would be at risk. They do not share my understanding that education is a right for all and that modifications can be made to the curriculum for individual children? What is my role, as her health professional, in a situation in which I see her life opportunities being severely restricted?

Investigations and interventions 'required'

On examination, Molly is significantly underweight and has signs of spastic quadriplegia with contractures, functioning at Gross Motor Function Classification System level V, Manual Ability Classification level V and Communication Function Classification System level V. She wears disposable napkins. The manual wheelchair in which she attends the appointment does not support her appropriately and is in a poor state of repair. Molly does not appear to be comfortable in it.

The parents come with a specific request, yet there is so much that could be done for this young girl, including efforts to determine an etiological diagnosis, addressing nutritional issues, organizing optimal seating and arranging a whole series of investigations that could include medical imaging, blood and urine tests. What are the ethical implications if the family refuses to address her nutritional issues, or chooses not to go ahead with investigations, or the appointments required for a new wheelchair? What is my responsibility if that occurs? How do I balance what I see as being best for my patient with my belief in respecting and supporting family autonomy? When do different parenting choices become child protection issues?

The child's right to communicate

Molly is alert, interactive and interested in her environment. She has no speech, nor does she have any formal communication system such as a communication aid or device. At one point during the consultation, her parents interpret her facial expression and body language as indicating she wants a drink. They are comfortable with her current level of communication, saying that they understand what she needs.

What right does an adolescent with functional impairments that include severe communication difficulties have to communication tools to optimize independent communication when this is not a priority of the family? The Convention on the Rights of Persons with Disabilities (United Nations 2006) makes two important statements that help me to determine what is right for Molly:

- First, Article 7 states that 'children with disabilities have the right to express their views freely on all matters affecting them, their views being given due weight in accordance with their age and maturity, on an equal basis with other children, and to be provided with disability and age-appropriate assistance to realize that right.'

- Second, Article 21 states that 'persons with disabilities have a right to freedom of expression and opinion, including the freedom to seek, receive and impart information and ideas on an equal basis with others and through all forms of communication of their choice.'

The priorities for Molly are clear to me at this time, but what do I do if the family sees the situation differently? Is this the time to raise the question as to how much she may understand even though she does not speak? What are the ethical implications if the family just does not believe it is worth exploring the issue of her communication abilities further? How can Molly's rights to independent communication, and the consequent agency this brings, be upheld if the family does not prioritize this goal?

A trainee doctor is present at the appointment. I can see the notes she is making and her priorities are to understand more about the cause of Molly's impairments by organizing a magnetic resonance imaging (MRI) brain scan, genetic and metabolic testing. She wants to institute a number of interventions including increasing the anti-seizure medication to an effective dose and organizing hip X-rays to check for hip displacement. In addition, she would like to discuss gastrostomy feeds to address Molly's obvious nutritional issues. These priorities are quite different from the family's priorities and I am concerned that if this junior doctor speaks out she might alienate the parents and they may not come to our service again. I feel we have not yet built the kind of trusting collaborative relationship with the family in which we could raise these challenging issues.

Whose priorities are paramount when the main concerns of the family differ substantially from those of the health professionals (or perhaps the child)? In what circumstances can and should the priorities of the family be over-ridden? What would be the implications for care of doing this? When could there be a case to consider a protective application if parents refuse a gastrostomy in the presence of severe malnutrition?

What opportunities exist in this situation for enhancing and enriching Molly's life and that of her family? To what degree are these opportunities Molly's rights?

The United Nations Convention on the Rights of Persons with Disabilities, to which Australia is a signatory, has a range of articles that are directly relevant to Molly's care (United Nations 2006). These include, in particular, her right to communicate (Article 7), community inclusion (Article 19), to go to school (Article 24) and optimal health care (Article 25). The dilemma is how to uphold her rights to these while respecting her home and family life (Article 23).

Molly

Her right to grow and develop as an independent young person
Molly is a young adolescent who, in her current circumstances, has very limited opportunities for agency and autonomy. She has never had the chance to form relationships with peers or to engage with her broader community. I recognize that she has a loving and protective family, but feel sad that her possibilities for developing independence and relationships outside the family have been so severely restricted.

Molly has had few opportunities to learn to trust people other than her family to provide the personal care assistance that she needs. Having paid workers assisting with these tasks could be initially awkward or embarrassing for her. I recognize that this will need to be introduced to Molly and her parents sensitively, and that every effort must be made to have a small number of workers provide this care each week to enable trust and confidence to be built. I feel that if she and her family could trust others to provide for her daily needs in this way, the foundation would be laid for a more independent life for Molly, and the care demands on her parents would be reduced.

Her right to healthcare: the importance of her doctor having the information required in order to make good treatment decisions
I need to know about her past history in order to understand the cause of her impairment and establish the best plan for her future care. I also recognize that, with this family, considerable time and several appointments will be required to gain a comprehensive view of her history and her current situation. The family needs to trust my team before they will reveal painful or sensitive past events, and I will have to wait and accept that it is not an immediate priority in this situation.

Her right to optimal seizure control
I know that improving Molly's seizure control will impact positively on her health, well-being, functioning and ability to learn and engage with others. I am impatient to address this, but recognize that the best time to attempt this discussion needs careful consideration. The risk of death may be higher when seizures are poorly controlled, so the timing of this discussion is also dependent on finding out more about the seizure types and frequency. Any change in anti-seizure medication will have to be implemented by the parents, and so it is crucial that they understand the need for the change and are partners in the decision. I know I need to take the time to engage them, as only then can I be confident that they will understand the need for and benefits of better seizure control and so implement my management recommendations. In some situations, a short hospital admission might be the most expedient way to assess the impact of increasing the medication to therapeutic levels, but this family has been reluctant to come to an outpatient appointment, and I strongly suspect they would be even more hesitant to even consider a hospital admission.

Her right to be included: to attend school and form relationships with peers and participate in her community
Molly has been cared for in isolation by her family. They perceive this care as loving, nurturing and protective of their vulnerable child. She has never been to school and so has not had the opportunity to learn and engage with other children, spend time outside the parental home and test her own abilities in different situations. She has been completely dependent on her parents, and has not had the chance to develop trust in

others to provide the personal care assistance she requires. The prospect of venturing into an environment outside of the home may engender feelings of both anxiety and excitement for Molly, and her parents may fear for her safety and be confronted by their loss of control. Molly will need their support to feel confident in embarking on this new adventure and so it will be vital that our team work with both Molly and her parents to support them to see the advantages for her of these new experiences, and encourage them to find and work with a supportive school to build trust in the school's ability to care for her.

Her right to have the investigations and interventions to enable her to achieve
the highest attainable standard of health and function
Molly's health, comfort and function are all high priorities. This includes the need for her to have appropriate bathing and personal care arrangements. Assessments and investigations are crucial to understanding Molly's needs, but focusing on pathology, rather than her abilities and strengths may be disempowering for this young woman, and may be perceived by her family as threatening and alienating. Investigations therefore will need to be carefully selected, prioritizing those that are most critical to her health, and with the reasons for them discussed sensitively with both Molly and her parents. I am very concerned about her nutritional status and her sitting posture, but improvement in these areas can be longer-term goals.

Her right to be heard
There is a pressing need to hear Molly's 'voice' in this situation. She has severe expressive communication impairment, but her receptive language ability is unknown at this point and it is wise to assume competence in such children. Assessments of her cognitive and communicative abilities are crucial to determining the best and most effective system of communication for her. Initial goals should be focused on ease of use and achieving successful communication to build confidence in this domain in both Molly and her family. More comprehensive and sophisticated communication options can be explored once a foundation of success is established. It is only through optimizing Molly's ability to communicate that her agency and autonomy can be developed and exercised. If Molly is able to build her ability to communicate independently, she will then be able to participate actively and increasingly in discussions and decisions about priorities in her care. Children's perspectives are vital in decision-making around priorities in care. They should be informed about and supported by healthcare professionals in the ways they can contribute to decisions regarding intervention (Anderson & Dolva 2014). When Molly reaches adulthood it will be important to involve her actively in decision-making as much as possible; opportunities for her to participate in discussions as a child will build her confidence and competence in this regard. Supported decision-making (rather than substitute decision-making) is now seen as a central mechanism to enhance self-determination and quality of life (Shogren & Wehmeyer 2015).

The parents and the extended family

The opportunity to share Molly's care

Molly's parents may be apprehensive about the cause of her impairment, perhaps believing that they are responsible in some way for it. The clinical setting may be unfamiliar and threatening to them and they may fear being judged by health professionals. Building trust over a number of appointments may enable the sharing of details and perhaps appropriate reassurance that they were not responsible, which may, in turn, relieve them of unnecessary guilt. I hope that this family comes to feel supported and relieved at the prospect of sharing responsibility for meeting Molly's complex needs.

The opportunity to work in partnership to control her seizures

There is the temptation to immediately adjust the dose of, or replace, the anti-seizure medication, as it is almost certainly subtherapeutic and therefore suboptimal for Molly. Informing the family about the value of keeping a log of the frequency, length and nature of the seizures, and showing them how this could be done, could start to develop a sense of partnership and lay the groundwork on which decisions about the medication could be discussed. Observing the seizures must be distressing for Molly's parents, as is their concern that the medication is making her sleep more. I share their concern and hope that my committing to work with them to address this issue together will build the foundation of a constructive collaborative relationship.

The opportunity to build a good life for Molly

Sometimes it can be hard to recognize that a family wants the best for their child, when their priorities are very different to those of our team. In Molly's case we acknowledge and value the family's dedication to her care over her lifetime. We are keen to encourage the family to consider and arrange schooling for Molly, but we know it will be challenging for them to do so. It is not a priority for the family; in fact, they had not even raised it as an issue at this point. We have to accept that it may take several appointments, further discussion and provision of information before they will be ready to visit schools in their neighborhood. Empowering them to consider schooling and to investigate which school might be most appropriate and welcoming for Molly will have long-term implications for the whole family, and the decision must therefore reside with them. Supporting and encouraging them through this process is critical to success. Their understandable concerns about Molly's safety must be addressed and gradual introduction to a supportive school setting may enable both Molly and her family to develop trust and confidence in the school.

The opportunity to understand Molly's needs better through investigations and assessments

The family may not understand why we feel that certain investigations or assessments are required, or see what benefit could eventually flow to Molly through subsequent interventions. Focusing on what is 'wrong' with Molly may be undermining and dis-empowering for the family, just as it could be for Molly. There are likely to be many 'deficits' found, for example in the levels of vitamins and other nutrients, abnormally developing hips and possibly a scoliosis. Treatment that is not currently being contemplated, let along sought, by the family, is likely to be recommended as the result of these investigations. I must ensure that my team and I work through the issues in a stepwise fashion so the family understands what is being suggested and why. We must provide the family with the team's clinical evaluation and discuss with them the options that might be available to optimize Molly's quality of life. The timing, order and priority of investigations and interventions must be jointly negotiated in the context of this partnership between the family and health professionals caring for Molly. Maintaining a focus on Molly's strengths and future health and life opportunities will help to develop common goals.

The opportunity for Molly's voice to be heard
The possibility that Molly may have the ability to communicate independently and may understand more than the family has assumed may generate disbelief, apprehension or even sadness at lost opportunities. The parents may need to revise their previously held views about Molly and this may be very challenging for them. On the other hand, enabling Molly to express herself will provide a new opportunity for them to know their daughter and enable her to have a voice in the family and in decisions about her life. With support, respect and trust, I hope our team will be able to assist the family in feeling the excitement inherent in this opportunity.[1]

The opportunity to share Molly's everyday care
The family have come to our clinic because they want assistance in providing the personal care Molly needs. This expressed need is a top priority for intervention and provides an opportunity to build trust and a collaborative partnership between our team and the family that will enable other issues to be dealt with over time (Smith et al. 2015).

The clinicians and other professionals involved

Every member of our team was touched by this story and reacted with emotion and passion. Some wanted to move quickly and make radical changes in Molly's life. In the end we decided that our approach should be a gentle and supportive one, seeking to understand what the family's experiences have been and acknowledging their love and care for Molly. This strengths-based approach was to be the first step in developing a trusting and positive relationship (Russo 2013).

---

1   The feeling of a person trapped in their impaired body without the ability to communicate is so vividly described in *Ghost Boy*, the book by Martin Pistorius.

The medical and allied health professionals wanted to have comprehensive information about this child and her family, and some felt frustrated that this had not been forthcoming. Some members of the multidisciplinary team felt sad and even angry to hear that Molly had neither attended school nor had allied health input. They were impatient for Molly to start school, receive the therapy she needed in order to develop her communication skills, to organize appropriate seating options and to support her to embark on a range of community activities. The challenge was for our team to focus on the 'positives' in this situation (the fact that the parents have attended the clinic, that they have lovingly cared for Molly over 14 years, and that they are concerned about her safety) and lay aside any frustration about perceived 'negative' aspects of this situation. All too often, health professionals tend to focus on a deficit or an area of obvious perceived need rather than looking at the overall care of children and families and how addressing a single issue might impact on the whole situation.

The trainee doctor was at first outraged at the lack of medical input in the past, but later acknowledged that the priorities for care rested with the family. Getting assistance with personal needs, including bathing, was, for them, a higher priority than organizing a hip X-ray and a brain scan. The team needed to respect this and address this priority first, knowing that these important investigations would be more likely to be followed through later when trust and confidence had been built.

Our team hoped that Molly's life and that of her family would be enhanced by developing partnerships with the healthcare professionals. We wanted to support them to take one step at a time, carefully building trusting, respectful, collaborative relationships that could be sustained long term. A careful balance needed to be struck between the family's right to privacy and our team's need to know in order to provide the best care for Molly.

Establishing a common commitment to and an expectation of the ongoing nature of this partnership between patient, family and professional created a context in which goals could be set, medical investigations performed and participation in school and community life could take place in a way that included and empowered the family (American Academy of Pediatrics 2012). This would have long-term benefits for all involved. We recognized that this approach would require patience, mutual respect and flexibility from all parties.

The healthcare system and society at large

There are many ways in which the lives of this family can be enriched through building the health, function, well-being, social connections and community participation of all members of the family. Many services may be available, but the ultimate goal is to achieve the best outcome for Molly through working with the family to set priorities for care.

The team decided to first attend to the explicit need expressed by the family. A local agency was contacted and personal care assistance was arranged for Molly and her family. Once this was put in place the family slowly felt able, one step at a time, to discuss and pursue the other medical and allied health issues.

The speech pathologist and occupational therapist visited the home at the family's request. They were able to assess Molly with respect to her communication and seating needs and prescribe a powered wheelchair for her to use, at first within the familiar and safe environment of her home. The chair would provide her with both independent mobility and the support she required to maintain good posture. In addition it would enable her to access an electronic tablet that would facilitate the development of independent communication, as well as providing access to music and games through switch access.

Less than 6 months later she had her chair and her tablet, incorporating her communication system. She was learning to make choices and greatly enjoying her favorite music and playing some interactive games.

With the support of the team's social worker, the family enrolled Molly in a local school. At first her parents were extremely concerned about her safety and had trouble leaving her there, but after several weeks they were delighted to see how Molly was enjoying the interactions with her age peers. The other children were envious of her tablet and gathered around her to explore the apps she had. Molly's mother decided to get a part-time job as an integration aide at the school (not in Molly's class), which further developed her relationship with and trust in the school.

Discussion of Molly's anti-seizure medication dose occurred soon after the family were receiving the personal care support for Molly. They started a seizure chart and when another anti-seizure medication was introduced and the dosages slowly increased, they were delighted to report that her seizures had become infrequent and she was not at all sedated. Control of her seizures also resulted in her being more alert and she was able to eat more efficiently and began to gain weight.

Molly's hip X-rays showed subluxed dysplastic hips. The prospect of surgery was most distressing to her parents, and a number of appointments were made to discuss factors important in that decision. The team offered to introduce the family to another child and family who had had the surgery and the family welcomed this opportunity.

Developing respectful and trusting relationships between health professionals, Molly and her family, and taking each step together in partnership, resulted in a greatly enriched quality of life for Molly and for her family.

Themes for discussion

- Does an 'ethical' framing of a story like Molly's differ from a 'legal' approach (where, e.g. the family might be reported for neglect) – and if so, in what ways? How does a different framing lead to different approaches to 'management'?

- How might professionals' personal responses of anger or frustration to a situation like that of Molly and her family have led to actions that ignore ethical principles – and what can professionals do to prevent this from happening?

- Time is a hugely valuable and limited commodity in the work of health professionals. In what ways might an ethically guided approach to a story like that of Molly and her family help – or interfere – with the provision of services to Molly and others in the clinic?

References

American Academy of Pediatrics (2012) Policy Statement. Patient- and family-centered care and the pediatrician's role. *Pediatrics* 129: 394–404.

Anderson CS, Dolva AS (2014) Children's perspective on their right to participate in decision-making according to the United Nations Convention on the Rights of the Child article 12. *Phys Occup Ther Pediatr* 35: 218–230.

Russo RJ (2013) Applying a strengths-based practice approach in working with people with developmental disabilities and their families. *Families in Society* 80: 25–33.

Shogren K, Wehmeyer M (2015) A framework for research and intervention design in supported decision-making. *Am Assoc Intell Dev Dis* 3: 17–23.

Smith J, Swallow V, Coyne I (2015). Involving parents in managing their child's long-term condition – a concept synthesis of family-centered care and partnership-in-care. *J Pediatr Nurs* 30: 143–159.

United Nations (2006) *Convention on the Rights of Persons with Disabilities* [Online]; www.un.org/disabilities/default.asp?id=150 (accessed 12 January 2015).

Chapter 10

The importance of patients' and families' narratives: developing a philosophy of care to support patient and family goals

Jean C. Kunz Stansbury and Scott Schwantes

Clinical scenario

Barbara S. is a 15-year-old girl with a history of cerebral palsy who has developed recurrent pneumonias due to chronic gastroesophageal reflux and aspiration. Barbara's overall level of impairment is significant. She functions at Level V on the Manual Ability Classification System (MACS) for Children with Cerebral Palsy (Eliasson et al. 2006) meaning she does not handle objects herself and has severely limited ability to perform even simple actions. She requires the total assistance of others in her daily activities. She also functions at Level V on the Eating and Drinking Ability Classification System (EDACS) (Sellers et al. 2014), meaning she is unable to eat or drink by mouth safely. She has a gastrostomy tube for feedings.

From a communication standpoint she functions at Level IV, able to communicate sometimes effectively with familiar partners (Communication Function Classification System, CFCS) (Hidecker et al. 2011). She does not speak (other than saying 'Mom') and uses augmentative communication with eye scanning in a limited way. Because this is tiring for Barbara and her device is not always available, she often prefers to use non-word vocalizations and facial expressions to communicate with others. From a gross motor standpoint, she is in Level V in the Gross Motor Function Classification System (GMFCS) (Palisano et al. 2008), meaning she has physical impairments that restrict voluntary control of movement and the ability to maintain head and neck position against gravity. She is impaired in all areas of motor function and cannot walk, sit or stand independently, even with adaptive equipment. Cognitively she appears to be functioning at about a 3-year-old level. Her mother has followed the pulmonologists' recommendations regarding airway clearance treatments, but ongoing deterioration is noted. The pulmonologists are adamant that further airway protection is urgently needed or the child may die. As instructed, Barbara's mother takes her to see an otolaryngologist, who recommends a laryngotracheal separation (tracheal diversion). The mother refuses the intervention. The pulmonologist continues to insist on the need for this intervention and the mother continues to refuse.

Autonomy, rights and respect: approaches to ethical thinking and behavior

Anyone who has been in clinical practice with patients and their families soon encounters situations that contain the potential for conflicts and disagreements. If the conflicts are not resolved, simmering resentments may occur, and each party may become increasingly entrenched in their position. Eventually, productive problem solving is nearly impossible, and a power struggle may develop, with each party trying to 'win' by imposing their will on the other. The real loser may be the patient, with collateral damage to the various staff (and family) members caught in the midst of the power struggle. If given the chance, the patient and the family can provide information about the aspects of their lives that are most important to them. The information about their roles, goals and values can be used to develop a plan of care and resolve conflicts. Each person's plan is unique to them, providing truly patient- and family-centered care.[1]

Listening to the patient and family's story
Taking a thorough history is a critical part of understanding how the patient's illness evolved, finding an accurate diagnosis and deciding on appropriate treatments. In the same way, understanding the patient's and family's stories, values and goals can help everyone develop a meaningful treatment plan that supports what matters to them. An integral part of this process is listening carefully to what the family says about their family member, who they are as a person, and how they function in the family. It would be easy to assume that a person with severe impairments has no function in

---

1   The editors recommend reading the autobiographical book *Ghost Boy*, by Martin Pistorius (2011), where the author tells his early life story of being 'locked in' inside an impaired body, and his wish and frustration to communicate that there is more to his personhood than the visible 'empty shell'. A healthcare worker, not his traumatized family, recognizes his cognitive potentials and arranges testing that leads him to receive an augmentative computerized device for communication.

the family and is merely a burden, but their care may be profoundly meaningful and their presence a comfort. On the other hand, a family may appear to reject a disabled member; it can be very easy for the healthcare providers to make judgments about the family based on their own values and experiences, and the limited exposures they have to patient and family.

Without asking, one has no way of knowing what the family's resources are, or the emotional or experiential context of the situation. This cannot be done well when the family is in a crisis state. They may be too distraught, or they may not want to tell healthcare providers something they think will negatively influence their loved one's care in some way. They also will not want to say something they think will reflect poorly on themselves or their family. Some adults will have completed a healthcare directive, but a dependent person – child or adult – may not have such a document in place. Even when available, such a directive does not give much information about family values and goals, and may not help much when the disagreement is not around life-sustaining treatments, but rather what constitutes quality of life, treatment burden and so on.

"An ounce of prevention is worth a pound of cure"

Goals, roles and values: identifying meaning guides treatment decisions

'An ounce of prevention is worth a pound of cure.' This proverb is especially applicable in cases like these. Many disagreements can be avoided by exploring these topics with the patient and family prior to a crisis. This might be done when first meeting the family, as part of the initial intake, but it is never too late to start collecting this information. Some providers find this can be woven into conversations during routine appointments. A child who sits quietly for long periods might still be an ideal companion to include on hunting, fishing or camping trips. The parent might still see the child as a good listener who understands everything going on around them. Knowing the nature of the relationship and activities the family enjoys can help in identifying what constitutes quality of life for them and later recognizing when this has changed, for better or worse.

The first step may be to assess how quickly a decision must be made. Next, one must listen to both sides of the story, looking for common threads. It is likely that all views have some truth to them. The hardest part will be asking everyone to step back, think about the patient, what is known about them, and try to figure out what is in their best interest. This can sometimes be done in a care conference format, but at other times it will take the shape of 'shuttle diplomacy'. Sometimes, disagreements can be defused by acknowledging that both sides may be partly right, that we might not know immediately which direction things are headed, and that it is alright to have short- and long-term plans. One can hope for the best but still be planning for the worst without somehow betraying the patient or 'giving up' on them. Likewise, the family who is rejecting a proposed medical intervention might be wanting to avoid what they see as needless suffering that will not have a meaningful impact on their loved one's quality of life. The consultant will need to affirm everyone's right to be heard, reinforce the value of mutual decision-making and possibly help salvage caregiving relationships that may remain needed over time.

In consulting with the family to help develop an agreed-upon philosophy of care to drive our medical plan of care, it is imperative to do a thorough benefit/burden analysis. In the above scenario, a surgery is proposed that cannot be reversed later. It will result in a permanent loss of Barbara's ability to vocalize and will impact her ability to communicate. She has very limited ability to use augmentative communication devices, and indicates her feelings and wants by facial expression and vocalizations. Her vocalizations are her only means of summoning help from someone in another room, someone working with their back to her and so on.

Benefit/burden analysis

What does this mean for Barbara?

- *Benefit:* possibly improved airway function; aspiration of oral secretions removed as a causal factor for pneumonia.

- *Burden:* unable to vocalize and will need to rely on facial expressions to communicate as her cognitive level and motor involvement makes use of augmented communication cumbersome; major surgery with risk of mortality and morbidity; not reversible; would not prevent continued challenges with pulmonary secretion clearance; may die prematurely.

What does this mean for the mother?

- *Benefit:* possibly improved or more stable airway and thus the potential for streamlining some aspects of care.

- *Burden:* Barbara will be unable to vocalize and will have to rely on only facial expressions to communicate when her device is not available; major surgery; she will not be able to return to her current school due to the medical technological burden; family will be obliged to have in-home skilled nursing, as mother is the only direct caregiver in the home; Barbara will have another in-dwelling medical device that is more obvious than her gastrostomy tube.

What does this mean for the clinician?

- *Benefit:* offering every available treatment; reducing risk of aspiration events.

- *Burden:* child will require hospitalization in the pediatric intensive care unit (PICU); care team expanded to include additional subspecialists; patient at increased risk for infection secondary to foreign body.

What does this mean for the healthcare system?

- *Benefit:* further lifetime hospitalizations might be minimized through decreased aspiration events.

- *Burden:* extensive major surgery; more expensive homecare.

After additional conversations to help lessen the tension between the family and the care team, and to help understand the goals and values driving the family's decision-making and care team's recommendations, the following details are uncovered:

- *Mother:* Barbara's mother has stage 4 cancer. She had long ago accepted that her daughter was going to have a shortened lifespan and would probably die from her medical complications before the mother would. Now, with her cancer diagnosis, she worries about what will happen to her child if she (the mother) dies first. Barbara's father and grandparents have already died and Barbara is her mother's main companion.

- *Pulmonologist:* The pulmonologist has treated this child for nearly her entire life. He believes a more stable airway will make it easier to care for the child and will eliminate one potential source of suffering. He does not think he has much else to offer from a treatment standpoint and does not want to 'give up' on her.

- *Community:* The school Barbara attends is nervous about her care. With her gastrostomy tube and nebulization treatments, she is one of their 'sickest' students. They also struggle with how to have open communication about her medical complexities with other students and staff. A laryngo-tracheal separation will increase her medical complexity to the point that they feel they will not be able to care for her safely in their rural school setting.

- *Barbara:* She is cognitively and physically quite impaired, but has appreciable interactions with her environment and can definitely experience both the benefit and burden of medical interventions. She has a sunny disposition and brings joy to the room with her happy vocalizations (including 'Mom', her only word) and facial expressions. Until her recent recurrent pneumonias, airway issues have not been a known source of discomfort for her.

Interview techniques

An open-ended conversation with the family and care providers can explore Barbara's past, current and possible future roles and functions in the family. One can explore what Barbara enjoys, what contributes to their quality of life and what the family thinks her health has been like. This is a good time to just listen to the family talk, although if they get off track gentle questions can redirect them. It is important to make sure to allow adequate time for this conversation, including allowing the family time to review and reflect.

Identifying family goals, values and roles

Identifying family goals, values and roles is an important part of defining who the patient is as an individual, what might help to give their life meaning, and help to sort out what might be an undue burden in the context of their life. Exploring the family's spiritual beliefs might also help sort out how they feel about life-sustaining treatments, the meaning of suffering, and beliefs about death and dying. The following are some of the important questions that might be asked:

• What is the family's understanding of their child's health?

• Ask the family what their goals are now and what they would be if things changed?

• What worries the family most?

• What does a good day look like?

• What do they care about most?

• What treatments/interventions might be negotiable and which are not?

• What are the essential elements of their child's personality? What do they enjoy doing and what impact might the proposed treatment have on their ability to enjoy life?

The ICF Core Sets can also be used to collect information on the patient's quality of life, body functions and structures, activities and participation, personal and environmental situation (Schiariti et al. 2015).

Identifying the problem

The exact nature of the problem will vary depending on the circumstances. In the case described above, there was disagreement about the benefit versus the burden of laryngo-tracheal separation. There was disagreement regarding the value of potentially prolonging life at the cost of ability to communicate vocally. The mother understood perfectly well what was being proposed, but did not agree that the benefit outweighed the burden/loss, including loss of a familiar and supportive community school setting. In other cases, the problem might revolve around resources, cultural issues or a lack of capacity on the part of caregivers. Clarity around the problem helps identify what may be necessary to resolve it. In this case, the provider was more distressed about the situation than the family was. Part of the solution was identifying what the 'next steps' might be and who would help provide them. A referral to palliative care was made regarding the identification of ways to relieve distressing symptoms. Involving the palliative care team gave the pulmonologist and the family someone with whom to collaborate for additional support and symptom management.

Finding consensus

Careful listening to all involved will allow the identification of commonalities that can be used to build consensus. In this case, all parties could agree that they wanted to avoid suffering and wanted to continue to offer care to Barbara and her family. It helped the pulmonologist to realize that the family was not expecting him to fix everything, but rather to continue to be their doctor, someone they knew and trusted. Adding the palliative care team provided new support, not only to the family, but also to the other providers. Arriving at this understanding decreased the distress around this situation significantly.

Developing a philosophy of care to drive the medical plan of care

Barbara's mother was not worried about prolonging life at all costs and had long ago accepted the likelihood that her daughter would have a shortened lifespan. While she did not want her daughter to suffer, if Barbara outlived her mother it would cause a new set of problems and another possible source of distress for the family as a unit. Recognizing that this was one of the mother's concerns, a 'backup' set of care providers was identified. They would function as guardians and take over Barbara's care when her mother became unable to do so.

Future action plans for symptom management (look for reversible causes of distress)

Recognizing that pulmonary/respiratory distress could be a significant source of suffering for Barbara, aggressive symptom management plans were put in place. Emphasis was placed on palliative care measures to relieve symptoms, including treating respiratory illnesses as they arose.

Decisions

The family and care team all agreed that all decisions made on behalf of Barbara needed to benefit her as an individual, using the family's goals and values to help drive their philosophy of care (maximizing the child's quality of life while minimizing burdens and maintaining her ability to vocalize). It was recognized that the laryngo-tracheal separation ultimately imposed too much burden without an assurance of equitable benefit. It was also reassuring to all that engaging in a model that focuses on the patient and continuing to employ interventions deemed beneficial was indeed continuing to 'do something' for the child.

Outcome

Seven years later, Barbara continues on supportive respiratory treatments, coordinating her complex care with her team of subspecialists supported through the palliative care team. Health-care and community relationships have been maintained, and Barbara and her mother – who has lived much longer than was predicted – continue to thrive in their home community. The 'backup' care providers stepped in once to assist when the mother experienced a temporary exacerbation in her own health condition. Because these people had previously been identified and were already 'in the loop', Barbara's care was not disrupted during this time and her mother could concentrate on taking care of herself during this setback.

Barbara follows up primarily with her pulmonologist and physiatrist, with the palliative care team available to assist in symptom management. If distressing symptoms begin to develop, the palliative care team will take on more responsibility for her care management. A plan is in place for the time when it is necessary to move on to the next steps, which could include end-of-life care.

Epilogue

Modern medical practice has resulted in a wide variety of treatments being available to patients, families and providers. Inevitably, there will sometimes be disagreements about the need for/value of these interventions. This is particularly true when no 'cure' for the patient's condition exists and the treatments involve increasingly aggressive or invasive attempts at symptom management.

One must use the known information about a patient and their family to resolve conflicts and move decision-making forward in a helpful direction. Increasingly complex treatment options require potential benefits to be weighed against potential burdens in light of the patient's and family's values and goals. This is particularly true for a patient whose issues are medically complex. These conversations take time and trust, and are best initiated prior to a crisis. Keeping the focus on the patient and what is meaningful to them can help direct care and decision-making. Clinicians should not hesitate to look for additional treatment options from other disciplines and keep communication open among all parties. In many cases, the supportive relationships with care providers are what the families need and want most.

Themes for discussion

- One of the bases for clinical decision-making in our field is prognostication, but we know that that is usually an imprecise process. How can we best counsel people when our knowledge of the 'natural' (or indeed the 'unnatural') history and course of a condition is so varied and vague?

- As illustrated by the story of Barbara, the 'best' management from a medical perspective may for many reasons not be the best in this particular situation. How do we feel when what is being recommended falls into this category? Do we communicate these feelings to families – and is that appropriate? If not, what can we do to be supportive to them when we might be uncomfortable?

- Many professionals in our field are now using the framework of the International Classification of Functioning, Disability and Health to think about the myriad factors that converge in any specific clinical situation. Can you discuss how the application of this framework might help the family and the clinical team to frame and consider Barbara's issues?

Further reading

Cohen E, Kuo DZ, Agrawal R et al. (2011) Children with medical complexity: An emerging population for clinical and research initiatives. *Pediatrics* 127: 529–538.

Ferrell B, Coyle N (2010) *The textbook of palliative nursing* 3rd edn. Oxford: Oxford University Press.

Hexem KR, Bosk AM, Feudtner C (2011) The dynamic system of parental work of care for children with special health care needs: A conceptual model to guide quality improvement efforts. *BMC Pediatr* 11: 95.

Schwantes S, Wells O'Brien H (2014) Pediatric palliative care for children with complex chronic medical conditions. *Pediatr Clin N Am* 61: 797–821.

References

Eliasson A, Krumlinde-Sundholm L, Rösblad B (2006) The Manual Ability Classification System (MACS) for children with cerebral palsy: Scale development and evidence of validity and reliability. *Dev Med Child Neurol* 48: 549–554.

Hidecker M, Paneth N, Rosenbaum P (2011) Developing and validating the Communication Function Classification System for individuals with cerebral palsy. *Dev Med Child Neurol* 53: 704–710.

Palisano RJ, Rosenbaum P, Bartlett D, Livingston MH (2008) Content validity of the expanded and revised Gross Motor Function Classification System. *Dev Med Child Neurol* 50: 744–750.

Pistorius M (2011) *Ghost boy*. New York, NY: Simon & Schuster.

Schiariti V, Selb M, Cieza A, O'Donnell M (2015) International Classification of Functioning, Disability and Health Core Sets for children and youth with cerebral palsy: A consensus meeting. *Dev Med Child Neurol* 57: 149–158.

Sellers D, Mandy A, Pennington L, Hankins M, Morris C (2014) Development and reliability of a system to classify the eating and drinking ability of people with cerebral palsy. *Dev Med Child Neurol* 56: 245–251.

Chapter 11

The ethics of patient advocacy: bending the rules on behalf of patients

Raymond Tervo and Paul J. Wojda

Prologue

It is commonplace in the diagnosis and treatment of childhood disability and developmental impairments that professionals are challenged by rules that appear to constrain them. In such situations, physicians are frequently tempted to 'bend the rules' or even lie outright in order to get third-party approval for the complex genetic tests both they and their patients' parents or caregivers desire. As is illustrated in a case scenario about Meghan (below) it can be easy for the physician to 'modify' one or two of the clinical findings in a way that makes the case for testing more compelling. However, many physicians understandably hesitate before doing so, wondering 'Can such deception ever be morally justified?'

In the following essay we examine this question in greater detail. We begin by looking more carefully at the case itself, identifying and analyzing the circumstances that give rise both to the temptation to deceive and the moral concerns about doing so. What makes cases like Meghan's especially challenging, we believe, is the combination of features that appear to justify deceit and on some accounts perhaps require it, in the name of patient advocacy. We then situate the argument that patient advocacy can sometimes justify deception of third parties within the long history of philosophical debate over the ethics of lying. While arguments justifying deception and what is often called 'beneficent lying' can be compelling, we do not find them persuasive. In our concluding section, we offer a case against deception and lying rooted in an *areteic*, or 'virtue-based', approach to ethics where normative evaluations are based on the character of the agent. Its roots go back to ancient Greek philosophy and the moral theories of Plato and Aristotle. By this account, the deception of third parties, whether with, or on behalf of, patients is wrong because it is contrary to the trust constitutive of the physician–patient relationship. This trust, we claim, is far more integral to the physician's identity as an advocate than is commonly observed. Thus, far from being in conflict with patient advocacy, a commitment to truth-telling is essential to it.

Clinical scenario: the denial of a request for complex genetic testing

Four-and-a-half-year-old Meghan was referred to the clinic by her certified nurse practitioner, who was concerned about both some emerging behavioral problems and Meghan's failure to meet developmental milestones. Born after an unremarkable pregnancy and delivery, Meghan was first diagnosed as developmentally delayed at the age of 7 months, and at 2 years 2 months she was seen in a neurodevelopmental clinic. Since that time she has been receiving special education services. At the current visit, an examination revealed that Meghan had pressure-equalizing tubes (PE tubes) in her ears and generalized hypotonia. Otherwise, examination was unremarkable. A developmental assessment showed global delay. All other investigations were normal, including magnetic resonance imaging (MRI), chromosome microarray analysis and single nucleotide polymorphism screening, molecular analysis for fragile X, MECP2-related disorders and sequence analysis, metabolic studies and thyroid function tests. Audiology assessment and an ophthalmology opinion were also unremarkable. A neuropsychology assessment noted Meghan's developmental delay (she was judged to be functioning like a 2-and-a-half-year-old) and attention problems.

Meghan's mother was still very concerned about the cause of her daughter's delay and wanted Meghan to have the most advanced genetic testing. This request was a recurring appeal, and Meghan's mother's sense of urgency gave emphasis to her persistent grieving and her bargaining: she hoped that finding a cause would help with further interventions on Meghan's behalf and perhaps identify something that was treatable with medication or diet such as specific medications, currently under development, that improve synaptic transmission to enhance cognitive functioning and behavior. A promise was made to help find a cause and an order was thus written for whole exome sequencing. The request was denied by the hospital laboratory, which cited a policy requiring an institutional review for all advanced genetic testing orders. It was possible to get the testing done at a nationally regarded genetic testing laboratory; however, Meghan's family's insurance would not cover the cost and the out-of-pocket expense was prohibitive. Nor would genetic counseling be available to help interpret the results if the testing were done at another laboratory. Meghan's mother was irate and the ordering physician was despondent. The physician shared Meghan's mother's wish for more testing. It occurred to him that embellishing Meghan's story and her physical findings would get her mother the testing that she wanted and that he had promised. Would it be ethical for the physician to bend the rules on behalf of the patient?

Vulnerable patients, motivated parents, powerful tests

The primary moral question raised by Meghan's case – whether lying on behalf of a patient is ever justified – is not entirely novel. However, we believe that the combination of features that gives rise to this question *is*. What are those features? There are essentially three: (1) a vulnerable and needy child with a perplexing set of symptoms; (2) a highly motivated and desperate parent/caregiver with limited financial resources; and (3) a powerful arsenal of complex genetic tests whose results appear to hold the promise of both narrowing the family's uncertainty about the reason for their child's condition and increasing access to a range of healthcare resources for the vulnerable child and her family. Together, these three features may augment a physician's self-understanding as a patient advocate, to the point where deceiving third parties can appear justified, perhaps even obligatory. May advocacy ever justify deception in such cases? The question has received far less attention than it deserves.

Doctors rightly understand themselves as advocates for their patients, all the more so when the patient is a child, like Meghan, with impairments or developmental delay. This was not always the case. As recently as 30 years ago it was not uncommon for medical professionals to advise parents to institutionalize their impaired children, often arguing that caring for a disabled child at home would be too time-consuming and difficult, or unfair to any typically developing siblings. (Sadly, this attitude still prevails in many parts of the world in varied cultural settings.) Families of children with impairments were characterized in the psychiatric literature as enveloped in 'chronic sorrow' and told to expect nothing of their disabled children (Solomon 2012). All of this has changed, of course. Today, parents are encouraged to love and care for their children with impairments at home, public policies are enacted, and public revenues made available to help them do so. For their part, physicians are now keenly aware of their role in promoting the full dignity and protecting the civil rights of children with special needs, among other things by providing their parents with access to these resources (Picker & Walsh 2013). Hence, obstacles to that access, such as the denial of genetic testing by third parties, can strike the physician as a blatant injustice.

A physician's sense of advocacy is also dramatically augmented by parents' and caregivers' advocacy for their child. As in Meghan's case, parents of children with impairments are typically well informed, highly motivated and passionate advocates for their children. Devotion to and promotion of their child's well-being is a full-time job and thus shapes their identity as parents more profoundly than usual. Searching for the causes of their child's impairment is a crucial part of being and becoming the parent of a child with a neurodevelopmental impairment. For some parents, as Andrew Solomon puts it, 'The sadness of a poor prognosis is vastly easier than the chaos of no prognosis. Once the course is clear, most people can accept it. Since knowledge is power, syndromes associated with dire prospects are borne more nobly than those of which little can be understood. Identity is a function of certitude' (Solomon 2012). Thus the denial of testing can seem to the physician to be a strike against the parent's identity and with it, his or her own. It is hardly surprising that the denial of testing left Meghan's mother irate and the physician despondent.

Finally, physicians usually present their requests for complex genetic testing based on recommendations of professional societies such as the American Academy of Neurology and the American College of Medical Genetics. These recommendations are themselves based on a deeper dynamic involving the implicit promise inherent in these technologies, which might be expressed in the motto/belief 'If you can find a cause you can find a cure.' Until fairly recently, physicians operated without much third-party oversight or constraint in the ordering of tests and/or the use of other costly resources that physicians judged were necessary for patients' life and health. Insurance companies and other third parties paid and asked few questions. 'Managed care' has made those days a fading memory. As Morreim observed more than 20 years ago, the physician today finds himself or herself '… increasingly trapped between traditional mandates to deliver unstinting resources to patients and a progressive loss of the power to do so' (Morreim 1991). Hence, regardless of how well-founded a denial of testing may be from the perspective of third parties, from the perspective of the requesting clinician, such denial can seem directly contrary to good medical practice. Indeed, such denial might even seem to the clinician like an abrupt and unjust abandonment of his or her patient.

Vulnerable patients, motivated parents, powerful tests – these elements constitute a potent mix. Together, they can augment a physician's sense of professional responsibility, of being an advocate for his or her patient, even to the point that the deception of third parties in pursuit of that patient's good seems not only excusable, but perhaps even required.

Lying for others

Is lying to third parties on behalf of a patient always wrong? Can patient advocacy ever justify such deception? These questions take us to the heart of the debate over the ethics of lying in the Western tradition. In this long tradition there are essentially three positions (Kemp & Sullivan 1993): the 'rigorist' (or absolutist) position, which prohibits all deliberate deception; the 'rejectionist' position, which, in reaction to the rigorist position, denies that lying is always and everywhere wrong, and seeks to establish general rules for when lying might be justified; and the 'revisionist' position, which shares with the rigorist position the conviction that lying is always wrong, but redefines what it means to lie in order to address some of the more common-sense objections to the rigorist position (e.g. that one may not lie even to save a third party from probable harm)

Table 11.1   Classic positions on the ethics of lying

Rigorist	Rejectionist	Revisionist
Lying, that is, speaking a falsehood, with the intent to deceive, is always and everywhere wrong, regardless of one's aim or intention	Lying is not always wrong. It may be justified in some circumstances, that is, to avoid a greater evil; or other duties, for example, to do good, may override the duty to not lie	Lying is always wrong, but not every intentional speaking of a falsehood constitutes a lie; for example, a lie can only be told in a situation where a hearer has a right to hear the truth

(Table 11.1). In thinking through these questions, a physician will find him or herself occupying one or more of these positions.

In Meghan's case, a physician inclined towards rigorism would simply deny outright that deception of third parties could ever be justified, much less required, on the grounds of duty or professional responsibility. He or she might recall the straightforward lessons of his or her youth: never tell a lie! The classic ancient statement of the rigorist position is that of St Augustine of Hippo (354–430 CE), for whom lying is not only contrary to a divine command but also an abuse of the faculty of speech. Lying, in which what is spoken (i.e. what is on one's lips) contradicts what is thought (i.e. 'on one's heart'), devalues language – the medium of communication – much as counterfeit bills devalue a currency (Kemp & Sullivan 1993). Among modern philosophers, Immanuel Kant (1724–1804) is the most famous representative of the rigorist position. For Kant, lying constitutes a violation of a universal and hence exceptionless principle of truthfulness. Acknowledging this principle is fundamental to our dignity as rational, self-legislating moral agents. For both Augustine and Kant, the lie is contrary to our nature as human beings, and what is contrary to our nature as human beings must also be contrary to any identity subordinate to it, such as our professional identity as doctors, lawyers or teachers. Advocacy cannot justify deception.

Many physicians will not be persuaded by such an austere and seemingly impersonal approach. Surely what matters most in our moral evaluation of deception, they might think, is not whether we are breaking a universal law (whether of divine or human origin), but what sort of consequences we are seeking, or seeking to avoid, in lying. In moving to this position, a physician will find him or herself in the company of 'rejectionists', that is, those who reject the rigorist claim that the prohibition on lying is absolute and exceptionless. Foremost among rejectionists are utilitarians, who think a lot about consequences, and 'prima facie duty' theorists, who think we have a general duty not to lie, but that it is not an absolute or exceptionless one. Neither utilitarian nor prima facie duty theorist would deny that a physician who passes on false information about a patient to a third party tells a lie. However, both would argue that, in such cases, a lie could be morally justified. For example, in Meghan's case, a utilitarian physician might argue that the deception is so minor as to involve practically no harm to the third party, while it brings great good to Meghan and her family. Of course, this reasoning cuts both ways, for if it *could* be shown that such deception involved more than minor harm, or that the harm did not outweigh the intended good, then the utilitarian would be forced to reconsider that judgment. A prima facie duty theorist acknowledges that the physician in such cases has a duty to be truthful, a duty in this case to third parties, but that where that duty conflicts with another, more central duty – in this case the duty to advance a patient's good – then the more important duty trumps the lesser. By this account, a 'prima facie duty' physician might reason that he or she does have a duty to be truthful to third parties, such as review boards and insurance companies, but that his or her primary duty is to the patient's good and thus a deception can be justified.

Not every physician who disagrees with the rigorist position will find these rejectionist arguments persuasive. For one thing, they seem too susceptible to abuse, or to 'slippery slope' objections. The old cautionary phrase might come to mind: 'Oh what a tangled web we weave, when first we practice to deceive' (Scott 1910). Is there then a 'middle way', one that avoids the stringency of the rigorists, but avoids the looseness of the rejectionists? Revisionists think there is.

A revisionist agrees with a rigorist that the prohibition against lying is absolute and thus finds the rejectionist positions unpersuasive; however, the revisionist seeks to avoid the difficulties raised by the rigorist position by redefining what it is to lie. The most common revisionist move is to argue that truth is owed only to those who have a right to it. Thus, in the most common example, a Nazi in occupied France who asks whether a householder is harboring any Jews has no right to the truth and so the householder does not lie in telling him, contrary to fact, that there are no Jews hiding on the premises. Kemp and Sullivan have proposed a more refined version of the revisionist position by arguing that a lie is not simply *any* linguistic utterance (locution) but an assertion, and that one of the key conditions of an assertion is that it be recognized as such in the context. In some contexts there is, in fact, no expectation that the truth will be told, or at least fully told, and thus assertions in these contexts are impossible.

International diplomacy and used car sales may be two such contexts. Could medicine be a third? That is, could it be the case that falsehoods told to third parties such as review boards and insurance companies do not constitute assertions, because in such situations it is understood that hardly anyone tells the truth, or at least the full truth? The analogy here might be to letters of recommendation. While a given letter may not contain explicit falsehoods about a candidate, most readers understand the degree to which hyperbole often overshadows reality in this literary genre and interpret accordingly.

In sum, a revisionist physician in Meghan's case might conclude that deceiving the insurance company or review panel, while a falsehood, does not constitute a lie properly speaking, either because the third parties are not owed the truth, or the 'full truth', in such situations, or because the request for such testing is recognized by all parties as a context in which assertions are not possible.

Deception, advocacy and trust: a virtue approach

It is easiest to justify lying – or to redescribe our speaking falsehoods as something other than lying – in those situations where doing so is the only conceivable way to avoid causing a great(er) harm. The appeal of both the rejectionist and revisionist positions is, in this respect, obvious. It may be just as easy, perhaps even easier, however, to justify deception when doing so will not simply avoid a harm, but significantly advance another's good: that is, lying for a good cause. If presented with an opportunity to benefit another and the only obstacle to furthering that benefit is a 'little white lie' told to a third party, we might well ask, 'Why not?' What good reasons are there to not lie?

This situation and hence this question are far more common to the medical profession than is sometimes observed. Physicians, like other professionals, are in fiduciary relationships, central to which are the duties to protect and pursue (i.e. advocate for) another's good. Because they generally disregard such role-specific elements within human relationships, none of the three positions briefly outlined above seems adequate to address the ethics of deception in cases like Meghan's. We propose, instead, an argument that begins here with an account of the doctor–patient relationship. Such an approach has been described as 'aretic' or 'virtue-based'. In this approach, the key questions have less to do with whether a particular act of lying is ever justified than with the sort of character-states ('virtues') that are (or might be) commensurate with being a good physician. Following the work of Pellegrino and Thomasma (1993), we argue that the virtue of trust, or, if you will, personal truthfulness, is essential to articulating why we ought to reject the suggestion that lying on behalf of patients can ever be good. How so?

First, it is crucial to recognize that medicine is a public profession. Physicians are publicly committed to the welfare of others. The profession of being a physician is 'affirmed' (i.e. 'professed') every time a physician asks a patient 'What can I do for you, what is wrong, what is your concern?' In doing so, the physician pledges his or her competence (i.e. having the knowledge and skill to help) and tries to apply that competence in a patient's best interests. By its very declaration, this 'profession' or commitment necessitates trust. The doctor, of his/her free will, *promises* that they can be trusted and incurs the moral obligations of that promise (Pellegrino 2002 p. 379). Whatever uncertainties there may be in relationships, to be effective in helping a child and family there must be some trust, and a physician must be faithful to that trust.

Secondly, lying, even to third parties about genetic testing, is a social activity, because it includes other people. It is mistaken because it is a breach of trust in a very particular and personal relationship among people, in this case, a physician, a child and family, and an insurer. In the end, what makes lying in these cases most objectionable is that it happens in a circumstance where the truth is expected, most noticeably in answer to a direct question such as 'Can I have the test for my child?' A physician who lies damages trust, regardless of how well established a relationship they may have with a patient. No matter how well intended, a lie sullies their reputation and undermines relationships with a patient and a third party. At one extreme, without trust, no interpersonal exchange is possible, no matter how well intentioned.

Pellegrino and Thomasma ground their argument for the necessity of trust in the profession of medicine in a more broadly phenomenological account of the nature of trust in all human relationships. The fifth (of five) elements they identify as operative in all trusting human relationships is '... an act of faith in the benevolence and good character of the one trusted' (Pellegrino & Thomasma 1993). What Pellegrino and Thomasma's description underscores is the essential relationship between beneficence and truthfulness in fiduciary relationships. Few would argue that the relationship proper to a doctor and patient has broken down, perhaps irreparably, when, because of deception, neither doctor nor patient can trust the other any longer. What we are claiming here is that the same holds for the relationship between doctor, patient and *all third parties* to the healing relationship, including such impersonal actors as insurance companies and review boards. For better or worse, these actors are (and really have been for quite some time) part of the 'extended' doctor–patient relationship. To engage in deception of these actors constitutes a breach in the understood truthfulness constitutive of the doctor–patient relationship. At such a point that a doctor deceives a third party, therefore, he or she actually ceases to be an advocate.

Finally, it is worth noting that deceiving third parties does nothing to correct the potential injustice of testing denial and arguably only makes matters worse for the next time. Even more profoundly, deception constitutes a grave threat to the very idea of evidence-based medicine upon which the effective diagnosis and treatment of patients like Meghan rests. Medicine is not *and cannot* be like international diplomacy or car sales where trust is compromised by an expectation of deception. Integrity and trust in the clinical relationship is fundamental. This remains true regardless of how unjust a practice situation becomes. Medical care that is not oriented towards the truth ceases, in that instance, to be medical care. Hence, *true* advocacy obliges a doctor and patient to engage in practices that make denial of testing less likely.

Outcome

One year later, at 5 years and 6 months, Meghan and her mother returned to clinic. Her mother was cheerful and cordial. She did not mention a current interest in advanced genetic testing and when prompted she did not want an appointment with medical genetics to discuss the option. She did not appear to be angry about being denied testing after the previous visit. Currently she saw the test as too costly and offering little to help her daughter or to aid in understanding the reason for Meghan's delayed development. She recognized that the potential for testing was not lost and waiting could mean an improved test at a lower price or choosing an option covered by health insurance.

She appeared to accept her daughter's functional limitations and she was more interested in moving on to know the best way to support Meghan. She was more concerned that her daughter was making very slow progress at school and that Meghan's ability to attend to task was interfering with her learning. A psycho-educational plan, behavioral intervention and medication management were discussed. Meghan's receptive and expressive language skills were still delayed and it was decided that she would continue to benefit from speech and language services. Meghan and her mother plan on returning to clinic in one year for an updated assessment.

Themes for discussion

- Think of a situation in which you have lied (or 'bent the truth'). Do the arguments in this chapter lead you to think differently about that situation? On the basis of these arguments, in this situation might you do things differently in future?

- How do you feel about the apparently absolutist views presented in this chapter? Are you likely to discuss them with colleagues (or indeed with families) when a situation like this arises in future?

- If there is an absolute prohibition against 'bending the rules' how else might one advocate on behalf of one's patients and their families without risking the trusting relationships we strive to create and maintain?

References

Kemp K, Sullivan T (1993) Speaking falsely and telling lies. *Proc Am Catholic Philos Assoc* 67: 151–170.

Morreim H (1991) Gaming the system: Dodging the rules, ruling the dodgers. *Arch Intern Med* 151: 443–447.

Pellegrino E (2002) Professionalism, profession, and the virtues of the good physician. *Mount Sinai J Med* 69: 378–384.

Pellegrino E, Thomasma D (1993) *The virtues in medical practice.* New York, NY: Oxford University Press.

Picker JD, Walsh CA (2013) New innovations: Therapeutic opportunities for intellectual disabilities. *Ann Neurol* 74: 382–390.

Scott W (1910) *Marmion: A tale of Flodden Field.* New York, NY: MacMillan.

Solomon A (2012) *Far from the tree: Parents, children, and the search for identity.* New York, NY: Scribner.

Chapter 12

Responding to requests for novel/unproven alternative and complementary treatments

Edward A. Hurvitz and Garey Noritz

Prologue

The popularity of complementary and alternative medicine (CAM) raises several challenging issues for healthcare providers working with children with disabilities and their families.

CAM treatments are difficult to characterize, as the definition shifts with each person's training, experience, culture and belief system. The National Center for Complementary and Integrative Health (NCCIH) in the USA describes them as '… the array of healthcare approaches with a history of use or origins outside of mainstream medicine …' (NCCIH, https://nccih.nih.gov). This obviously changes when a clinic in an urban North American center is compared to one in rural China. CAMs are popular in the treatment of conditions for which there is no cure. Over 50% of individuals with neurodevelopmental conditions such as cerebral palsy (Hurvitz et al. 2003), autism (Levy & Hyman 2015) and epilepsy (Doering et al. 2013) may be exposed to these treatments during childhood (Akins et al. 2014). Although many CAM modalities do not pose ethical dilemmas for the medical/ therapeutic providers (e.g. prayer or massage combined with standard care), others can create significant challenges related to autonomy, beneficience/non-maleficience and the obligation of the clinician to their patient. The following scenarios illustrate these issues.

The family of a child with cerebral palsy asks for an opinion and a letter of support, for travel and costs for a treatment program in Europe that has gained a reputation for its 'miraculous' effects. It uses a variety of techniques that sound unusual to the clinician and are based on highly questionable neurological theories. However, there are multiple testimonials on the Internet and great pressure from the extended family to pursue this treatment. There is talk of mortgaging the home, and community fundraising events may be undertaken to support the effort if insurance funding is not available. The parents note that the child has been resistant to the idea of spending several weeks in this program during the summer break from school. He does not want to miss summer camp and swimming at the community pool with friends. In general, he does not like the idea of 'intensive therapy', as he is not all that pleased with the stretching and strenuous activities of his current therapies.

The family of a child with contractures wants an opinion about the use of turmeric to relieve contractures. They have seen multiple Internet testimonials that this works and they bought some from a website promoting this use. They would like to know your thoughts on the safety of this herb, as well as what dose they should use. You note that while the family has often tried unconventional therapies that have provided no objective benefit, these interventions seem to increase the family's engagement with the child, which benefits the child's overall care. You can envision, for example, that trying turmeric will encourage the family to be more compliant with a range of motion exercises.

A family is bringing their son, a young adult with autism, to you for traditional treatment, and also to a naturopath for CAM treatment. The family asks you to work with the naturopath to find the best treatment for their son. You receive a message from the naturopath that he would like you to call him to discuss stopping the young man's risperidone and instead starting a regimen of glutathione and other antioxidants for detoxification. During the examination, the young man speaks joyfully about recent social experiences that he has had. The parents confirm that he has had increased ability to participate. You believe that the risperidone is contributing to this outcome and that stopping it will cause worsening behavior and less social participation.

Evaluation framework

The scientific nature of medicine demands an evidence base, or at least the experience of a trained clinician who understands the importance of the scientific method in evaluating interventions. Scientific evidence related to medical interventions has a hierarchy. The randomized controlled trial is considered the definitive proof of effect of intervention, followed by uncontrolled trials, case series and finally clinician experience. Despite 25 years passing since the founding of the Office of Alternative Medicine at the National Institutes of Health (NIH) (which grew into the National Center for Complementary and Integrative Health), the 'evidence' supporting most CAM interventions is at the lower end of the evidence spectrum, ranging from case reports in peer-reviewed journals to unverified testimonials in the lay press (see also Chapter 13 by Mann et al.). Most reports of success in mainstream medicine *"extraordinary claims require extraordinary evidence"* describe relatively incremental improvements with a measured review of side effects, while CAM testimonials are notable for their glowing reviews and lack of harm. It is thus easy to see why families are drawn to CAM when researching on their own. However, 'extraordinary claims require extraordinary evidence' (Sagan 1980), which is not forthcoming in the arena of CAM.

However, there is no question that the history of conventional medicine is rife with well-intentioned disasters that were based on 'high-level' evidence. The use of COX 2 inhibitors, estrogen therapy for postmenopausal women, immobility following myocardial infarction and many other 'innovations' tell us that wide acceptance within mainstream medicine does not mean that evidence is accurate; we must constantly test what we believe to be true. On the other hand, some treatments that started as CAM techniques – such as the ketogenic diet in refractory epilepsy – have become evidence-based standard care. As it is commonly said about evidence-based-medicine, 'The absence of evidence is not necessarily the evidence of absence' (Sagan 1997) of therapeutic effects. In fact, often the absence of evidence reflects the lack of resources and investigators to conduct the needed trials, or the poor quality of those investigations. This is particularly relevant in neurodevelopmental conditions, where efforts to perform clinical trials are often complicated by limited subject pools, heterogeneity of the conditions, complexity of interventions and lack of funding for research into these conditions.

Although evidence-based medicine is a well-accepted framework for the evaluation of interventions, other frameworks also influence clinical decision-making. Culture and history play a role in the evaluation process in many places and cultures, such as in traditional Chinese medicine and Indian Ayurvedic medicine. In many religions, clergy or other spiritual leaders participate in the process of evaluating treatments based on religious teachings and their own understanding of the interventions offered. Clinician experience often takes the place of evidence-based medicine, especially in places that have not yet developed a strong culture of research. For example, in one Eastern European country, there are arthritis clinics where the physician prescribes mixes of minerals for mud baths, using different mixtures based on the symptoms.

The absolute and (often) arrogant belief in the infallibility of science and evidence-based medicine embraced by many in the Western medical establishment – generally accompanied by an equally arrogant feeling that many cultural and religious beliefs are wrong, primitive, backwards and dangerous – can easily lead to a decrease in trust in science and of clinicians and a tendency to weigh other types of evidence equally or more strongly. If the clinician is not willing to accept the limits of science and to try to understand the framework in which their patient is working for decision-making, we are not going to succeed in aiding the patient to make the best decisions regarding choices for their care.

Doing what is right for the child

In guiding the family in making their decisions, the clinician must consider the costs and benefits to the child of pursuing treatments that may have no effect. First, the clinician should make an objective assessment of potential harm. Most CAM modalities have no measurable effect, so while providing no benefit, they also cause no bodily harm. However, 'harm' may be defined in other ways. The patient may have a loss of benefit from other treatments that the parents put off or refuse due to the involvement in CAM. Interventions that involve travel or large time or cost commitments will probably interfere with other activities such as play, socialization, academics or similar activities. For a child who will never achieve ambulation as a functional goal, a 4-week trip to Europe to work on this skill will take time and resources away from attainable (and perhaps child-preferred) goals, such as improved communication through the use of an augmentative communication device. Even the time taken away from socialization should be considered potential harm (or at least loss). Many adults with neurodevelopmental impairments report that their most valuable experiences in childhood were not therapies and surgeries, but times when their families opened up avenues of participation for them. Families that take frequent forays into CAM interventions, or use various remedies over long periods of time, place emphasis on abnormalities and deficits that reinforce an image of the child as sick or poorly functioning and needing to be 'fixed'. If the desired improvement is not achieved, there may be the additional grief of failure for the family and patient, although the outcome may have been completely predictable based on knowledge of the CAM. All of these factors should be considered along with any potential physiologic harm that may occur.

There are aspects of 'harm' that extend beyond the child and family to the community and perhaps even society as a whole. Resource limitation is always an issue. Even a wealthy family has limitations on their time and energy. Extensive focus on the child with the impairment can lead to family disruption, including lengthy trips for one parent and that child; extensive time and energy spent on the one child; and reduced financial resources to support the needs of other siblings. The community may be affected by being pulled into fundraisers to support CAM modalities, or even being asked to spend time working with the child, as is common with the patterning therapeutic method.

There are also cases in which government entities have been strongly lobbied to support CAM modalities by mandating insurance coverage, which takes away resources for more established interventions (Sheppard 2015).

On the other hand, the possibility of benefit must be considered. The placebo effect is strong and known to be stronger when the patient is actively involved in the intervention, or is being touched, or has a belief system that contributes to the effectiveness. Conversely, families interested in CAM may be prone to the nocebo effect (Bingel 2014) when it comes to mainstream medicine: with the expectation that a medicine may have adverse effects, adverse effects are more likely to become apparent. This may further enhance the probability that CAM will be more acceptable to the family.

Sometimes CAM time is family time. Some families report wonderful experiences of swimming together with dolphins or traveling to new places and gaining new experiences. In 1988, a study was published comparing neurodevelopmental therapy (NDT) to family time together playing games for children with cerebral palsy. The family time was no worse, and may have been better, than the therapy (Palmer et al. 1988). There may be CAM treatments with benefits that will eventually find their way into the mainstream armamentarium, such as has happened with the ketogenic diet for seizures, as mentioned above, or melatonin for insomnia. Other CAM modalities are rooted more firmly in a healthy lifestyle than the actual powder or herb that the patient is asked to take, and this approach has positive effects. In addition, the clinician must take into consideration that the family will be involved with this child throughout their lifespan. As the family sees how the individual's developmental impairments interfere with their societal participation, they will always wonder if they 'did everything they could for their child'. Providing this CAM treatment now may help alleviate that feeling in years to come.

Patient/family autonomy versus societal responsibility
A core tenet of current Western medicine is that patient autonomy should be respected. In the case of children (or adults with developmental impairments severe enough to warrant a guardian), decision-making for the patient is performed by the parent (or other caregiver), who is expected to act in the patient's best interest. Although patients with guardians cannot act autonomously, their wishes are often part of the decision-making process by both clinician and family. There are only rare occasions in which the medical team will believe that the parent is not meeting this best interest standard and ask a court to intervene. Usually, this will happen when the family has declined a highly recommended evidence-based medical intervention such as first-line chemotherapy for pediatric leukemia.

Occasionally, as suggested by the first vignette, the tension will be between parental autonomy and societal justice. The clinician in the first scenario is asked to write a letter of support for a CAM treatment program with which they are not familiar. After reading the testimonials on the website and quickly reviewing traditional medical literature around the treatment (and finding none), the clinician concludes that the proposed therapy is probably not harmful, but unlikely to produce the effects touted by the website.

However, 'harms' are not limited to damage to the body; there can be financial and societal harms as well (see also Chapter 28). Society depends on clinicians to be good stewards of insurance resources and to recommend treatments that are of good value – that is, have the greatest benefit for the least cost (e.g. AMA n.d.; CMA 2015, see also Chapter 11). This holds true whether the family is insured by private or public insurance.

Even if the family does not intend to use insurance resources to pay for the therapy, it could be argued that the commitment to non-maleficence could extend to non-medical spheres as well. The money the family will spend on the proposed therapy might (in the judgment of others) have a better use for the family with more long-lasting positive effects, such as additional mainstream therapy or home modifications, or could be placed in a special-needs trust for the care of the individual in adulthood. In Scenario 1, for example, the child might benefit significantly both socially and physically from participation and engagement in activities that are meaningful to him. Indeed, such exposures might well have downstream effects on body structure and function that could outweigh the possible benefits from the intensive therapy about which the parents are asking – and at a considerably lower cost.

If the clinician does not feel that the therapy is likely to be beneficial, they should advise against it and decline to write the necessary prescriptions. This can, of course, place the physician–family relationship in jeopardy, but if there is no common ground in regard to such treatments, the family would do well to find other sources of medical care. In addition to declining to write prescriptions or letters of medical necessity, are there more active measures that should be taken to discourage the family? If the clinician feels that the proposed treatment is dangerous, a report to children's services might be warranted, and mandatory reporter laws would protect the clinician.

Clinician responsibilities to the family that uses CAM
In the first vignette, the clinician decided to investigate the treatments proposed by the family. They searched the treatment's 'official' website, as well as traditional sources of information, such as PubMed. This consumed a very precious commodity, the clinician's time. What responsibility does the clinician have to protect their time? This is a justice issue.

In the second vignette, although the family is specifically asking about the use of turmeric to reduce contractures, the astute clinician may hear 'My child has increasing contractures and I want to do everything I can to prevent them.' The family may not necessarily distinguish turmeric as CAM and different from stretching or the use of botulinum toxin (which is not considered CAM despite its 'natural' origin). Once the physician has reviewed, for the family, the lack of evidence for turmeric, they may no longer be interested in giving it to their child, or they may decide to use it in addition to mainstream methods of stretching and bracing.

In the third scenario (collaboration with the naturopath in the treatment of the patient with autism), there is a conflict between the duty to treat the patient and the time that might be consumed in a fruitless effort to collaborate with a professional who does not share the scientific world view as understood by the mainstream clinician. Within reason, it seems prudent for the medical clinician to investigate any proposed treatment with which they are not familiar, whether promulgated by a non-physician professional, the family or another physician. Just as the family would expect the neurodevelopmental specialist to collaborate with a traditional physician colleague, such as a neurologist or psychiatrist, an attempt should be made to collaborate with a CAM professional. However, this cannot be one-sided. If neither mainstream physician nor CAM professional is willing to meet in the middle, no collaboration is likely to be possible and instead will be a waste of time for the neurodevelopmental specialist, who has other patients who might make better use of that time and attention. When both clinicians can agree that there are many areas where evidence is lacking, there can perhaps be collaboration in areas of uncertainty. If the family sees that the traditional physician is open to exploring CAM treatments but ultimately advises against them, this may help steer families away from unproven, perhaps dangerous, treatments.

Based on many years of clinical experience with pediatric onset disabilities, the authors suggest that people consider the following principles when evaluating CAM therapies in light of the issues noted above:

- *Be open-minded.* The clinician should put aside prejudices for or against the treatment based on their own training and cultural background, and attempt to make a judgment based on best available facts. For example, acupuncture has a very weak body of scientific evidence and a theoretical basis (meridians and the flow of qi) that is outside Western medical training. The clinician working with a patient who is asking for an acupuncture referral should consider that this treatment has been used for thousands of years, is very common in a nation comprising one-fifth of the world's population and is gaining popularity in Western medicine as well. As medical evidence changes over time, the clinician should approach each situation with humility and a commitment to try to understand the patient's point of view, even if they will not agree (Noritz 2015). On the other hand, clinicians in societies with a strong culture of treatments based on experience rather than evidence should have a willingness to challenge long-held beliefs and traditions, helping their patients to pursue the interventions with stronger scientific basis.

- *Be non-judgmental.* The clinician must assess the family, but not judge them. They should not judge the use of resources or a family interaction based on how they themselves believe that they would act in the situation, but rather on what is best for this family and child. Despite this, in all situations, injury to the child must be avoided, even if to do so involves child protection services (e.g. a family giving inadequate calories based on a CAM method). Resources, time, family cohesiveness and family stress should be considered, but above all the clinician must fulfill the role of an advisor with training and experience.

- *Set priorities.* The clinician should decide what issues to prioritize in crafting a response to a request for CAM. The care of children with impairments, with their myriad challenges, frequently involves an ordering of priorities. In the office, the stated medical problems are usually only the obvious reason for the visit. These problems may be accompanied by unstated distress, which often has longstanding provenance. No matter the age of the patient, even well into adulthood, the family may still be grieving the loss of the 'normal' child. They may bear the scars of various experienced medical traumas, or careless remarks by previous clinicians. By the time they have presented to the neurodevelopmental office, the clinician may be challenged to change a family's attitudes about the nature of mainstream medicine and its practitioners.

> *"The expert clinician recognizes that when there is a patient and a doctor (or other service provider) in the room, there are two people with problems"*

The expert clinician recognizes that when there is a patient and a doctor (or other service provider) in the room, there are two people with problems (Personal communication Dr David Greer 1991). Without self-awareness of the clinician's own needs and biases, they can be only superficially helpful to the patient. It is important for the clinician to recognize the pressures that remove attention from the patient at hand, such as having a waiting room full of patients, all with similarly complex problems. This creates a tension in the ethical realm of *justice*, namely that resources should be equally available to all who need them. The time of the neurodevelopmental specialist is a finite commodity and choices must be made to share this resource rationally. Discussion of CAM may, at times, be a stressor for the physician, but its request can be seen as a signal of other important issues that need to be covered. These can include a full exploration of impairments that the CAM is purported to treat, a feeling of hopelessness in the family, and shame or guilt over having a child with an impairment (Grossberg 2008).

A broader issue of priorities relates to effectiveness research. Some CAM proponents are interested in having their modality put through scientific testing, which they are certain will prove its efficacy. Many in the scientific community advocate for randomized controlled trials (RCTs) for the opposite reason – they hope that a demonstrated lack of efficacy will quell the desire for the treatment. However, RCTs are generally highly complex and very expensive. They are well worth doing to determine if a plausible treatment is actually effective. They are generally ineffective in stopping the desire for a popular treatment, especially when the treatment proponents are savvy enough to point out the flaws in the study design (and there are always some). Putting resources into research on CAM draws away resources for research into promising treatments – is it really worth the effort to do this? Is it not the responsibility of the people promoting the CAM to do the studies and do them well?

Understand the unspoken agenda: what is behind the request for CAM?
As described above, the request for CAM can be taken as a signal of family frustration, perhaps with the current limitations of medical science. In this era of patient empowerment and the democratization of information via the Internet, patients may view CAM as a liberating factor in their attempts to parent a child with an impairment.

In these cases, and when the parents remain rational consumers of Internet information, investigation into CAM can be considered a mature coping mechanism. At other times, often when parental stress is prominent, interest in CAM can be more dysfunctional, and the clinician must unravel the unspoken agenda, which often includes grief, helplessness, anxiety and depression.

Rarely, there are more sinister factors at work. We have seen instances where there was a specific request for CAM by a guardian, where the guardian was selling the product in question. She thus would directly profit from the use of CAM by the patient, who would pay for it (at that guardian's direction) through their disability income. As these products are often sold in pyramid-type schemes (a seller recruits others to sell for them, keeping a portion of their profits), there is enticement for families to 'talk up' such products within their communities and networks. Cases such as this, with financial incentives, can easily cloud the judgment of parents and guardians who are expected to act in the best interest of the patient (see also Chapter 23 by Wright et al.).

Epilogue

When families request advice and support related to CAM methods, the clinician must be objective and open-minded, but must fulfill their ethical obligations. They must put aside prejudices based on their training and cultural biases. Requests for CAM are deeply rooted in the reality that currently available evidence-based treatments for developmental disabilities are limited. Approaches to a request for CAMs will vary, depending on potential harm to the child, the required resources and family needs. Even where there is disagreement, the clinician should seek to maintain a trusting, working relationship for the sake of the patient.

Themes for discussion

- 'Complementary and alternative therapies' (CAMs) often raise concerns and perhaps anger among health professionals working in mainstream services. In what ways are we, perhaps, threatened by these CAMs and what are our ethical challenges when responding to questions about them from families, colleagues, program managers and policy-makers?

- If a family chooses to pursue a CAM against the advice of their clinicians, what options should the clinician consider? Viewed from an ethical perspective, what principles can be brought to the issue? For example, should the clinician discharge the family from follow-up?

- At times, mainstream practitioners are drawn into debates with CAM providers. What approaches are ethically appropriate and which are inappropriate?

- What are the similarities and difference between pursuing CAM and rejecting immunizations?

References

Akins RS, Krakowiak P, Angkustsiri K, Hertz-Picciotto I, Hansen RL (2014) Utilization patterns of conventional and complementary/alternative treatments in children with autism spectrum disorders and developmental disabilities in a population-based study. *J Dev Behav Pediatr* 35: 1–10.

AMA (n.d.) *Opinion 9.0652 – Physician stewardship of health care resources*; http://www.ama-assn. org/ama/pub/physician-resources/medical-ethics/code-medical-ethics/opinion90652.page (accessed 27 May 2015).

Bingel U (2014) Avoiding nocebo effects to optimize treatment outcome. *JAMA* 312: 693–694.

CMA (2015) *CMA code of ethics*; http://policybase.cma.ca/dbtw-wpd/PolicyPDF/PD04-06.pdf (accessed 27 May 2015).

Doering JH, Reuner G, Kadish NE, Pietz J, Schubert-Bast S (2013) Pattern and predictors of complementary and alternative medicine (CAM) use among pediatric patients with epilepsy. *Epilepsy Behav* 29: 41–46.

Grossberg RI (2008) Psychoanalytic contributions to the care of medically fragile children. *J Psychiatr Pract* 14: 307–311.

Hurvitz EA, Leonard C, Ayyangar R, Nelson VS (2003) Complementary and alternative medicine use in families of children with cerebral palsy. *Dev Med Child Neurol* 45: 364–370.

Levy SE, Hyman SL (2015) Complementary and alternative medicine treatments for children with autism spectrum disorders. *Child Adolesc Psychiatr Clin N Am* 24: 117–143.

Noritz G (2015) How can we practice ethical medicine when the evidence is always changing? *J Child Neurol* 30: 1549–1550.

Palmer FB, Shapiro BK, Wachtel RC et al. (1988) The effects of physical therapy on cerebral palsy: A controlled trial in infants with spastic diplegia. *N Engl J Med* 318: 803–808.

Sagan C (1980) *Encyclopedia galactica,* 14 December 1980; http://www.imdb.com/title/tt0759806/.

Sagan C (1997) *The demon-haunted world: Science as a candle in the dark* 1st edn. New York, NY: Ballantine.

Sheppard MK (2015) The paradox of non-evidence based, publicly funded complementary alternative medicine in the English National Health Service: An explanation. *Health Policy* 119: 1375–1381.

Chapter 13

A miracle cure for neurological disability: balancing hype and hope for parents and patients in the absence of evidence-based recommendations

Paul C. Mann, Russell P. Saneto
and Sidney M. Gospe Jr.

Clinical scenario

Sarah M. is a 5-year-old girl we have followed since 2 years of age. She first developed seizures in the context of a febrile illness when she was 6 months old. Her initial events, diagnosed as complex febrile seizures due to their length, were thought to be benign. An electroencephalogram was normal at that time, there was no family history of epilepsy, and symptoms resolved with rescue medications alone. Unfortunately, her next febrile illness at 9 months of age provoked a very prolonged seizure event that required anesthetic medications to terminate status epilepticus. Subsequently, she developed afebrile seizures intractable to numerous antiseizure medications either as monotherapy or in combination. Hospitalization for a second prolonged febrile status epilepticus event prompted genetic testing which revealed a pathological mutation in the SCN1A gene. Although she had developed normally until 18 months of age, autistic behaviors have now arisen and she is demonstrating significant cognitive delays.

Topiramate, levetiracetam, zonisamide, clonazepam and a ketogenic diet have all failed to control this patient's seizures. Despite a current therapeutic regimen of valproic acid and clobazam at moderate dosages, her seizure semiology remains complex with frequent photic-stimulated myoclonic seizures. Numerous interventions have been tried by her parents aimed at reducing these episodes, including darkening all car windows. Review of her seizure calendar, however, indicates she is still having >10 days a month with 100 or more myoclonic seizures. Additionally, she has 20–30 atypical absence seizures monthly along with 2–3 rare hemiclonic seizures.

At her office visit today, her mother uses her smartphone to show a video from CNN of Charlotte Figi, a child who had a remarkable response to marijuana extracts with a high cannabidiol (CBD)-to-cannabinol (THC) ratio (Maa & Figi 2014; Young 2013). Our local jurisdiction has legalized marijuana so that parents can go to a local dispensary, purchase a high CBD product, and give their children the extract if they wish. This patient's mother and father are in a social media group with parents of children with Dravet syndrome and whose symptoms are similar to those of their daughter. Some of these parents have been providing their children marijuana extracts for seizure control and most tell them the response has been very favorable. Currently in the USA, marijuana is a Federal Food and Drug Administration (FDA) Schedule I drug, which does not exist in the Pharmacopeia and cannot be legally prescribed. However, this hospital has not formulated an official policy statement, and providers can authorize the use of medical marijuana in minors. The father is an active member of the US military and is against trying this intervention because of possible ramifications on his career, but the mother is crying as she tells us that she is desperate for anything to help her daughter. They are looking for guidance on what to do next, a challenging ethical dilemma – to endorse or dismiss a new approach to a clinically formidable condition.

Making sense of incomplete evidence

In recent years, particularly in jurisdictions where dispensing medical marijuana is permitted, medical providers have been inundated by requests similar to this case. The dramatic increase in parent interest for obtaining medical marijuana to treat refractory seizures in children has been largely impelled by prominent media reports of anecdotal successes and widespread accessibility to parent-to-parent support groups on social media outlets (Cilio et al. 2014; Porter & Jacobson 2013) (see also Chapter 12 by Hurvitz & Noritz). As a result, some child and adult neurologists are daily finding their personal convictions about what is in the best therapeutic interest for their patients to be in conflict with parent desires and media exuberance regarding this alternative medical therapy.

Providers encountering parents wishing a trial of marijuana for their child should first familiarize themselves with the scholarly work of their peers. At the time of the presented scenario, the American Academy of Neurology had stated that oral cannabinoids were of unknown efficacy in treating epilepsy, highlighting a 1% risk of serious adverse psychopathologic events in studies where patients were treated with marijuana (Koppel et al. 2014). Early uncontrolled studies demonstrated conflicting results for controlling seizures using high-ratio THC-to-CBD marijuana extracts in animals, with one study showing a proconvulsant effect and the other an anticonvulsant effect (Carlini et al. 1973; Keeler & Reifler 1967). A Cochrane review on this topic emphasizes the paucity of high-quality studies that demonstrate reliable efficacy for medical marijuana in seizure control (Gloss & Vickrey 2014).

However, more recent uncontrolled studies using marijuana extracts with high ratios of CBD to THC show pronounced anticonvulsant effects for patients with medically intractable seizures (Hussain et al. 2015; Press et al. 2015). Additionally, a published abstract studying the CBD extract Epildolex™ (recently given orphan drug status by the US federal Drug Enforcement Administration) reports that after three months of treatment, seizure frequency was reduced by 54% in all patients treated with the drug and by 63% in the population with Dravet syndrome (Devinsky et al. 2015). Although these results may be promising for some patients with severe seizures, they are also preliminary and nonrandomized, which leaves providers in the quandary of cautiously trying to interpret the potential benefits of CBD for their individual patients.

Authorizing alternative medications like medical marijuana to treat pediatric patients can be ethically challenging for clinicians (Committee on Children with Disabilities 2001). The ability to review objective and unbiased data providing evidence for efficacy and safety is essential for providers prior to prescribing new medications. In the case of many alternative therapies, purported benefits are based on limited data, or data that have not been scientifically validated by placebo-controlled studies. Anecdotal successes, although potentially informative, cannot provide substantive evidence for therapeutic efficacy. Randomized controlled and comparative effectiveness trials of alternative therapies are rarely available to guide clinician decision-making, and nearly impossible to get funded and completed. Therefore, providers are unable to offer truly informed advice to parents and patients that would meet the ethical burden of nonmaleficence were an alternative medical therapy they prescribed ultimately be found harmful.

First do no harm versus autonomy

Clinicians have fiduciary obligations to educate and inform parents about the potential risks that alternative drug therapies may pose to their patients. In the case of medical marijuana, there is the potential for unanticipated drug interactions (e.g. increasing or decreasing blood levels of prescribed antiepileptic medications) and/or toxicity from unregulated and variable product qualities (e.g. inconsistent levels of cannabinoids) (Gilmour et al. 2011a). Additionally, the lack of regulation and oversight of the medical marijuana industry poses significant safety concerns for patients, including risks of product contamination (fungal products, pesticides) (Associated Press 2013). The provider in this case must therefore impel continued close follow-up for this patient, even if the parents elect to begin such alternative therapies against their physician's medical recommendation. Providing a safe environment that allows parents to discuss openly all of the alternative therapies they are providing their children without passing personal judgment is an essential safeguard for the pediatric population (Gilmour et al. 2011b).

Although the provider in this case may not believe it to be in this patient's best interest to be given medical marijuana, taking legal measures to override parental authority – were they to seek out this independently – is probably not indicated by the current lack of evidence for substantial harm. There are, however, notable exceptions to non-intervention against parental autonomy in such cases involving minors (Zarzeczny & Caulfield 2010). Specifically in this case, if the parents were to decide to discontinue all current conventional seizure medications and treat with alternative medications alone (putting the child at risk for a potentially life-threatening seizure exacerbation), the clinician may be obligated to report this to local child safety authorities. However, physicians electing to override parental authority must be careful to research the available medical literature comprehensively to substantiate the potential risks and serious harms for the proposed alternative therapeutic interventions and/or parental actions. Professionals must also examine themselves for potential biases that may cloud their personal judgment and objectivity.

Turning to CBD-enriched cannabis or CBD oils to treat severe refractory seizures may be consistent with acting in their child's best interest from a parent and family-centered viewpoint. This is especially true if the neurodevelopmental risks of frequent seizures and/or current standard medical therapies for epilepsy ultimately outweigh the potential harms of CBD and other cannabinoids on neurodevelopment. This presupposes, however, that CBD is ultimately found efficacious in the treatment of intractable seizures, or is at least therapeutically inert, without significant side effects. Unfortunately, the available data on the safety of high-concentration THC extracts raise concerns for substantial detrimental effects (Hall & Solowij 1998; Radhakrishnan et al. 2014) and there are limited long-term data on the safety of high-concentration CBD-to-THC extracts (Bergamaschi et al. 2011). Any risk-versus-benefit analysis of the long-term effects of CBD therapy on neurodevelopmental outcome is therefore at best premature and necessarily speculative.

The parents' overwhelming desire for a seizure 'cure' in this case shares similarities with alternative medical therapies that families seek for other childhood neurodevelopmental diseases (e.g. autism, cerebral palsy etc.) (Bell et al. 2011). Desperation for an abatement to a chronic illness can lead parents to subject their children to potentially harmful interventions with no long-term or uncertain short-term benefit. However, the provision of medical marijuana by parents to their children is unique, because its social and legal implications differ greatly from other complementary or alternative therapies that families may seek. In the USA, as an example, medical marijuana is currently legal in only 23 states; physicians cannot legally prescribe the drug and can only recommend its use (Gregorio 2014). In states where medical marijuana can be obtained legally, many disallow the provision of the drug to minors. Similarly, there is great variation in the legality of marijuana possession worldwide, regardless of its intended use. Parents have committed criminal acts in order to procure and provide medical marijuana to their child with epilepsy, including illegal transportation of the drug, imperiling their entire family (Pickert 2014).

Clinical complexity can be encountered when children receiving marijuana at home are hospitalized. Patients can have clinical worsening of seizures and neurological status, or fluctuations in the blood levels of prescribed medications as a result of rapid withdrawal from cannabinoids and other therapies, both conventional and alternative (Bushra et al. 2014). Medical institutions almost universally forbid drugs with recreational abuse potential to be brought into hospital. Therefore, secure storage and safe distribution of marijuana in the inpatient setting require overcoming significant administrative and legal obstacles. Hospitals have an additional obligation to ensure the safety and integrity of the medications and therapies they provide, which is not possible in the current unregulated climate of medical marijuana and other alternative medications.

Ethical responsibility of the media

An important societal and ethical aspect to this case is how favorable media coverage surrounding potential curative alternative therapies can impair parental (and perhaps professional) judgment, remove protective safeguards and potentially introduce unnecessary harm to children. Parents seeking alternative medical therapies are frequently portrayed in the media as heroic in taking on the established medical community to act in the best interest of their child (Gonzalez 2015). Parents may see these depictions and be motivated by the anecdotal reports of efficacy where benefits are unchecked against potential harms (Sanderson et al. 2006). The increasing influence of social media on health decision-making can exacerbate this problem, as friends and relatives, online blogs and 'tweeting' celebrities are mistaken for credible sources of medical information (Moorhead et al. 2013). Additionally, known predilections for patients and parents to believe that 'natural' remedies are healthier and more efficacious than standard medical therapies may cause them to disregard warnings of potential harm from healthcare providers.

The population at large has significant difficulty understanding the results of clinical trials and media reports about medical advances (Pector 2007). As a result, clinicians may need to challenge misperceptions when explaining to parents the applicability of clinical studies about promising new therapies for an individual child. The substantial differences between evidence gathered from well-controlled double-blind placebo-controlled studies versus open-labeled, Internet-reported or chart-review studies are not likely to be easily understood. Parents (and professionals) may fail to recognize placebo effects and differences between association and causation when beginning alternative medical therapies for their child. Placebo effects are believed to have influenced reported seizure frequency rates in a recent cohort of patients with intractable seizures who began CBD therapy (Press et al. 2015). In that study, families who moved to Colorado seeking access to medical marijuana were more than three times as likely to report that CBD use resulted in a greater than 50% seizure reduction in their children than families with established residency and care in Colorado.

Promoting health

The numerous documented reports of 'miraculous' cures that were trumpeted by the media but later found to be inefficacious or even harmful should provide ample cautionary pause to providers and parents about rushing to embrace new alternative therapies. It is therefore essential that physicians stay engaged in the public sphere to educate families about the potential unknown risks and benefits of both novel alternative and conventional medical therapies, such as medical marijuana for refractory seizures (Devinsky 2015). Physicians should both demonstrate and encourage prudence before accepting news about scientific discoveries and should be vocal advocates for properly designed clinical research to provide the scientific evidence needed to validate or refute the claims of benefits of new mediations and treatments.

Finally, the provider in this case should make an altruistic argument to the parents, encouraging them to consider enrolling their child in clinical trials (if available in their region) studying the efficacy of CBD therapy in a scientifically rigorous manner. Such trials provide opportunities to advance medical knowledge and benefit future generations of children with epilepsy. These trials are also critically important, because if CBD is ultimately found to be beneficial for the treatment of refractory epilepsy in children, reproducing safe and predictable clinical responses in patients will probably result from purified, titratable CBD extracts, rather than whole-leaf marijuana preparations available at local dispensaries (Saper 2015).

Resolution

A detailed discussion with the M. family ensued, in which we described our hesitancy to recommend a therapy for which medication purity cannot be guaranteed, batches lack dose standardization, and long-term efficacy is uncertain. We advised them that if they chose to move forward in purchasing this product for Sarah we would be willing to monitor levels of CBD and THC, but that the optimal levels of CBD for seizure control are not known and medication contaminants cannot be screened. We provided reassurance that if they decided not to purchase CBD extracts, we would continue our efforts to reduce Sarah's seizure frequency using approved medications at our disposal. We also discussed the possibly of enrollment in an upcoming FDA-approved clinical trial using a proprietary CBD product if eligibility criteria are met. The parents appreciated our open stance in this conversation and unwavering support of their daughter. They decided to take some time to talk over next steps and know that they can call us at any time with further questions.

Themes for discussion

- In an era in which 'evidence-based medicine' is the touchstone, what are the clinical and ethical dilemmas facing practitioners when there is either (1) no evidence or (2) significantly conflicting evidence, and families are seeking our advice and guidance?

- How can we use arguments based on ethical principles to work with parents and colleagues who are swayed by media hype and request our support when we cannot comfortably offer it? And would it make a difference if the patients are receiving palliative care?

- There seems to be an important bias in the media (both mainstream news outlets and the informal communications networks) towards reporting and celebrating the 'big news' (anecdotes of the 'miracles'), while the 'sober second thought' resulting from studies and 'failures' is usually elegated to the 'back-page' reports (if any). What is our role as professionals to hold the media ethically responsible for the stories they tell, especially when these are anecdotal rather than evidence-based?

References

Associated Press (2013) Marijuana may be contaminated with mold, mildew. *CBS News* [Online] 2 December; http://www.cbsnews.com/news/marijuana-contaminated-with-mold-mildew/ (accessed 6 February 2015).

Bell E, Wallace T, Chouinard I et al. (2011) Responding to requests of families for unproven interventions in neurodevelopmental disorders: hyperbaric oxygen 'treatment' and stem cell 'therapy in cerebral palsy. *Dev Disabil Res Rev* 17: 19–26.

Bergamaschi MM, Quiroz RH, Zuardi AW et al. (2011) Safety and side effects of cannabidiol, a *Cannabis sativa* constituent. *Curr Drug Saf* 6: 237–249.

Bushra A, Mahfooz N, Farooq O (2014) Withdrawal of medical marijuana. *Pediatr Neurol* 51: e15.

Carlini EA, Leite JR, Tannhauser M et al. (1973) Letter: Cannabidiol and *Cannabis sativa* extract protect mice and rats against convulsive agents. *J Pharm Pharmacol* 25: 664–665.

Cilio MR, Thiele EA, Devinsky O (2014) The case for assessing cannabidiol in epilepsy. *Epilepsia* 55: 787–790.

Committee on Children with Disabilities, American Academy of Pediatrics (2001) Counseling families who choose complementary and alternative medicine for their child with chronic illness or disability. *Pediatrics* 107: 598–601.

Devinsky O (2015) Commentary: Medical marijuana survey and epilepsy. *Epilepsia* 56: 7–8.

Devinsky O, Sullivan J, Friedman D et al. (2015) Epidiolex (Cannabidiol) in treatment resistant epilepsy. *Neurology* 84 (Meeting Abstracts): 005.

Gilmour J, Harrison C, Asadi L et al. (2011a) Natural health product–drug interactions: Evolving responsibilities to take complementary and alternative medicine into account. *Pediatrics* 128: S155–S160.

Gilmour J, Harrison C, Cohen MH et al. (2011b) Pediatric use of complementary and alternative medicine: Legal, ethical, and clinical issues in decision-making. *Pediatrics* 128: S149–S154.

Gloss D, Vickrey B (2014) Cannabinoids for epilepsy. *Cochrane Database Syst Rev* 13: CD009270.

Gonzalez D (2015) For children's seizures, turning to medical marijuana. *New York Times*; http://lens.blogs.nytimes.com/2015/03/26/medical-marijuana-eases-childhood-seizures/?_r=0 (accessed 24 May 2015).

Gregorio J (2014) Physicians, medical marijuana, and the law. *Virtual Mentor* 16: 732–738.

Hall W, Solowij N (1998) Adverse effects of cannabis. *Lancet* 352: 1611–1616.

Hussain SA, Zhou R, Jacobson C et al. (2015) Perceived efficacy of cannabidiol-enriched extracts for treatment of pediatric epilepsy: A potential role for infantile spasms and Lennox–Gaustaut syndrome. *Epilepsy Behav* 47: 38–41.

Keeler MH, Reifler CB (1967) Grand mal convulsions subsequent to marijuana use. Case report. *Dis Nerv Syst* 28: 474–475.

Koppel BS, Brust JC, Fife T et al. (2014) Systematic review: Efficacy and safety of medical marijuana in selected neurological disorders. Report of the Guideline Development Subcommittee of the American Academy of Neurology. *Neurology* 82: 1556–1563.

Maa E, Figi P (2014) The case for medical marijuana in epilepsy. *Epilepsia* 55: 783–786.

Moorhead SA, Hazlett DE, Harrison L et al. (2013) A new dimension of health care: Systematic review of the uses, benefits, and limitations of social media for health communication. *J Med Internet Res* 15: e85.

Pector EA (2007) Save patients from media hype. *Med Econ* 84: 37–38, 41–42.

Pickert K (2014) Pot kids. *Time* [Online]; http://time.com/pot-kids/ (accessed 28 January 2015).

Porter BE, Jacobson C (2013) Report of a parent survey of cannabidiol-enriched cannabis use in pediatric treatment-resistant epilepsy. *Epilepsy Behav* 29: 574–577.

Press C, Knupp K, Chapman KE (2015) Parental reporting of response to oral cannabis extracts for treatment of refractory epilepsy. *Epilepsy Behav* 45: 49–52.

Radhakrishnan R, Wilkinson ST, D'Souza DC (2014) Gone to pot – a review of the association between cannabis and psychosis. *Front Psychiat* 5: 1–24.

Sanderson CR, Koczwara B, Currow DC (2006) The 'therapeutic footprint' of medical, complementary and alternative therapies and a doctor's duty of care. *Med J Aust* 185: 373–376.

Saper CB (2015) Up in smoke: a neurologist's approach to 'medical marijuana'. *Ann Neurol* 77: 13–14.

Young, S (2013) Marijuana stops child's severe seizures. *CNN* [Online] 7 August; www.cnn.com/2013/08/07/health/charlotte-child-medical-marijuana (accessed 11 April 2015).

Zarzeczny A, Caulfield T (2010) Stem cell tourism and doctors' duties to minors – a view from Canada. *Am J Bioethic* 10: 3–15.

Chapter 14

Terminology in neurodevelopmental disability: is using stigmatizing language harmful?

Lisa Samson-Fang

I grew up with a sister with an intellectual disability. At that time, intellectual disability was referred to as mental retardation (MR) and individuals with it were referred to as 'retarded'. As a kid, I really didn't understand what she had or why, just that she was 'slow', had difficult behaviors and at times embarrassed me. I never thought about how hard it was for her, but rather focused on how hard it was for me: disruptions in my home life resulting from her challenging behaviors and the not-so-rare remarks of schoolmates that made me feel like being related to someone 'retarded' implied there was something wrong with me and my family. It didn't affect all the children in my family the same way; my older sister seemed never embarrassed but rather our sister's proud defender. I recall no role models on how to be a sibling of someone with 'special healthcare needs', no books that describe the experience and no one offering guidance, including my parents, who were overwhelmed with their own adaptations.

As an adult providing healthcare for children with neurodevelopmental impairments, I grew to understand the power of the words 'mentally retarded' to create stigma. A parent told me that the diagnosis of mental retardation was overwhelming for her, not because it confirmed her child's disability, but rather because it triggered her memories of how children with 'MR' were teased and excluded in her own childhood and hence her fears of how her child might be treated. As a parent, I watched my child give a presentation about himself to his third grade class. It was a humorous presentation on his birthday and the children gathered around. As some point, he made a joke and one of the kids said, 'That's retarded'. Several of the other children reflected his response using the 'R' word several times. The teacher acted as if nothing had happened. I was quite sure that, had the child sworn, the reaction would have been swift and decisive. I began to tell my children that I didn't care if they used swear words but I never wanted to hear them say the 'R' word. There were many other disability-related stigmatizing words I tried to get them not to use (e.g. mute, dumb, spastic, midget, crippled) although in general to no avail.

One day, my now 40-year-old sister was riding in the car with us. My husband commented that the political process surrounding some issue was 'retarded'. In his mind, this was an adjective that didn't relate to a condition or to people. However, my sister's reaction was swift. Wrestling tears, she told him that it was a cruel word that she had been called and that she didn't think he or anyone should use it. I was proud to see her become her own spokesperson and reflected back to the realization that whatever stigma it created for me as a child, it was a mild inconvenience compared to that with which she had struggled. My sons are now entering college and as I wrote this chapter I discussed it with them and asked if they or their friends used 'the R word'. My son responded with dismay that I would ask the question, saying, 'Of course not, it would be pejorative toward a group of people.' Perhaps the kids in the back seat had listened.

When a clinician evaluates a patient with a neurodevelopmental impairment, often the first goal is to make a diagnosis. A diagnosis may identify a developmental pattern or category (e.g. autism, intellectual disability, Tourette syndrome, cerebral palsy) or may identify a specific etiology (e.g. a genetic condition such as fragile X syndrome, brain injury, fetal alcohol effects). The goals of diagnosis include a better understanding of an individual's condition, identification of appropriate treatment and management, and qualification for community-based resources or research protocols. However, diagnostic categories and terminologies also may carry with them stigmas that can result in stereotyping and potential prejudice (Garrand et al. 2009).

For the individual, their family, those that provide services to the individual, and the society in which the individual resides, diagnostic terms have the power to communicate intense positive or negative images. Why these terms come to have such power is multidimensional, including misunderstanding, misconceptions, judgment and fear. Stereotypes are knowledge structures that the public learns about a marked social group. Stereotypes generate preconceived impressions and expectations of the individual. When a stereotype is negative, the distinguishing characteristics of a social group become stigmatizing and in turn trigger individuals to think using the negative stereotype. Negative expectations and impressions can result in prejudice. Any diagnosis has the potential to create stereotypes, stigma and prejudice, depending on the notions and beliefs of the society in which the individual lives. Individuals with neurodevelopmental disabilities such as intellectual disabilities (IDs) and those with mental health challenges are consistently found to be among the most socially excluded populations and they continue to face substantial health, housing and employment disparities due to stigma, stereotyping and prejudice (Ditchman et al. 2013).

The use and misuse of diagnostic terms (and their slang alternatives) can have secondary consequences beyond the mere identification of an individual's condition:

- For the individual, a diagnostic label impacts their power of self-determination through self-stigma and social categorization (seeing oneself as a member of a specific group) (Corrigan 2004). The stereotypes associated with a specific condition become personally relevant, resulting in some cases in an altered self-concept (e.g. a child with specific learning impairment viewing themselves as 'stupid') and/or defensive behavior that may impact adherence to treatment (e.g. a teen's refusal to take medication for ADHD in order to normalize their sense of self). The extent to which the labels impact an individual depends in part on the degree to which the individual internalizes the label. The individual's prejudice may impact their expectations of self and thus outcomes (e.g. an individual with a learning disability might assume that they are not capable of attending college).

- Caregivers and families experience similar stigmatizing impacts (All et al. 2012). This is referred to as 'affiliated' or 'courtesy' stigma. In some cultures, parents who birth a child with a developmental or health issues are assumed to have done something bad that resulted in their misfortune. Additionally, individuals outside the family may view the burden of such a child as a devastation from which the family will never recover (Green 2007). In families of children with autism, the level of affiliated stigma has been correlated with the caregivers' or families' sense of well-being, with greater levels of stigma resulting in lower ratings of sense of well-being. Efforts at avoidance of stigma may result in a parent denying a diagnosis or rejecting a child.

- A parent who internalizes a negative stereotype of their child's condition through their actions, statements and behaviors may teach the child to internalize the negative stereotype. This is referred to as 'stigma coaching' (Jacoby & Austin 2013). In addition, the stereotypes that a parent or caregiver associates with a particular diagnostic group can result in the family having altered expectations for their child's future. These altered parental expectations also impact the child's internalized sense of self.

- On a societal level, the stigma and stereotypes associated with a particular condition may result in reduced compassion toward an individual when mediated through prejudice. Diagnostic terms can be harmful when used to bully or when their use results in discrimination or exclusion from societal participation. The use of a stigmatizing label might impact the resources a society is willing to delegate to support a particular group of individuals, whereas these same individuals' function and societal participation will be optimized if they are provided with the supports and services they need, thus reducing societal burden.

There are medical terms whose use is now avoided because the words have come to embody the stigma that a condition experiences within society (e.g. words like cripple, midget, mute and moron). As a clinician, it is a challenge to stay up to date on what is currently 'politically correct' and it can feel like the changes in terminology that occur are inconvenient and unhelpful. For example, telling a parent their child has an intellectual disability often creates a response of confusion and subsequently requires an explanation of the meaning of 'intellectual disability', only to ultimately have the family say 'so you are saying my child has mental retardation'. However, it would seem that the negative impact of these words ('MR') justifies the transitions in terminology and all the efforts needed to implement change.

Regardless of stigma, diagnostic terms may become pejorative by being used in a dehumanizing context, for example, when referring to a child as 'autistic'. The clinician has been encouraged to use People First Language (Snow 2009), in which an individual is identified first and then his/her condition presented secondarily (e.g. a child with epilepsy as opposed to an 'epileptic child'). By changing the word order, the condition is viewed as a secondary attribute, not part of the person's identity.

There is not always agreement regarding what terms are stigmatizing, and the issue is complex and multidimensional. Interpretation of words and phrases varies based upon experience (Streeter 2010). For example, clinicians have been encouraged to say 'The child utilizes a wheelchair for mobility' as opposed to 'wheelchair-bound (or confined)' when describing a patient's level of motor function. This is to avoid the negative image of a child literally tied to a wheel chair. The term 'wheelchair-bound' also emphasizes the individual's impairment rather than focusing on the wheelchair's ability to liberate and empower independent mobility and enhance function. However, I recently heard a young adult with severe cerebral palsy say he found the term somewhat humorous as the image he sees when he hears 'wheelchair-bound' is himself 'bounding across the room to his chair'. Some individuals in the deaf community have indicated that they prefer the term 'deaf child' over the people-first 'child with deafness', because they view deafness as a culture and community, similar to saying an 'Asian child' (Gallaudet University n.d.). Others have criticized people-first language because, by attempting to de-emphasize a condition, it may inadvertently create emphasis. Consider a manuscript where a 'child with blindness' is written repeatedly. Could the awkwardness and repetitive nature of the phrase create more emphasis on the disability than the individual? Might 'blind child', by being less cumbersome, allow more emphasis on the child?

It has been demonstrated that medical training of clinicians can negatively impact attitudes towards those with impairments, given that many interactions in the healthcare setting occur when the person is in a setting of vulnerability and not demonstrating their strengths (e.g. when they are unwell in hospital). It is also notable that many of the images used in the medical setting to teach clinicians promote stigma, as they often represent a condition with a dated picture of a child with a condition of which the degree of impact is on the severe end of the condition spectrum, shot in unflattering light, with a medical background (or none at all) and sometimes naked or in a medical gown.

A better understanding of the variability among individuals with any particular condition and enhanced understanding of the competencies and strengths among individuals, regardless of diagnosis, may result in less stigmatization and stereotyping. While attitudes towards individuals with impairments can be enhanced through education of individuals and society, advocacy and protest, the most effective and enduring way to enhance attitudes towards individuals with impairments is through shared experiences and positive interaction in school, employment and community settings (Morin et al. 2013; National Disability Authority 2007). In the USA, The Education for All Handicapped Children Act (Public Law (PL) 94-142) was enacted in 1975 to ensure participation of all individuals in the public school setting. While enacted to ensure the rights of individuals with impairments, it also allowed children without impairments to have more shared experiences with children with impairments, ideally reducing the bias of society as these children grow up. Similarly, enhanced employment experiences for individuals with impairments secondarily allow for more positive interactions in the workplace.

For the child with neurodevelopmental impairment, building resilience and a sense of coherence and self-esteem may help to mitigate the extent that the child internalizes a negative stereotype. Mechanisms to build resilience and self-esteem may include strong family support with open communication, counseling, peer support and make it possible to involve the child as a partner in their healthcare or educational decisions. In the healthcare setting, engagement of the individual and family in all aspects of care, focusing on strengths (as opposed to impairments) and facilitating empowerment may help to diminish self-stigma and its impacts upon self-image, adherence behaviors and outcomes (Smith & Schonert-Reichl 2013).

In summary, although diagnostic terms often impart helpful information to guide prognosis and care, they may also result in stigma, stereotyping and prejudice toward the individual and their family. These effects in turn may impact the individual's sense of self and their goals, as well as the family's views and expectations and society's treatment of them. The clinician can help a person cope and reduce internalization of negative stereotypes by encouraging strategies that enhance resilience and support positive self-esteem. Education, advocacy and protest can be used to alter stereotypes, but ultimately contact between individuals with and without neurodevelopmental conditions may have the most significant and enduring impact on society's attitudes. In the healthcare setting, evolving diagnostic terminology, people-first language and positive imagery are other strategies that may be employed to reduce stigma.

Finally, one might posit that an ethical responsibility of all healthcare providers is to be both attentive to the language we and our colleagues use, and to help families understand the ways in which the language of 'disability' can be used either well or badly. We can become engaged in these issues when we ask families how they talk to others about their child, what has been said to them by professionals, family members and community people, and whether the language used about their child and themselves creates challenges for them. There would appear to be considerable opportunities for preventive counseling to address some of the hurt and damage that can too easily be done with careless, thoughtless labeling.

Themes for discussion

- When discussing a child's impairments with a family – perhaps including the extended family (such as siblings and grandparents) – do we discuss the language of impairment and disability? Do we emphasize – as is illustrated here – how personal strength and resilience can be developed and expressed? Should we know how these conditions are thought about and talked about, in an effort to address possible misconceptions?

- Besides the general expectation for professionals to 'watch our language' – is there an ethical responsibility to become engaged with community people (teachers, parents, policy-makers, the media) when language about neurodisability is used pejoratively or is a potentially stigmatizing manner?

- Given that language, terminology and labeling are constantly changing and evolving, is it likely that the 'correct' use of today's language will matter 'tomorrow'? Isn't this simply political correctness gone mad?

References

All A, Hassiotis A, Strydom A, King, M (2012) Self stigma in people with intellectual disabilities and courtesy stigma in family carers: A systematic review. *Res Dev Disab* 33: 2122–2140.

Corrigan, P (2004) How stigma interfere with mental health care. *Am Psychol* 59: 614–625.

Ditchman N, Werner S, Kosvluk K, Jones N, Elg B, Corrigan PW (2013) Stigma and intellectual disability: Potential application of mental illness research. *Rehabil Psychol* 58: 206–216.

Garrand L, Lingler JH, Conner KO, Dew MA (2009) Diagnostic labels, stigma, and participation in research related to dementia and mild cognitive impairment. *Res Gerontol Nurs* 2: 112–121.

Green SE (2007) 'We're tired, not sad': Benefits and burdens of mothering a child with a disability. *Soc Sci Med* 64: 150–163.

Gullaudet University (n.d.) Terminology describing deaf individuals in resources for mainstream programs. A practical guide; http://www2.gallaudet.edu/ (accessed 22 May 2015).

Jacoby A, Austin JK (2013) Stigma: A pervasive contextual barrier. In: Ronen GM, Rosenbaum PL, editors. *Life quality outcomes in children and young people with neurological and developmental conditions*, pp. 154–165. London: Mac Keith Press.

Morin D, Rivard M, Crocker AG, Boursier CP, Caron J (2013) Public attitudes towards intellectual disability: A multidimensional perspective. *J Intell Disab Res* 57: 279–292.

National Disability Authority (2007) Literature review on attitudes towards disability; http://nda.ie/Publications/Attitudes/Literature-Review-of-International-Evidence-on-Attitudes-to-Disability/ (accessed 22 May 2015).

Smith V, Schonert-Reichl K (2013) Contextual facilitators: Resilience, sense of coherence and hope. In: Ronen GM, Rosenbaum PL, editors. *Life quality outcomes in children and young people with neurological and developmental conditions*, pp. 120–135. London: Mac Keith Press.

Snow K (2009) People first language; http://www.disabilityisnatural.com/explore/people-first-language (accessed 22 May 2015).

Streeter L (2010) The continuing saga of people-first language. *Braille Monitor* 53: 58–63.

Chapter 15

Everyday ethics in Rwanda: perspectives on hope, fatigue, death and regrowth

Emily Esmaili and Christian Ntizimira

'Death of death, who will give us medicine for death? Death knocks at your door, and before you can tell him to come in, he is in the house with you.'

(Grace Ogot, 1968)

Prologue

Rwanda is a stunning country that is staggering back to its feet following the wake of the 1994 Genocide. This dark event in history took the lives of about 1 000 000 people and made another 2 000 000 refugees in this small landlocked country (Human Rights Watch 2014). The health sector was also affected, with most health professionals killed and the national health infrastructure destroyed. Although great progress has been made in overcoming this massacre as well as the subsequent onslaught of HIV/AIDS, tuberculosis and malaria, Rwanda has remained in rehabilitation mode (Farmer et al. 2013; McCarthy 2015). The nation continues to be disabled by poverty, inequity, orphans and widows. As we consider questions of ethics in childhood disability, a few clinical vignettes from a country riddled with handicaps may provide a unique perspective. And, as we will suggest, such a country is also ripe with opportunities for rehabilitation and reconstruction.

Clinical scenario

Espérance is a 9-month-old girl weighing 4kg who presented to our referral hospital with dyspnea, hypoxia and failure to thrive. Physical exam revealed an impressive cardiac murmur with hepatomegaly, and chest X-ray demonstrated cardiomegaly with pulmonary edema. We made the presumed diagnosis of congestive heart failure due to congenital heart disease. As echocardiography was not available, we treated her with furosemide, digoxin, oxygen and nutritional support for 3 weeks, until a visiting cardiologist from abroad was able to confirm our diagnosis (large ventricular septal defect [VSD], small atrial septal defect [ASD] and pulmonary hypertension). We adjusted medications and continued oxygen and nutritional support. Her mother was tirelessly attentive and dedicated. She breastfed until she couldn't afford to feed herself well enough to produce milk. She patiently watched as Espérance's clinical course waxed and waned. We explained how Espérance badly needed cardiac surgery, which was not available in Rwanda. As the weeks progressed she developed increasingly severe hypoxia and hypotension, despite our interventions, and she eventually developed apnea and cardiopulmonary arrest. She was successfully resuscitated and placed on bubble continuous positive airway pressure (CPAP) for respiratory support. Soon after, her mother asked us to remove 'this machine that was keeping Espérance alive' and let them go home. By that time, she already had no money left. Our Head of Department did not agree with letting her go home to die, so we urged the mother to allow her child to stay for minimal oxygen support through nasal cannula. While making these negotiations, Espérance had another cardiopulmonary arrest. After 20 minutes of resuscitation and three rounds of adrenaline we could not recover her heartbeat. We asked her mother for direction and she requested that we please stop. We stepped away, cleaned and wrapped Espérance's small body and gave her to her mother to hold.

Questions, challenges, ethical dilemmas

This case scenario, although not mainly about a neurological impairment, illustrates how discussions of withdrawing life support typically take place during intense, pivotal moments at the bedside. Currently, advance directives such as 'Do Not Resuscitate' simply do not exist in Rwanda. Deciding to stop life-sustaining measures is highly stigmatized by health practitioners and usually avoided until the latest possible moment, even when chances of recovery are minimal. How might the healthcare team approach these discussions in a way that is sufficiently anticipatory, but still sensitive to the medical and social culture of Rwanda?

Given Rwanda's history of profound loss and grief, most Rwandese are exceptionally sensitized to death, which contributes to the stigma around the end-of-life issues mentioned above. Within this context, how can Rwandan doctors approach end-of-life discussions in an ethical but sensitive way?

- Could the mother's voice and perspective on these decisions be heard by the Head of Department, again considering the medical and social context?

- In this authoritarian medical setting, how might voices of nursing staff, who are charged with watching over and tending to this critically ill child, be heard by the physician staff?

- Should the hospital use its resources (human resources and medical technology such as CPAP) to prolong the suffering of a critically ill child who cannot receive curative treatment in this setting?

- Does this further deplete resources in an already low-resourced setting?

Financial and socioeconomic factors contribute an additional dimension to such dilemmas in these low-income countries. Quite often, children from wealthier families will be pushed through an assortment of desperate, intrusive attempts at curative treatment, despite our better medical judgment. Does this unnecessarily prolong the suffering of the child and the vicarious suffering of the family? And does this give the family a message of false hope, suggesting that recovery is still a strong possibility? In such bleak circumstances as Espérance's case, how else might we offer the family hope, in a way that would not prolong the suffering of the child, or of the family that is watching vigilantly at the bedside?

From death to disability

In developing countries such as Rwanda, death and disability exist not only because of neurodevelopmental conditions, congenital cardiac anomalies, genetic syndromes and rare neuromuscular disorders, but also from the inability to treat common pediatric emergencies and serious medical conditions efficiently. Therefore meningoencephalitis will more frequently result in chronic neurological impairment, and sickle cell disease will more often lead to debilitating anemia, osteomyelitis and stroke than in resource-rich countries (Farmer et al. 2006). As an example, a common presentation to our emergency room is a child with fever and coma. We cannot extract historical details from the care-giver, who is rarely the biologic parent and rarely at home actually caring for the child. We cannot rely on our substandard microbiology results and the family cannot afford a computerized tomography (CT) scan. We therefore use our bedside clinical skills and limited armamentarium of antibiotics and antimalarials, and hope for the best. In the days to follow, we anxiously check the child's pupils, reflexes and fever curve for some hint of response. We begin feeding high-calorie formula through a nasogastric tube, as these children are usually wasted as well, and we treat seizures as they arise. Perhaps they will fully recover consciousness and slowly sit, walk and eat again. Perhaps they will partially recover, but require nasogastric feeds, seizure control and lifelong bedside care from some committed caregiver. Perhaps they will not survive.

Between these unknowns, nurses may not know how much effort to put into caring for this child. Doctors may not know how to counsel families. As the healthcare team succumbs to fatalism and apathy, the child may be left in pain, unfed and unmedicated, developing bedsores that become infected. The uninformed family may try to feed them porridge by mouth, and the child may aspirate and develop cardiopulmonary arrest. When we call our intensive-care unit (ICU) during resuscitation, the on-call senior may see this disabled child and refuse ICU admission based on poor prognosis. Do we fight this decision, arguing that we should do as much as we can? Should we in fact do as much as we can, with what information and resources we have? Does the family have a voice in that decision, especially in a medical culture where highly respected attitudes of physicians override the unspoken choices of patients and families? We recognize that by challenging this cultural norm of giving senior physicians ultimate ruling power, we would rock delicate professional relationships. Furthermore, we recognize that we ourselves may not fully understand what it might mean to stop resuscitation. Can we therefore expect the family to understand what this might mean, well enough to have an opinion on the matter?

We constantly face these challenging questions, and we often face them alone. Similar to the Head of Department not wanting to allow Espérance to go home in her final hours, we do not want to demonstrate to families, colleagues and ourselves that we are giving up. We allow the stigma of death and impairments to impact our clinical decisions. We avoid being likened to genocidaires at all costs.

Similar challenges exist in neonatology in Rwanda. With a high prevalence of hypoxic ischemic encephalopathy (HIE) resulting from suboptimal peripartum care, we are frequently stabilizing babies with recurrent apnea or refractory seizures from extensive anoxic brain injury, knowing that if the child survives, chronic neurodevelopmental impairment may be the most likely prognosis. Mothers themselves are often starved and cannot produce sufficient breast milk, with several other children at home and financial obligations to work the fields most days. Understandably, they often resist staying in hospital for palliative care of these chronically oxygen-dependent newborn babies with feeding problems. Also, many newborn infants are sent to us with congenital malformations such as gastroschisis or diaphragmatic hernia, although we do not have the surgical expertise to treat these conditions. A baby like Espérance with congenital heart disease stands no chance in this setting. These technical inadequacies impact the morale and clinical confidence of healthcare workers. Nurses will assume – from experience – a grim outlook, and slowly back away from the babies. The healthcare team makes an unspoken decision to withdraw care indirectly, leaving their patients hypothermic, irregularly fed and unmonitored. We sheepishly dismiss the babies and their families and avoid confronting the heavy discomfort of the situation. We avoid updating the family on as much as we know or do not know. We fail to suggest a basic plan for pain and symptom control, or simple anticipatory guidance when sending them home. We fail to offer a mother the opportunity to hold her dying baby. We forget to do those things we can do and we forget our strongest asset in these settings: our humanity.

We may therefore conclude that healthcare workers are charged with creating a new standard, both at home and abroad. In resource-poor settings such as ours, where death and impairments are so frequently encountered, health workers must remember always to respect the dignity of a dying child and always advocate for the rights and needs of children with impairments. In these pockets of the world where even many healthy children struggle for basic human rights, one can imagine the difficulties in obtaining speech therapy and physical therapy, crutches and daily medications. There are not many options for a child without means who cannot chew and swallow, or sit without support. Home healthcare is not yet a part of the national healthcare scheme, and most caregivers are already overtaxed. In such settings, survival of children with complex medical needs often means slow death because of the absence of support services.

However, this is precisely where we are given the novel opportunity to show caregivers a different and perhaps more compassionate alternative. We find creative solutions for the child's unique needs. We take the time to explain in detail the clinical condition and prognosis – to the very best of our ability. We listen to families' concerns, desires and needs, and also listen to the children themselves. Ultimately, in order to help families embrace their child's situation – be they terminally ill or permanently impaired – we ourselves must also accept these realities. Recognizing and accepting the limitations of medicine is the challenge of every healthcare practitioner.

In studying these ethically challenging situations, perhaps we should thus begin with questioning ourselves. Facing one's own limitations and one's own grief is particularly loathsome for those whose country is still recovering from genocide and who have faced deep suffering and loss in their personal lives. Rwandan healthcare workers therefore face a tall challenge in this movement to provide fully comprehensive medical care over the background of tremendous suffering, using very limited resources. They face emotionally charged ethical dilemmas every day. Without the luxuries of diagnostic imaging, sophisticated laboratory investigations, subspecialists and an ethics board behind them, rarely can they counsel a family on prognosis with as much confidence as those in the developed world. Moreover, in a country with limited medical technology and non-existent disability services for children, what do we actually have to offer? How do we fight fatalism in our colleagues and ourselves?

We should come to recognize that we, as healthcare workers in the developing world, are at the forefront of an emerging paradigm shift in the care of chronically and terminally ill children. As we continue to make advances against the communicable diseases common to impoverished populations, non-communicable diseases and conditions are gaining more and more public attention. We must now advocate for competent, comprehensive rehabilitation and palliative care services for children, and we must begin by offering such quality care ourselves, immediately. In a country such as Rwanda with a developed public health infrastructure, we must integrate these services into the national healthcare scheme, from academic referral centers down to the community level. This level of care should not be the exception at certain tertiary institutions, but rather the expectation of workers at all levels of health facilities.

According to the United Nations Convention of the Rights of the Child and the UN Convention on the Rights of Persons with Disabilities (both of which Rwanda has signed), every child is entitled to adequate and equitable healthcare, including disability and palliative care (United Nations 2006). This is a basic human right of every child. In settings such as ours with such pervasively limited resources, every healthcare worker should personally fight the systemic shortcomings and cultural norms that interfere with these basic rights, and confront the inner reticence that may be standing in the way of availing these rights to each child we treat. One should personally accept that every child has all the same rights and privileges as a wealthy adult, even when they are an 800g neonate born preterm to a young destitute mother. We must advocate for such rights every day, even when this means advocating for a peaceful death. Every healthcare worker must also be a palliative care specialist and an 'everyday' ethicist.

We can therefore begin with ourselves. We should listen vigilantly for those voices in ourselves saying there is no hope, no purpose to addressing the pain, no need to stay with challenging situations long enough to offer a child or family some solace and relief. These defiant voices are even more difficult to differentiate in the developing world, where so many neglected voices compete for attention. We must recognize the limitations that ultimately stem from inequality, poverty and neglect, as well as our own limitations, perhaps from fear of death and pain. Once we learn to see and accept these darker realities of medicine and humanity, once we shift our own view of chronically and terminally ill children, we may begin to care adequately and ethically for the living and dying children of countries like Rwanda. Limited resources must not also mean limited quality of care. Modeling such quality care and open, accepting attitudes is the only way forward. It is upon each of us to build this new, more equitable paradigm – even in the face of war wounds, cultural barricades and disabling destitution. Rwandese people demonstrate this way forward with their exceptional resourcefulness and tireless daily efforts to rebuild their economy, homes and families. This country, littered with mass graveyards and generational grief, has much to teach us about human resilience, regrowth and the revival of hope.

"Every healthcare worker must also be a palliative care specialist and an 'everyday' ethicist"

Hope and regrowth can take many different forms in countries such as Rwanda. On the national level, we might hope and advocate for any number of policy changes that would benefit children in need of disability support or palliative care services. For example, integrating home care services into the national healthcare scheme and providing services such as occupational, speech and physical therapy would hugely enhance the quality of life of these children who may have a limited lifespan. Also, easy and equitable access to pain-relieving drugs such as morphine is imperative. This multilevel, multidisciplinary approach implemented on the national level would thus minimize the suffering of all children – regardless of wealth or status – and perhaps make the way for a dignified death. On the international level, raising awareness of the gaps, needs and negligence in Rwanda would help push for these imperative policy changes. Building a global web of proactively ethical healthcare workers would help build new paradigms and standards for the care of disabled and terminally ill children. This strongly interwoven web would reach down to the community level – to the district hospitals and health centers where front-line health staff are given daily opportunities to model this new, more comprehensive and more compassionate approach. They would stand as a united front to challenge the outdated norms and traditions of their medical culture, and the personal powerlessness and despondency that so often results. They would ultimately build a new culture of medicine from the rubble that is so often left behind by poverty, war and postwar exploitation.

This brings us back, finally, to the individual level, where we are each responsible for spinning our portion of this web, with care and meticulous consistency. We must stand ready for fatigue and fatalism as we face our daily dilemmas and ethical challenges. Whether we are in Africa or America, we must continue to ask questions that probe deeply yet carefully into our patients and their needs, as well as questions that examine and challenge our current medical culture. It is our personal responsibility as healthcare workers, in developing and developed worlds alike, always to ask how we may quell suffering and inspire hope, even in the most seemingly morbid of circumstances.

Themes for discussion

- In the context of clinical medicine, what do we mean by the idea of 'suffering'? How does a consideration of suffering translate into our clinical activities? (We have in mind the excellent and thought-provoking writing of Eric Cassell (1982) and the challenge for us to be aware of caring and trying to alleviate suffering, whatever else we do.)

- What lessons can we in the developed world learn from an impoverished, war-ravaged country where services are so much less well developed than in the 'Western' world?

- What are our ethical responsibilities to ourselves and to our patients, to recognize and deal with and manage our own despair regarding clinical situations that are beyond our capacity to manage?

- Readers may be moved emotionally by this account but may also feel a sense of 'outsiderness' and might perceive this as a foreign story from faraway lands; however human suffering (and our inability to relieve it) is, of course, on our doorstep, everywhere. How can we use an account like this as a jumping-off point to contemplate the universality of the human condition and how these challenges also exist at home?

References

Cassell E (1982) The nature of suffering and the goals of medicine. *N Engl J Med* 306: 639–645.

Farmer PE, Nutt CT, Wagner CM (2013) Reduced premature mortality in Rwanda: Lessons from success. *BMJ* 346: f65.

Farmer P, Nizeye B, Stulac S, Keshavjee S (2006) Structural violence and clinical medicine. *PLOS* 3: e449.

Human Rights Watch (2014) Leave none to tell the story: Genocide in Rwanda; http://www.hrw.org/reports/1999/rwanda/Geno1-3-04.htm.

McCarthy B (2015) United States Agency for International Development: Global Health, Rwanda, 31 March 2015; http://www.usaid.gov/rwanda/global-health.

United Nations Convention on Rights of Persons with Disabilities (2006) http://www.un.org/disabilities/convention/conventionfull.shtml.

Chapter 16

When expectations diverge: addressing our cultural differences differently

Laura S. Funkhouser
with contributions by Suzanne Linett

Prologue

When medical and allied health practitioners used to sophisticated healthcare see children in parts of the world with fewer resources, they may drastically re-evaluate their goals for the patient in front of them. In the case of a child with motor impairment, that might include putting aside hopes for great mobility in favor of a basic wheelchair. Rather than seeking improvements in the special education plan, they may be trying to find *any* school for the child. We bring to mind a boarding school in Kenya for children with physical impairments where the students often stayed on past childhood as helpers. Back in the villages it was nearly impossible for families to keep even the youngest of such children at home. The expectation was lifetime segregation and dependence.

Many of us have never practiced in such different settings, yet even in our home countries with potentially more access to medical and educational supports we may work in an environment of low expectations for children with significant impairment. The view that the lives of these children will always be 'less than' can surface, not only in our conversations with friends and colleagues (Rosenbaum 1998) but also in our clinical encounters with families. How this difference in understanding can distress the individuals involved was learned painfully during the care of a young girl in a US-based program. The clinical team's reliance on cautious intervention, when her parents declined a recommended beneficial surgery, may not have given this child her best chance at well-being. The family had brought their daughter to clinic voluntarily, so should the professionals have needed to tread so lightly? In this chapter, we will conclude that an optimal ethical practice, from the first encounter forward, would have included not only being attentive to what was discussed during the decision-making process, but also acting on our professional ethical duty to achieve the best results for her. An important strategy would have included communicating the truth about a child's potential for a life well lived and the duty of all parties (clinicians, family and society) to hold and champion the greatest expectations for this child and others like her.

The story of 'Cami'

A number of years ago Cami, a 12-year-old Asian-Pacific Island girl with cerebral palsy (CP), moved with her family to the USA and went to school for the first time. She presented to a public clinic, where children with orthopedic impairments were brought for evaluation, direct therapy and planning meetings with pediatricians and orthopedic surgeons. Public health nurses and social workers often attended, to help with further medical care and support services.

Cami was a playful girl whose interactions were those of a child less than 6 years. Her dysarthric speech sounded like happy chatter, particularly with her friend at school, also a girl with CP. She seemed comfortable with the clinic and staff. It was not known whether she had intellectual impairment, as she had not been formally tested. Reconstructing the situation, the therapists recall her Gross Motor Function Classification System (GMFCS) level to be V. Her family carried her everywhere. She could only manipulate simple toys and could not feed herself. She was very thin, and due to chewing issues was fed mostly homemade fish and rice soup. She had all childhood immunizations, but had never had any specialized medical care. Although such care was available it was at a distance and difficult to access.

Her family consisted of her father, who had not found employment in the USA, his wife, who was marginally employed, Cami and several older siblings, who lived with them. From what the clinic staff could tell, only Cami and the siblings had made friends.

The clinic initially provided a customized wheelchair, ankle-foot orthotics and physical therapy. The occupational therapist, making a home visit to the tiny apartment, saw that there were fewer places to sleep than the family probably needed. Cami was fed in her wheelchair, bathed on the shower floor and always used diapers. There were sparse furnishings and décor, and Cami did not have toys. No one in the family expressed frustration or sadness with the situation. The siblings were tender towards Cami and stayed close by during the visit.

Cami was brought to clinic by her father, but her mother was never able to come because of her job. An older teenaged sister, with adequate conversational English, came to the pediatric and orthopedic meetings to translate, sometimes missing school. Even with a translator present, she gave a childlike description of Cami's birth, more so than staff expected for her age and education. When the pediatrician discussed what foods Cami needed to thrive, her sister answered that Cami's low weight made her easier to lift. She said that the family had always anticipated caring for Cami 'just as she was' for her lifespan. They were not interested in nursing visits, nor in respite care.

Cami's therapy attendance was initially satisfactory. When she was 13, she developed a 45-degree rotary scoliosis. The consulting orthopedic surgeon then recommended spinal fusion with placement of a posterior rod to prevent increasing deformity, to allow comfortable positioning and to maintain respiratory function and health. He showed Cami's father and sister drawings of the procedure as well as before-and-after photos of other patients. He said that the timing was right for her skeletal maturity and that cognitively Cami seemed to be a good candidate to tolerate the procedure and cooperate with rehabilitation. He described the significant risks of surgery, as well as postoperative care and pain control at home. The family adamantly declined surgery. The clinic staff felt that the family was having difficulty conceptually with the discussion.

Arrangements were then made for a nurse who could translate to attend the next conference. A surprised staff thus learned that the father thought the rod would be placed on Cami externally. That idea dispelled, the nurse explained that the family was saying they did not understand the necessity of surgery – to them doctors are to be visited after someone becomes ill and surgery is provided to fix something, not to prevent further decline.

The father said respectfully that the family did not understand the American push for educating Cami. He said they had never read to her. The father did ask for a walker, which was not indicated. He saw no point to a stretching program, or further clinic appointments, much less surgery, if Cami were never to walk. The family definitely did not want her to experience pain.

Soon after that visit, the family moved, which required a change of schools. Cami begged her family to take her back to her previous school to see her friend. Her sister admitted to feeling guilty that she could not take Cami on outings, due to lifting and wheelchair issues. After a few months, Cami stopped attending the orthopedic and pediatric consultation clinics. She was reported to be taken to intermittent appointments at a regional medical center, regarding weight loss, seizures and spasticity. Eventually the team lost contact with Cami and her family.

Our differences

In some ways, the story seems extraordinary in terms of the understanding of two cultures: a family who views CP as crippling, to be endured without help, versus a clinical team realistic about ambulation, but wanting a more comfortable and better quality life for their patient. A child whose first dozen years were isolated meets a community striving to give her education, inclusion and some independence. A family whose history of visiting doctors was essentially limited to acute illness is told surgery for their child is

Table 16.1   Ethical challenges for treatment decisions for a child with impairment

Appropriate balance of child versus family needs and wishes
Incorporation of a family's culture and story: forming a narrative
Truthful communication about outcome and resources

'preventive medicine.' Had this same family experienced more than a few months in a society where perhaps more people expect habilitation of individuals with special needs, there might have been a more closely matched vision.

In other ways, the feeling of this story may be quite familiar, as beliefs about the potential of children with impairments, although changing, are not changing universally. For example, some medical insurance policies disallow appropriate 'wheels' for toddlers with paralytic spina bifida. The existence of such policies speaks to decision-makers who are not only being misinformed but are also working within a culture that may believe these young children to be 'less than' or have less need for exploratory play than other children. In the field of childhood neurodisability practice, having seen and heard many powerful life stories of people with disabilities, we can imagine that in every child with severe functional limitations there is an inner world yet to be tapped. To help them live life to their fullest, we must influence outcomes that will allow these young people unrestricted participation. This chapter presents an account of what well-intentioned professionals experienced, in contrast to what they believe they could have done better for Cami. The discussion includes specific steps to take when children cannot speak for themselves, but are facing a treatment that their family does not want.

The challenges of divergent expectations

Certainly there were core ethical practices that each team member would have felt immediately, such as choosing best practices (Table 16.1), without causing harm and speaking truthfully about the proposed surgery, but there were other challenges germane to a family's major treatment decision for their child with impairment. Had the team recognized them, they could have developed a plan to elicit a more family-centered dialogue, to have more conscious ethical discussions and to act more assertively. (See Chapter 24 on an orthopedic surgeon's analysis of this kind of situation.)

Balance of child versus family
The initial impression of the occupational therapist (OT) was that the family seemed to be living almost in 'survival mode', but that the household seemed to reflect imbalanced priorities, as if the family did not take into account Cami's developmental needs. The OT confirmed how close the siblings were to each other and to Cami. The mother was

not there. The OT also noted that the father seemed depressed about *his* situation, possibly contributing to his seeming failure to show interest in 'giving Cami a childhood'.

Asking first 'What can we do for you?', the OT wanted to set the tone that the family would start the visit with their needs and wishes discussed. She hoped to gain trust that she was there to help, not to cause more burdensome care. For example, at school, toileting for Cami was carried out within standards for privacy and developmental appropriateness, while the same method could not be achieved at home because of environmental limitations. So, despite better expectations for the quality of Cami's activities of daily living, the matter was dropped.

At no time did the medical social worker, who had the longest relationship with the family, refer Cami's case to child protective services. Her ongoing impression was that they were catering to a child who manipulated them, for example, into shortening therapy sessions. She felt that the deference Cami's parents gave to her fear of pain essentially led to a form of medical neglect, but, with no immediate harm, did not cross her threshold to report. These cases are difficult to prove and the family's actions did not reflect any general lack of caregiving, or dysfunction leading to lack of compliance. They said that 'they would always take care of Cami'. Their evident plan was to keep her at home. They may never have considered residential placement when she became a young adult. *They* called the social worker constantly for assistance with applying for financial support for their caregiving.

The attending pediatrician expressed feeling disheartened by what the team perceived as severe family stressors: a mother absent from the discussion, a father who primarily transported his child and signed papers, and a not-fully-mature teenage sibling as translator. It was hard to imagine their life, and the pediatrician accepted that there was nothing one could do to get better information. The family did not want a public health nurse visit at that time and the team did not insist on one.

At that time a laissez-faire attitude toward nutrition in patients was common in some communities, with stories of physicians telling families that their children with CP should stay thin 'for a reason'. The evidence about the harm this causes was just reaching the awareness of general practitioners. A decade later, an approach to lessen a caregiving burden to the detriment of a child's nourishment would likely be considered immoral in mainstream culture and subject to a child protective service report. In the years that the team was seeing Cami, the estrogen-produced growth attenuation of Ashley, a 6-year-old girl in Washington State with significant developmental disability from static encephalopathy, had not yet occurred, much less raised a public debate over the ethics of parents and physicians using pharmaceuticals to render a child 'easier to lift' in adolescence and adulthood (Gunther & Diekema 2006). (See also Chapter 29 by Samaan, where this issue is discussed in detail.)

The pediatrician's insistence on informing Cami's family about how more typical food choices could benefit her did not allow for acceptance of their 'efficient' feeding style, which had developed over 12 years. A semi-liquid diet seemed neglectful both nutritionally and developmentally. As the family had probably developed this style by trial and error in their home country and were doing what they felt was best for Cami, it would have been insensitive to start a conversation about whose needs this feeding strategy was serving. Referral to a feeding clinic, with a more assertive approach, might have driven the family further away from the clinic and from nutritional supplements that the team could obtain for them.

A family's culture and story

Most of the team could only make assumptions about Cami's home environment. During her home visit, the OT had her standards for activities of daily living, but the family could have felt her to be judgmental, were she not empathetic to their culture and the stress of immigration. Any suggestions that came to mind would have to be adapted to the family style. While she may have wished for the parents to have bought toys for Cami or taken her to the park, or arranged for a visit with her friend from school, the sparse household and very limited community activities may have been the norm from the family's previous life.

In encouraging scoliosis repair, could the team have used a different approach to address the family's expectation of receiving only the basic medical care they knew in their homeland? What knowledge did the family have of surgery in children? If they had experienced pain from surgery themselves, what was their experience of therapeutic pain control? This situation also required assessing the family's ability to handle postsurgical care. Beyond the two weeks that her mother would be allowed to take off work, Cami's daily care would be by a father with virtually no personal community supports and by a teenaged sibling.

The pediatrician discussing the surgery may have been operating from assumptions about 'what is in the best interest of children generally' (Robinson 2002) rather than learning about this particular family's goals. The physician had only envisioned Cami's potential progress in a story she could have in the USA, not what her family had experienced in their homeland, and thus was not convincing to the family. A report to child protective services could harm the family's fragile cultural balance, especially if the child's removal from home was set into motion. Beyond the major trauma of separation, it would have been very difficult to find specialized medical-care foster home parents who would understand the family's culture any better than the clinical team had.

Truthful communication

Translation issues significantly affected all the team's actions on Cami's behalf. The importance of what good experiences could happen for Cami after surgery was lost in the major effort to describe the biomedical rationale and procedures for it. One problem was how to determine if the family was more unwilling than incapable to understand how surgery could help: it was almost as hard to 'read' their minds as to imagine Cami's preferences.

The clinical team relied on an older teenage sister, but did not know whether she was, consciously or unconsciously, editing the translation based on what course of action she thought would be the most palatable to her parents. It was also apparent that she was naïve about health issues, much less medical ones. Although the father had the responsibility to sign papers for surgery, he presented as anxious and was probably not processing the information. Once the team found a health professional to translate, they learned that the family did not understand how any surgery could be preventative.

The family would probably have accepted surgery if the team had been able to say that surgery could improve Cami's mobility. As neither the natural history, nor possible future treatment options, was fully predictable, no-one could even have said, 'This surgery could help Cami benefit from treatments for CP that may be developed later.' The truth was that without scoliosis repair, deterioration in health and well-being was predictable.

To hold a truthful discussion would also include admitting that even if she were to benefit from surgery, Cami still might need to live at home in the family's care. Although vocational services and group living were available, not everyone with developmental disabilities could access them. In contrast to the seemingly unlimited support services, there was the ironic situation that medical care, equipment, nutritional supplies and other health supports that were free to most children who came to the clinic disappeared on their 21st birthday when program eligibility stopped (see also Chapter 30). In addition, no one could be certain about Cami's long-term opportunities for inclusion and participation.

Staying conscious of expectations and our influence

The team's approach to trying to improve Cami's quality of life was based on clinical knowledge of child growth and development, taking little of the family's understanding or ideas into account (Table 16.2). This situation seemed similar to the same lack of cultural review that occurred with the case of Lia, the Hmong baby with epilepsy who immigrated with her family to California and whose parents and physicians were in grave conflict. In that well-known story, her family believed that her convulsions were part of the process of spiritual healing and could not fully accept the medical imperative to reduce their frequency. In a medical record of more than 400 000 words, the decisions of the family were documented, but not their perceptions of her illness (Fadiman 1997).

Table 16.2   Essential conversations with families about values

The influence of expectations for a life course

Placing the family's narrative in perspective

Ensuring the child's 'voice' is heard

Expectations for a life course

The team could have explored more thoroughly how the family's values and decision to decline surgery were determined by their understanding of the life course for their daughter. The team did not know what the parents were told at birth about her future development. Over the years, the family had experienced her changing as she responded to them and they to her when she developed language and play. Presumably they knew her best, yet they did not appear to help her experience new activities. For them, going to school was purely pragmatic, and as they did not foresee Cami working at a job, they did not agree with the value of education that the clinical staff emphasized. The staff, on the other hand, experienced that Cami was learning and making friendships, valuable regardless of future occupational activities, employed or not.

Had the team, from the outset, elicited her family story, or narrative, 'with sensitivity and compassion' to understand what was 'not stated' about her family's life (Robinson 2002), they might later have had more discussion about what was in Cami's best interest. The 'providers' story' needed to be told also, as a basis for mutual reflection on the best choice for Cami. Had people recognized the size of the gap between the family's expectations and the team's, they might have thought to describe their experience with the social milestones attained by many people with impairments.

In regard to their expectations for Cami's physical growth and development, the team fell short in identifying her family's issues about lifting her while concentrating on her skeletal correction, and so did not initiate much of a discussion about changes in puberty and adulthood, which can cause added stressors. It was only a few years later that the discussions around growth attenuation brought awareness of these important parenting issues to the community (Gunther & Diekma 2006).

The team members did not ask about any religious beliefs that might have had an impact on this family's decisions. This omission may have stemmed from previous encounters with other families – what others have experienced with immigrants who are reluctant to disclose their religion because of caution around public authorities (Lach 2013) or because it was usually the practice not to raise the question unless the family did. It is difficult to be 'mini-ethnographers' in clinic, and most professionals do not really have the training, much less do they know whether the conclusions they would draw would be valid (Kleinman 1998). The team did not ask the question, 'How long do you expect Cami to live?' or provide them with an estimate of her life expectancy. There was little communication with her primary community pediatrician, except shared records, so the team did not know if such a discussion occurred beyond their clinic.

Had staff explained to parents that disallowing surgery could pose a barrier to a more desirable quality of health regardless of longevity, would the parents have made a different, better balanced decision? Although detailed, relatable examples of the experiences of other families could be exactly what a family longs to hear, privacy standards limit such discussion in a community where the children attend the same schools and clinics. With enough time and flexibility of personnel resources, a team can bring in consenting patients and families who have positive stories about 'life after scoliosis repair' or other procedures.

A family's narrative: with limitations
In this case, the decision about surgery was neither dire nor needed immediately. Without that pressure, is a clinical team justified in silently assenting to a family following their own values when there is great divergence? Was the family declining surgery on Cami's behalf, or on their own? There could have been an important conversation with the family about basing their decisions on their daughter's current situation, not on her previous story, which was greatly changed by moving to a different country and culture. The team took direction from the parents without determining whether the parents' sense of inevitability of a reduced life experience for the whole family was influencing their decision more than their uncertainty of Cami's future. It is likely that Cami's mother would have contributed importantly to this discussion had she been able to come to appointments, but the team did not make creative efforts for out-of-hours arrangements to include her. Cami's family did not ask 'What would you do if she were your child?', as so often occurs when the parents can relate to the cultural values of the clinical team.

It was clear that the siblings were expected to spend a lot of time with Cami. Having no experience with developmental disability support services in the USA, those siblings might have been envisioning even more years of caregiving. They were nearing adulthood and would legally, but perhaps not culturally, have been able to lessen their day-to-day responsibilities for Cami. Medical appointments were clearly a burden to this family, and the team needed to let them know which were the most important. If the clinicians had noted objections to her care that were based solely on inconvenience or low priority, they could have pursued more aggressive support. There were secondary prevention programs available through child protective services for families at risk of abuse and neglect.

Table 16.3 Steps to take when expectations differ

Keep an 'ethical problem-oriented record' for major treatment decisions
Recognize and discuss differences promptly
Clarify the decision-making authority, including the court system
Identify resources that may influence decisions, and bring them into the process
Support the decision-makers after treatment or non-treatment

The child's 'voice'

The team was focused on their priorities for Cami, while the family seemed satisfied in a number of areas (e.g. feeding and nutrition) to passively let her condition run its course, including, ultimately, isolation from society when her school years were over. Faced with a decision about surgery with significant expected pain, they were actively choosing against it. This child with language delays seemed unlikely to show the capacity to participate in full discussion for years, if ever. Practically, Cami was not even assenting to physical therapy when it caused pain. Their professional judgment that a good outcome would be worth the pain (a different matter from the risk of surgery) was the team's responsibility to present clearly. It was also incumbent on the team to share (and hopefully elicit) more hopeful expectations for Cami's life based on their understanding that quality of life is not limited by physical boundaries. 'Few would think to say that a good quality of life is … clapping to your favorite song … giving joy to your parents and caregivers' and experiencing beauty' (Kittay 2010). Although Cami's parents were not seeing the point of education and inclusion, the team was seeing a young girl make friends and *enjoying* going to school. When the family tried to keep her in their own *status quo*, the team needed to be her voice for 'I want to grow up healthy and happy.'

> "In the context of divergent expectations for a disabled child, there needs to be an 'intensive, systematic, imaginative empathy' from a multidisciplinary team"

Addressing differences differently

In the context of divergent expectations for a disabled child, there needs to be an 'intensive, systematic, imaginative empathy' from a multidisciplinary team (Kleinman 1998). Preparation for such situations is not only appropriate, but helps a team to know it has done its best (Table 16.3). Some clinics have preclinic conferences. These are ideal to look at the possibilities for differing expectations and how to address them and ask each other the right questions. It is important that the team understand that the 'reason for referral' may very well not be the *family's* reason for coming to clinic. An outside clinician who is not one of the patient's providers

may be able to offer more objective suggestions. At the very least, making sure that a few steps are always in place could permit deliberate ethical decisions instead of reactive ones.

Keep an 'ethical problem-oriented record'

Social history is frequently lost in the first volume of medical records, or hidden in pages about eligibility, income and reimbursement, but it could be brought to the foreground at each visit. Has the family's situation changed significantly since the last encounter? Are major treatment decisions pending? How will this family provide for and nurture the child regardless of the decision? What external supports are needed? What effect will treatment have on the other members, especially children?

'From both an ethical and empirical standpoint, adherence to a family-centred approach is not negotiable' despite our need to speak strongly for the child (Lach 2013). This approach, which has been promoted for more than 25 years but implemented in a patchwork fashion, starts with the healthcare providers being intentionally responsive to the family. Ideally, one member could be watchful, on behalf of the whole team, that open-ended questions are used to begin history taking. This team member could also follow up on any discussions held about treatment decisions, by reviewing the family's experience a few days later and regularly after that, particularly to learn whether 'the family's voice' is becoming lost. Depending on how the team is organized, the choice of who would be *ethical* case manager might be different from the team member who is the clinical case manager.

Outpatient clinics may not have codes of practice such as those seen in hospitals. Clinics could adopt a record for patient discussion about treatment decisions. A chart that states only 'the risks and benefits were discussed' misses key ethical details of the child's age and presumed competence to be part of the decision and what each parent (and the child) has heard and asked. Clinical staff could outline, from the point of view of their specialty, the expectations for health, comfort and rehabilitation after a proposed treatment, versus potential problems. For example, a social worker could document the contrast between the predicted benefits to a child of using a stander at school after an Achilles tendon procedure and the predicted trauma of temporary placement in a medical foster home if the parents were not able to perform postoperative care.

"From both an ethical and empirical standpoint, adherence to a family-centred approach is not negotiable"

Recognize and discuss differences

As important as accurate translation and adequate quantity of communication are, they are not as important as the quality of the dialogue. In the care of children with disabilities, it is important to avoid the assumption that the issues are too complex for a family to describe their priorities. Conventional social history questions do not necessarily elicit what areas of *life* are really important to the family members, or how different their ideas about the child may be from ours. What drives their decision process may be totally unexpected for the team. How families cope with their child's disability may reflect 'ethnic or cultural values unfamiliar to the professional[s]' and any expected stages – and timing – of 'theoretical [family] adaptation' are probably 'neither mandatory nor experienced universally' (Hostler 1991). An added dimension of great value occurs when the clinician or other team members may have had personal experience with impairments and disability, and while not necessarily speaking of it, can move from empathy to a role of caring resulting in action. The 'right questions and the precise listening' required to find out about differences in expectations will lead to an 'ongoing process of engagement from which decisions will emerge' (Weiner & Auster 2007).

Clarify decision-making authority

A sensitive topic that may require an objective and trained 'third party' concerns who is making decisions in the family. If the child can participate in the discussion but is not considered mature enough to decide, it is important to listen to them and document their opinions, especially if there could be a lengthy delay until the decision legally becomes theirs. In some instances, families or health providers can readily access bioethics consultation as outpatients. As professionals, we can advocate for increased visibility of this resource.

> "How families cope with their child's disability may reflect 'ethnic or cultural values unfamiliar to the professionals'"

Juvenile court judges can be sought for proxy decisions when there is a major treatment decision for a child, but such a step can risk a serious disruption in the therapeutic relationship with the family. Although it is unusual for clinic staff to report to child protective services because parents are not allowing elective surgery, it must be reported if there are other indicators of medical neglect. Reference can be made to the 1970 case of Kevin, a 15-year-old boy in New York State with neurofibromatosis, whose mother would not allow blood transfusion and thus facial reconstruction. This suggests that the act of declining surgery can be considered neglectful of a child's basic interests (Miller 2003). Even though the boy's eyesight and hearing were not at immediate risk, the judge felt he had a right 'to live and grow up without disfigurement' (*Matter of Kevin Sampson* 1970). The judge took the decision from the mother, ruled for surgery and notably placing a high value on the family unit, allowed the boy to continue to live with her. The surgery in that case was also considered preventative – for emotional health.

Identify resources

The team members have a responsibility, just as they identify vendors for medical equipment, to know the 'vendors' for family supports and bring them into the process to impart information about available benefits. In Cami's case, the government agency responsible for lifetime support services, including housing, employment, social activities and group residence, was not involved in the discussions. The clinical team explained what might be available, but her parents might have made a very different decision had they been encouraged to visit a neighborhood group home where Cami could be comfortable and cared for in adulthood. This might have led to different expectations – that their other children would not necessarily have lifetime physical responsibilities for Cami.

Based on Federal law, Cami was eligible for educational services through age 21. This fact would have been beyond the family's imagination when they initially moved to the USA. It would certainly have been prudent to include teachers in the discussion, as they might have encouraged the family to proceed with the surgery so Cami could sit better at the school she enjoyed so much.

Beyond the obligation (and basic humanity) of finding translators when there is a language barrier, there is an opportunity to look for cultural connections for families where this does not occur naturally by neighborhoods. The team social worker can certainly justify the time required. The translators themselves very well may have transitioned from different cultures and have information about local events and community groups that could ease the isolation and contribute to the family well-being.

Support the decision-makers

Medical and surgical procedure outcomes can be unexpectedly burdensome, even devastating. One of the often-stated reasons for upholding parental consent is that the family has to live with the consequences of their decisions (Forman & Ladd 1991). When the decision has been hard and the events are perhaps life-altering, the family should not be left alone with the results. The team, crucial to the decision process in clinic, needs an external care plan. Best practice would put safeguards into place concerning physician and nursing follow-up, and also home visits by rehabilitation therapists. More often than not, the treatments take place in a distant hospital with other clinicians. A trusted team member could visit – it is predictable that the family at the hospital will feel both terribly 'responsible for their child, yet personally vulnerable' (Iverson et al. 2013). It would also be important to check that the family members' roles had not undergone dramatic changes, such as a primary caregiver starting employment.

If treatment is not accepted, close follow-up of the child still needs to continue, and if treatment is still indicated, it should be offered at each encounter with a focus on understanding the parents' current reasons for declining and discussion of the reasoning behind the medical recommendation.

Regardless of the decision, when parents might feel the experience as a 'turning point', it is important to review with them their child's and family's strengths, much as reviewing these was – or should have been – an integral part of disclosing the diagnosis of childhood disability. Additionally, the recognition that the family may be in a stage of grieving unique to that family or culture could guide health practitioners how to show compassion while each stage evolves. For example, after a decision that a procedure is not indicated because it will not result in walking or talking, the timing of informing the family of changes in therapeutic activities or a reduction of hours for physical therapy or speech services should be chosen with sensitivity. Unfortunately, in a climate of need for efficiency in healthcare services, proceeding at a gentler pace – while clearly the 'right' thing to do – can be challenging. (See also Chapter 8.)

Our duty to influence

We enter into the life of a child and family when the parents initiate a therapeutic relationship on behalf of their child. In the clinic, we can feel that we are on familiar ground where we can draw upon our expertise and experience to help a child, but when the family leaves there is uncertainty as to whether they will follow the team's (or more appropriately, mutually developed) recommendations, or 'be compliant'. If they are not and there is concern that the child may not thrive physically or developmentally, team members may have to become surrogate family and argue for treatment for the child, but they need to do so in an effort as careful and caring as if that child were theirs. We strive to keep promises to the family to do what is best to help the child improve their function and to make every effort to bring to them the best resources available.

As professionals we reach a point when we need to decide whether to seek external authority, to help our patient be all that we believe they can be. 'The enduring dilemma, if we really believe children are separable from their parents, and ideally should be entitled to a free and open future' is whether we should take legal action if those parents are narrowing the child's prospects (Sayeed 2010). While we have empathy for the family's story, we must care for the child who has a *new* story when they become connected to us. Although we do not expect families always to make perfect decisions, we want the decision to *surpass* an 'acceptable standard' for a child who has years to grow and develop.

In 'the story of Cami', the important responsibility of influencing for the best outcome got lost in the details of 'patient management'. The team could not see that the family's position against surgery and the team's reluctance to push them would result in the therapeutic relationship fading. They reported that they did not feel acutely the ethical challenges they faced, but rather the frustrations of the complex social situation. When the clinic lost Cami and her family to follow-up, they missed an opportunity to make deliberate choices about their own ethical behavior and to allow the family the same privilege.

Epilogue

Almost 2 years after the clinical team experienced the family's apparent permanent refusal for surgery, the parents agreed to the scoliosis repair. Postoperatively, Cami refused to be out of bed for many weeks and developed a decubitus ulcer. She recovered fully and then had successful placement of a baclofen pump to reduce spasticity. Her posture stabilized, she was beginning to feed herself and had clearer speech. The older sister had married and moved out of the home and had her own baby, but was still Cami's primary caregiver along with their father. Cami was seen in clinic with a different team, to address new cardiac issues and ongoing nutritional problems, among others. Chronic non-adherence with medical care follow-up prompted that team to file a report with adult protective services shortly after her 18th birthday.

Themes for discussion

- One of the problems we may face as service providers is the reality that our patients' and families' lives are often 'complicated' in ways that frustrate us.
  What are some of the ethical challenges in dealing with our own feelings?

- People often say of families whose grasp of English is limited 'They don't speak English' (or whatever language is prevalent in our community). This might be considered very arrogant of us and begs the question: What else might we
  say – and do – to address this bidirectional communication gap?

- When a family is clearly struggling and 'non-compliant' we may have to refer to Children's Services for 'protection'. As noted both here and elsewhere in this book (see, e.g. Chapter 18), this can be a complex and emotionally challenging decision. What can we do to make this decision less painful for all or even avoid it, and is this really our responsibility in the first place?

- How do we converse with a family realistically about both our divergent and our shared values for the best life for their child when societal behavior reflects inconsistent willingness-to-pay for taking care of the complex activities and changes that habilitation, participation and inclusion require?

References

Fadiman A (1997) *The spirit catches you and you fall down: A Hmong child, her American doctors, and the collision of two cultures.* New York, NY: Farrar, Strauss and Giroux.

Forman EN, Ladd, RE (1991) Parents' rights. In: *Ethical dilemmas in pediatrics: A case study approach,* pp. 7–10. New York, NY: Springer-Verlag.

Gunther DF, Diekma DS (2006) Attenuating growth in children with profound DD: A new approach to an old dilemma. *Arch Pediatr Adolesc Med* 60: 1013–1017.

Hostler SL (1991) Family centered care. *Pediatr Clin N Am* 38: 1545–1560.

Iverson AS, Graue M, Raheim M (2013) At the edge of vulnerability – lived experience of parents with children with cerebral palsy going through surgery. *Int J Qual Stud Well-being* 8: 20007.

Kittay EF (2010) Rationality, personhood, and Peter Singer on the fate of severely impaired infants. In: Miller G, editor. *Pediatric bioethics*, pp. 165–172. Cambridge: Cambridge University Press.

Kleinman A (1998) *The illness narratives: Suffering, healing, and the human condition*, p. 230. New York, NY: Basic Books.

Lach L (2013) The family does matter! In: Ronen G, Rosenbaum P, editors. *Life quality outcomes*, pp. 136–151. London: Mac Keith Press.

Matter of Kevin Sampson (1970) 65 Misc. 2d at 658.

Miller RB (2003) Basic interests. In: *Children, ethics, and modern medicine*, pp. 119–145. Bloomington, IN: Indiana University Press.

Robinson WM (2002) The narrative of rescue in pediatric practice. In: Charon R, Montello M, editors. *Stories matter: The role of narrative in medical ethics*, pp. 97–108. New York, NY: Routledge.

Rosenbaum PL (1998) But what can you do for them? *Dev Med Child Neuro* 40: 579.

Sayeed SA (2010) The moral and legal status of children and parents. In: Miller G, editor. *Pediatric bioethics*, pp. 38–53. Cambridge: Cambridge University Press.

Weiner SJ, Auster S (2007) From empathy to caring: Defining the ideal approach to a healing relationship. *Yale J Biol Med* 80: 123–130.

Chapter 17

Service provision for hard-to-reach families: what are our responsibilities?

Michelle Phoenix

Cinical scenario

I was standing at my colleague's desk trying to decide whether or not to plan a treatment session for little Nicole and her family. This was not an uncommon scenario in our children's treatment center – trying to guess 30 minutes before a session whether the family would come in. The occupational therapist (OT) and I, the speech language pathologist (SLP), had scheduled a joint therapy session for this 2-year-old with cerebral palsy. Nicole typically came in with her father Jeff and they both participated enthusiastically. Our goals included increasing functional play and imitation skills, and teaching parents ways to engage Nicole in play at home to promote her development.

Things seemed to be going well until that first missed appointment. We recognized that this can happen to anyone. We called and spoke to Jeff who said the appointment had been forgotten, but he would be there next week. Next week they came in and we seemed to be

------

Author's note

Please note that the opinions expressed in this chapter are those of the author and not of the program in which she works.

back on track. In discussing home practice, we learned that Jeff and his wife had recently separated. He said he was coping well with the change and they were sharing custody. Sensing this was a chaotic time for the family, we offered to postpone therapy. We did remind him of the center's policy that if two appointments were missed without prior notice the child would be discharged from services. However, Jeff chose to continue with the appointments we had scheduled. We printed out a schedule and gave it to him … which brings me back to my colleague's desk a week later.

It is hard to describe the premonition that warns you not to expect that family you ought to be expecting. We decided to prepare the room and materials anyway, but that day the family did not arrive. With sinking hearts my colleague and I knew this meant discharge from the center and the OT and SLP services that might be of benefit to Nicole and her family. We were still working on feeding, early sign language and accessing daycare. In accordance with the center's policy, we charted the second 'no-show', recorded the discharge due to 'declined intervention' and notified the family via a discharge report.

I continue to question whether we did everything we could to engage this family in service and also whether it is ethical to discharge families when they are having difficulty making it in for appointments.

This scenario describes a so-called 'hard-to-reach family', often defined as a family who is eligible for services but for a variety of reasons does not use them (Boag-Munroe & Evangelou 2012; Cortis 2012). Within a pediatric rehabilitation context, clinicians identified reasons at the child, parent, family and organizational levels that contribute to making a family hard-to-reach (Phoenix & Rosenbaum 2015). These reasons may occur in isolation (e.g. having a child who is medically fragile) or co-occur (e.g. having a lengthy wait list for service, no childcare for siblings and a parent with mental health impairments). The ethical dilemma explored in this chapter concerns how pediatric rehabilitation services are provided to hard-to-reach families. Specifically I examine the practice of discharging families if they miss appointments without prior notification, so-called 'no-shows'. First, this issue is discussed at the parent-therapist level to explore whether and how missed appointments could be avoided. Second, I explore the issues at a systems level to question whether discharging families after missed appointments is an ethically acceptable practice.

Can parents and therapists work together to avoid missed appointments?
The term 'hard-to-reach families' implies that problems with service use are the family's fault; therefore many authors recommend reframing the term as 'hard-to-access services' (Barrett 2008; Boag-Munroe & Evangelou 2012; Cortis 2012). This change in language suggests that organizations and therapists bear some responsibility in helping families to access their services. There is strong evidence to suggest that using the principles of family-centered services and cultural competence can help families to access care

(Kuhlthau et al. 2011; Rosenbaum et al. 1998; Tseng & Streltzer 2008). By communicating clearly with families, listening to the families' needs and priorities, and allowing families to make decisions about their care it might be possible to engage these apparently hard-to-reach families and avoid the missed appointments that result in discharge.

Therapists are responsible for providing both general and specific information to families (King et al. 2010). This may include general information about childhood development, a particular condition, or resources and services that are available. It is important that this information is presented in a way that helps parents to understand their options and to make informed decisions regarding their child's goals and services (Rosenbaum et al. 1998). In studies evaluating parents' perceptions of family-centered service in pediatric rehabilitation programs, parents consistently rate therapists poorly in their provision of general information (Dyke et al. 2006; King et al. 2010). This can have major implications for service use; for example, families are unlikely to access a service if they do not understand what is on offer (Winkworth et al. 2010).

In thinking back to my experience with Nicole and her family, I wonder how clearly we had communicated the goals of therapy. Given that we were focused on developing play and early imitation skills, perhaps it appeared that we were simply playing with the child. We may have taken for granted that parents knew that play was the way that children learn about and experience the world around them. When the family was trying to cope with a separation, it may not have seemed important to come in and play. Alternately, the family's attendance may not have been a reflection of the value they placed on therapy; rather, the missed appointments may have been due to logistical difficulties of scheduling and transportation. In this family's case we did not know the precise reason that they missed appointments. An essential skill in family-centered service is listening to and valuing parents' information about their own strengths and needs in addition to those of their child. It is possible that by improving the quality and timeliness of the information we provided to this family and by being better listeners, we could have avoided the missed appointments and resulting discharge.

When working as a pediatric therapist, it is easy to focus solely on the needs of the child; however, within a family-centered service approach we are expected to recognize the holistic needs of the family (Rosenbaum et al. 1998). This is because children develop within a family system, and the health and well-being of parents will impact the child. In hard-to-reach families, parents may have a multitude of challenges that need to be addressed (e.g. poverty, limited literacy, mental health issues, substance abuse, language or cultural barriers) (Barrett 2008; Boag-Munroe & Evangelou 2012). It is vital to ask parents about these areas of their lives and to help families to access resources and supports to address these challenges. Early intervention programs are of the most benefit to children once material security in the family is achieved (Turnbull et al. 2014).

Given the competing challenges for parents' time and energy, it is critical to encourage parents to determine the nature of intervention that would best suit their family's needs. Within a model of family-centered service, therapists should present families with options about the services that could be provided and allow families to determine how much control they want over decision-making (Rosenbaum et al. 1998). Some families may decide to ask the therapist what she would recommend for their child; other families may want total control over developing their service plan. Ideally, services would be individualized and flexible, able to adapt to the families' changing needs and strengths over time.

In the vignette described at the opening of the chapter, individual therapy was being offered in the center on a weekly basis, with the father bringing his daughter in and participating throughout the joint OT and SLP session. This therapy plan was developed with the parents to fit with Jeff's work schedule. Offering OT and SLP sessions together meant one less appointment for the family each week and also allowed for collaborative practice. At a surface level it appears that we created an individualized service plan together with the family to best fit their needs. Looking back now, I question if we could have done more. Perhaps the more pressing needs were related to the parents' relationship and social work help could have been offered. If the parents were overwhelmed by the appointments, we might have been able to dedicate more time and effort into supporting daycare enrolment and supporting the staff there. Although we offered to postpone therapy, we could have encouraged a richer dialogue about what a break in therapy might mean, or even discuss whether the family wanted to continue with therapy at all.

When parents assume responsibility for making therapy-related decisions for their child they may act in a way that is different from what the professional believes to be best. It is important for professionals to accept and respect these decisions, given that a basic assumption within family-centered care is that parents know their child best (Rosenbaum et al. 1998). This can be especially difficult in cases where the family chooses to decline therapy services. As therapists we often believe that we can help children to develop and we offer support to parents. There is evidence to indicate that participating in pediatric rehabilitation services can lead to positive outcomes for children with impairments (Chen et al. 2004). Therefore, it can be difficult to accept a parent's choice not to participate in therapy. Therapists might even overlook the option of 'discontinuing services' when discussing choices for therapy (e.g. group intervention or individual therapy). This makes it very difficult for parents to tell a therapist that they may not want to continue with services and to discuss openly the reasons for this choice. Parents may feel pressure to accept therapy and appear that they are being 'good parents' by doing what is recommended, as opposed to doing what they feel is right for themselves and their family.

There are some instances in which not following through with therapy might indicate harm or neglect and child protective services would need to be involved. These circumstances might be clear and include, for example, unsafe feeding practices for a child with swallowing difficulties. Yet there are many circumstances when it is not clear whether a child is in need of protection. For example, what if a parent does not want to take the child out of the house because they are afraid that child will be made fun of? The term 'child not brought' was suggested to replace 'did not attend' to indicate that it is the parents' responsibility to bring the child to appointments and that failure to do so might indicate safeguarding and welfare concerns (Arai et al. 2013). It can be challenging for therapists to decide when to trust parents as knowing the best and doing the best for the child versus making decisions that constitute harm or neglect.

In some cases, families are already involved with child protective services and attend therapy because this was recommended (or indeed ordered) by the agency as a mandatory part of retaining (or regaining) child custody. These families often attend because they have to, not because they want to. When these families miss an appointment the therapist is obliged to notify the family's caseworker. This practice may hold families who are known to child protective agencies to a higher standard of participation than is common for most families who use pediatric rehabilitation services.

In the scenario described, the family was observed to be loving and highly supportive of Nicole. They avidly watched her develop and cheered her on enthusiastically. Nicole appeared to be safe, stimulated and well cared for. When the family missed appointments we did not consider involving the child protective agency or approaching our manager. We followed the center-based policy that indicated a discharge from service was required for this little girl and her family.

Is the practice of discharging families due to missed appointments ethically acceptable?

The center's discharge policy directs clinicians to discharge a family following two missed appointments without prior notification. It is intended to promote equity for clients such that clinicians are consistent and unbiased in their discharge practices. However, this policy may unfairly disadvantage children whose parents did not commit to participation in therapy and families whom service providers had difficulty engaging. The policy is also intended to promote utilitarian justice, whereby resources are shared fairly among those in need of service. Thus by taking the therapy spaces from families who are not using them and offering the time, space and care to families who are awaiting service, program administrators are promoting justice. The ethical dilemma is how to balance the need to best serve each individual client (beneficence) while limiting harm (non-maleficence) with the need to use resources fairly for all (utilitarian justice) (Blackmer 2000).

In Ontario, Canada, the Ministry of Children and Youth Services funds pediatric rehabilitation services with the aim of ensuring 'all children and youth have the best opportunity to succeed and reach their full potential' (Ontario Ministry of Children and Youth Services 2010). Yet not all families may be served equally by the existing services. Hard-to-reach families have been described as isolated, often facing multiple challenges that impair their ability to access healthcare and early intervention programs (Barrett 2008; Boag-Munroe & Evangelou 2012). These families can be overlooked, potentially never accessing the services that are available to them (Coe et al. 2008; Winkworth et al. 2010). As in the case described here, families may try to use services but demonstrate difficulties by missing appointments. If some hard-to-reach families never access care and others are discharged because of missed appointments, organizations may be missing the opportunity to support the families – and children – who are probably most in need of support (Cortis 2012).

It is recognized that attracting and retaining hard-to-reach families takes additional time and resources (Barrett 2008; Boag-Munroe & Evangelou 2012; Cortis 2012). Time and skilled professionals are required to empower and build trust with these families (Cortis 2012). This can pose difficulties for publicly funded organizations that are often responsible for doing much more than their limited resources make possible. Organizations are concerned about their waitlists and may be evaluated on the number of children seen, the time periods spent waiting for care and positive client outcomes. 'Resource scarcity and pressure to achieve and demonstrate short-term results may lead providers to concentrate their efforts on those easiest to reach and engage, or those for whom change will be most evident' (Cortis 2012 p. 352).

At the center at which I work, the policy regarding discharge following missed appointments was developed and implemented in part due to high numbers of client 'no-shows'. Clients at this center missed over 4000 appointments in a 1-year period, 1367 of them without prior notice (Phoenix & Rosenbaum 2015). These appointments use clinician time and center resources. Retaining families on active caseloads who are not attending their appointments keeps clinicians from picking up children from the treatment program waitlist that can range from 3 months to over a year. Given the belief that services provided early in childhood provide the greatest impact on development, it can be considered unfair to increase the wait times for children while attempting to engage families that are not typically coming in for their appointments. In this service environment it is understandable that the organization would choose to implement a discharge policy based on missed appointments in an effort to promote justice via equitable sharing of resources for all clients.

This discharge policy can create tension for clinicians who want to promote justice for all clients, but also are concerned with beneficence – providing the best service for the client in front of them. This tension is increased when clinicians recognize that providing the best service for hard-to-reach families requires increased time and effort, resources that could otherwise be directed to clients awaiting care. In the case above, I was left with the unsettled feeling that there was more I could have done to engage this family and provide services better suited to meet the family's needs. I did not feel right following the center's discharge policy, but I understood the reasons the policy exists. I could have circumvented the organization's discharge policy, but thought this created unfairness for other families discharged when clinicians have followed the policy. The struggle to achieve balance between beneficence and justice within rehabilitation medicine is an ethical dilemma that is not easily resolved (Blackmer 2000).

The resolution

In this case we notified the family of the discharge via a mailed report that clearly stated that if the family had further concerns they were welcome to re-refer for service. It felt uncomfortable discharging Nicole when we knew there was so much more we could do to support her development. It was hard to inform the parents of the discharge knowing that they were going through a difficult time. We thought about circumventing the policy – no-one would be checking to see if this child had a previous missed appointment – but felt that wouldn't be fair to other families who were discharged after two missed appointments per the center-based policy. We hoped that Nicole's family would come back – and they did initiate a re-referral and returned for service. The family had great attendance when they returned and Nicole developed many of the skills needed for successful entry into a community-based junior kindergarten program.

In retrospect it is easy to think that we could have provided better service for this family. Perhaps we could have given more information about service options and the goals we were working on in therapy. It might have helped had we been better listeners and aimed to elicit more information about the whole family and not just the child. We assumed that therapy was doing no harm, but perhaps it was adding stress to the parents' lives. Discharge should have been discussed as an acceptable choice with this family prior to the missed appointments. We could also have negotiated a different schedule that fit better with family needs and might have avoided missed appointments. Once the appointments were missed we could have ignored the policy that specified discharge as a next step. Regardless of our decision to discharge the family or keep them on caseload, we would have struggled to balance our relationships with the employer and the client while acting ethically and doing 'what's right'. Perhaps the organization should revisit the policy to determine if there is an alternate way to support families who have missed appointments. Any policy changes would need to consider not just the needs of the family who is participating in care, but also the needs of the children and families who are awaiting service.

The big picture

The case above is used to illustrate the ethical complexity of providing pediatric rehabilitation services within the context of a Canadian children's treatment center.

This environment can be considered resource-rich when contrasted with the money and services available for children with impairments once they move into school age and adulthood. We must also consider that there are countries that do not publicly fund rehabilitation services for children. Furthermore, some countries do not have the professional support, infrastructure or money to provide comparable pediatric rehabilitation services. Limited funding can heighten barriers to service accessibility, making even more families 'hard-to-reach'. In the case of limited service it becomes even more important to consider which families are able to access care and whether certain families are being marginalized and disadvantaged by rehabilitation organizations.

Themes for discussion

- Does the program in which you work have a policy regarding 'hard-to-reach' (or 'hard-to-serve') families? On what basis was such a policy developed? Was there ever an explicit discussion of the ethics of such a policy?

- Most if not all the services we offer to families of children with developmental impairments are available during 'working hours' of weekdays. Is it ethical to expect busy families to march only to our drummers, or would it be more appropriate to offer evening and weekend hours as part of being 'family-centered'?

References

Arai L, Stapley S, Roberts H (2014) 'Did not attends' in children 0–10: A scoping review. *Child Care Health Dev* 40: 797–805.

Barrett H (2008) *Hard-to-reach families: Engagement in the voluntary and community sector.* London: Family and Parenting Institute.

Blackmer J (2000) Ethical issues in rehabilitation medicine. *Scand J Rehabil Med* 32: 51–55.

Boag-Munroe G, Evangelou M (2012) From hard to reach to how to reach: A systematic review of the literature on hard-to-reach families. *Res Papers Educ* 27: 209–239.

Chen CC, Heinemann AW, Bode RK et al. (2004) Impact of pediatric rehabilitation services on children's functional outcomes. *Am J Occup Ther* 58: 44–53.

Coe C, Gibson A, Spencer N, Stuttaford M (2008) Sure start: Voices of the 'hard-to-reach'. *Child Care Health Dev* 34: 447–453.

Cortis N (2012) Overlooked and under-served? Promoting service use and engagement among 'hard-to-reach' populations. *Int J Soc Welf* 21: 351–360.

Dyke P, Buttigieg P, Blackmore AM, Ghose A (2006) Use of the measure of process of care for families (MPOC-56) and service providers (MPOC-SP) to evaluate family-centred services in a paediatric disability setting. *Child Care Health Dev* 32: 167–176.

King S, King G, Rosenbaum P (2010) Children's health care evaluating health service delivery to children with chronic conditions and their families: Development of a refined measure of processes of care (MPOC-20). *Child Health Care* 33: 35–57.

Kuhlthau K, Bloom S, Van Cleave J et al. (2011) Evidence for family-centered care for children with special health care needs: A systematic review. *Acad Pediatr* 11: 136–143.

Ontario Ministry of Children and Youth Services (2010) *About the Ministry* [Online]; http://www.children.gov.on.ca/htdocs/English/about/index.aspx (accessed 14 May 2015).

Phoenix M, Rosenbaum P (2015). Development and implementation of a paediatric rehabilitation care path for hard-to-reach families: A case report. *Child Care Health Dev* 41: 494–499.

Rosenbaum P, King S, Law M et al. (1998) Family-centred service: A conceptual framework and research review. *Phys Occup Ther Pediatr* 86: 1–20.

Tseng W, Streltzer J (2008) *Cultural competence in health care.* New York, NY: Springer.

Turnbull H, Loptson K, Muhajarine N (2014) Experiences of housing insecurity among participants of an early childhood intervention programme. *Child Care Health Dev* 40: 435–440.

Winkworth G, McArthur M, Layton M, Thomson L, Wilson F (2010) Opportunities lost – why some parents of young children are not well-connected to the service systems designed to assist them. *Austral Soc Work* 63: 431–444.

Chapter 18

The obligation to report child abuse or neglect is more complex than it seems

Lucyna M. Lach and Rachel Birnbaum

Clinical scenario

Wanita is a separated mother of two children, Eli (10 years) and Ranee (6 years). She has been the sole custodian of both children since she left her husband 4 years ago; her only source of income is social assistance, as she receives no financial support from the children's father, who has had no contact with either of their children since the separation. Wanita believes that he returned to his home country in South Asia as he had wanted to go back and was ashamed of having a son with a 'condition'.

Eli was diagnosed with autism spectrum disorder (ASD) and epilepsy at 3 years of age. Wanita has accessed medical and support services at various times throughout Eli's life, but remains steadfast that he will 'get over it' and be just like his 'normal' sister, Ranee. Wanita is devoutly religious and relies on her faith to maintain her belief that Eli will grow to be the man she believes he can be.

Wanita was referred to the social worker, Ariba, by the neurologist who follows Eli for medication management of his seizures. The neurologist had expressed some concern about Wanita's expectations of her son. Ariba meets with Wanita and her son and observes Eli's behavior. During the interview, he paces around the room flapping his hands, making no eye contact with either his mother or with her. His mother repeatedly tries to get him to sit down and at one point, grabs his hand aggressively in an effort to try to get him to stay put. He responds by hitting her back. During the interview, Wanita acknowledges her frustration with Eli; at the same time, she reports that Eli will be fine if he would just get enough sleep and eat the food that she prepares for him. She reports that Eli has not been able to sleep through the night and while she finds him to be hard on her, he is very good with his younger sister. Eli does not attend a regular school program. Wanita reports that she keeps him at home because she does not want Eli to attend the specialized program recommended for him. She thinks that he should be in a regular program where he can interact with peers and learn how to behave properly. She is not interested in receiving any of the rehabilitation services the center offers, stating that this has not helped in the past.

During the interview, Ariba notes that Wanita is trying to manage a lot on her own. Wanita acknowledges that Eli takes more of her time and energy and she is not as focused on parenting Ranee as she should be. Ariba observes that Wanita seems to care a great deal about both of her children but is very unrealistic about Eli's capacity and future and is also concerned about Ranee.

Coming from the same cultural background as Wanita, Ariba understands the importance of a first-born son and how admission of any type of disability might cause a mother to be stigmatized by her community. At the same time, Ariba is concerned that Wanita's 'denial' is getting in the way of her decision-making and so contemplates whether to contact child protection services. What should she do?

The primary decision facing Ariba is whether to call child welfare authorities to report Wanita for suspected neglect and physical abuse. As a professional who is bound by her own code of ethics, Ariba must make a decision that requires deliberation with her colleagues, but for which, ultimately, she is professionally accountable. Furthermore, it is not her role alone to decide on the extent to which Eli might be at risk. If she reports the family to the local child welfare agency, trained child welfare professionals, who have been given legal authority, will conduct a thorough assessment. They will then determine the extent to which Eli might be at risk. It seems that Ariba could simply defer to the local child protection legislation for direction on how to proceed. However, there are other sources of knowledge that may assist Ariba in making recommendations for Eli – each of which represents an additional layer of considerations.

In this chapter, we draw on five sources of knowledge that inform social work practice: *principles, theories* (psychosocial and ethical), *legislation, research* and *self* (Fig 18.1). Our goal is to expand social workers' understanding of ethics by bringing to light different ways of thinking, including how to unpack the complexity of what at first appears to be a simple decision. Each of these ideas represents a unique source of information upon which social work and other healthcare practitioners can draw in order to critically analyze how Ariba should proceed. We have purposefully not tried to arrive at a resolution. Instead, we provide a framework or set of tools to add to a decision-making toolbox that we hope helps readers reflect critically on how to proceed.

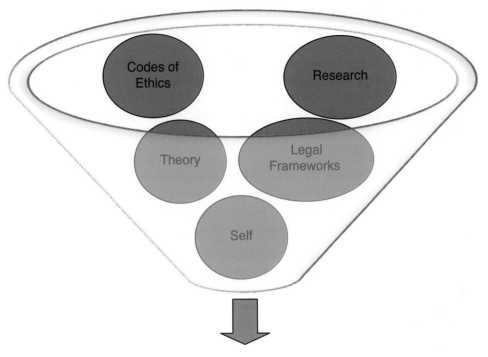

Figure 18.1 Principles, theories (psychosocial and ethical), legislation, research and self

The primary decision in any ethical dilemma is typically expressed as 'doing something' versus 'not doing something'.[1] In this case, the social worker's primary decision is whether to report the case to child welfare authorities. The social worker would like to do the 'right' thing, but the 'right thing' is not so simple to figure out. The model suggests that the social worker's decision should be uniquely informed by each of these sources of knowledge. Let us examine how each of these plays a role in her decision on how to proceed.

Principles and the professional codes of ethics

The decision of whether to call child welfare authorities or not is based on Ariba's concern that Eli *may* be at risk of neglect and physical abuse at home. Given that Wanita behaved in a frustrated and somewhat rough manner with her son in front of Ariba, Ariba wonders what Wanita does at home when there is no one to witness her behavior. She realizes that calling child welfare authorities will potentially take Eli and his family down a completely different path. An investigation would be conducted, questions will

---

1 Editors' clarification: Not all ethical questions or challenges are dilemmas. Dilemmas have a particular structure (two competing and defendable options with only one to be chosen).

be asked, and child welfare authorities will need to decide whether not sending Eli to school or for rehabilitation services is neglectful, as well as whether interactions between Eli and his mother escalate to a point of harmful physical contact and/or neglect. As a professional, Ariba is bound by a code of ethics that articulate principles, which, in turn, specify the values of the profession; these can be used to help frame the ethical dilemma.[2]

Social workers' professional and societal values associated with contacting child welfare authorities include, but are not limited to, the following:

- *Protection of vulnerable members of society.* Society has an obligation to protect its most vulnerable members. Given the intellectual impairment associated with both autism and epilepsy, Eli is not able to describe what is happening at home. He is non-verbal and isolated from others who would normally provide some level of monitoring regarding his well-being (e.g. teachers, therapists, other parents).

- *Maintaining the best interests of the child.* Ariba and the child welfare authorities must always keep this principle at the forefront of their decision-making. Is it in Eli's best interests to be at school, or at home with his mother? Considerations may include evaluation of where he is more likely to receive beneficial therapies, engage with peers and improve his social and communication skills if he is at one place or the other.

- *Beneficence.* This principle refers to Ariba's 'moral obligation to act for the benefit of others' (Beauchamp & Childress 2013 p. 202). The decision about whether to contact child welfare authorities must consider not only Eli's best interests, but also the best interests of Ranee and Wanita. Although initially intrusive, engagement with child welfare may also turn out to be a supportive experience for Wanita. Child welfare agencies have a mandate to protect children, but they also have a mandate to prevent, if possible, placement of the child outside of the family. If Wanita is able to accept the support they have to offer, it may benefit her as well as her two children.

Principles and values associated with not contacting the child welfare authorities include, but are not limited to, the following:

- *Respect for autonomy.* Social workers and other healthcare providers have an obligation to respect the rights of their clients and patients, who are entitled to set the course of their clients' lives as they best see fit. Wanita is Eli's mother and knows him best. Her resistance to recommendations made by educators, health and social care providers is consistent with her beliefs about Eli's best interests. The case study does not identify what these beliefs are. Therefore, instead of calling child welfare, Ariba could decide to spend more time gaining a better understanding of what Wanita's beliefs about Eli are, what they are based on and how she sees them unfolding over time.

---

2   Editors' note: *Principles* help to achieve what is *valued*.

- *Non-maleficence.* Engagement of child welfare in a person's life is rarely a welcome experience for families. Although some may purposefully seek out that kind of support, most experience it in a non-voluntary manner and regard it as an intrusion into their private life. The principle of non-maleficence refers to one's obligation to prevent harm to the child, to the mother and to the family unit. Therefore, not calling child welfare is aligned with a desire to avoid Wanita having to expose her life story and experience the distress that this exchange would inevitably bring. It is also potentially aligned with preventing harm to Wanita in the context of her community; should others find out, she may feel stigmatized.

- *Confidentiality.* Ariba may be very conscious of the fact that Wanita disclosed information about her private life to her in the context of a trusting relationship. Limits of confidentiality are rarely explained on a routine basis in hospital settings. Therefore, Wanita may not have understood the limits of consent when meeting the neurologist and social worker. Ariba may also believe that because she has developed an alliance with Wanita, she may be able to work with her and over time will be able to convince her to get Eli to school and to receive rehabilitation services. Calling child welfare would significantly decrease the likelihood of this alliance continuing.

Each of these principles can be located in a professional code of ethics. In Canada, each province has a professional college or association that has a code of ethics guiding its members' conduct; it is the standard against which the public may hold the professional accountable. The Canadian Association of Social Workers has a Code of Ethics (2005) and Ethical Guidelines for Practice (2005) have been adopted by some provinces; some provincial professional associations such as in Ontario have elaborated their own Codes of Ethics (2008) (ocswssw.org/wp-content/.../Code-of-Ethics-Standards-of-Practice).

Articulating an ethical dilemma as a conflict between two principles is a key aspect of this deliberation. For example, in this case, the principles of *protecting vulnerable members of society* versus *respect for self-determination* conflict with one another. Protecting Eli and ensuring that he has access to programs that will support his development both at school and through the rehabilitation services conflict with the principle of respecting Wanita's role as a parent and her right to establish what is in his best interests. Similarly, framing the conflict between the principles of *maintaining the best interests of the child* versus *confidentiality* identifies how difficult it is to uphold both principles simultaneously. It is in Eli's best interests to achieve his developmental potential, but that may be difficult to

> "Articulating the tension between ethical principles may start the process of critical reflection that highlights complexities but also helps to move towards a resolution"

achieve if Ariba decides to maintain in confidence what Wanita has told her. Naming the conflict between principles is a way of externalizing what practitioners may intuitively be sensing and begins a process of critical reflection that highlights complexity but also assists in finding a way forward.

Theory

Theoretical frameworks can bring a fresh perspective to a situation where certain aspects are highlighted, while others are either minimized or not emphasized at all. There are two sets of theories upon which practitioners can draw to further reflect on this case. The first are psychosocial theories and the second are ethical principles and theories.[3] An example of a psychosocial theory is the strengths-based perspective (Nash 2005; Saleeby 2002), while an example of ethical theory is utilitarianism (West 2004). We have chosen these two theories to illustrate how adherence to a particular theoretical lens highlights particular aspects of the case.

Psychosocial theory
A strengths-based approach to practice is collaborative and focuses on the assets and abilities of clients. Central to this approach are key principles such as empowerment, respect for cultural diversity, an emphasis on social justice and self-determination, and achieving an understanding of the client's narrative through their eyes (Saleeby 2002). Adherence to these principles would cause Ariba to take time to better understand Wanita's beliefs about her son, about services with which she has come into contact, and about her wishes for his improvement. She would learn more about what goals Wanita has for her son's future and how she thought he would get there if he was not attending school or rehabilitation. Instead of calling child welfare authorities immediately, she would wait to develop a stronger alliance with Wanita. Doing so would provide her with an opportunity to better understand the basis for Wanita's parenting decisions and to perhaps engage her in a different way of parenting. At the same time, a strengths-based approach is not counter-indicated when situations of alleged abuse or neglect arise. At all times, Ariba would maintain a respectful stance, even if she decides to contact child welfare to investigate possible neglect. In a strengths-based approach, her belief that Wanita was doing the best she could, under the circumstances, would be retained.

---

3   Editor's clarification: It is common for ethical analysis to include a *specification process* where the principles derive meaning from being specified, that is, understood according to scholarly and societal context/knowledge. In this process of specification, different theories and pieces of knowledge can be mobilized to define what the principles mean.

Ethical theory

Utilitarian/teleological approaches to moral questions and dilemmas emphasize an evaluation of the pleasure/pain associated with a course of action itself, as well as its consequences. *Act* utilitarianism applies to an individual and assumes that an act is right if it maximizes utility (greatest pleasure/least pain). Here the focus is on the consequences of an act being performed. *Rule* utilitarianism applies to classes of acts by an individual where the main consideration to determine whether an act is right or wrong concerns the consequences of a rule that everyone should follow in similar circumstances. An action is considered right or wrong depending on the consequences if everyone who had the occasion to do the act did it (West 2004).

Applying an act utilitarianism approach to this case study, Ariba must weigh the consequences of calling child welfare to report that Eli *may* be in need of protection against the consequences of not calling child welfare; consequences refer to both positive and negative potential impacts and consider the principles of maximizing pleasure and minimizing pain. Contacting child welfare will initiate a process that will clearly be painful for Wanita; perhaps it will only be painful in the short term, but that is unclear. Surveillance and scrutiny in child welfare investigations are inevitable and there is a risk that Eli might be removed from his mother's care. It is also possible that engagement with child welfare will initiate supports that Eli needs in order to thrive. Should Wanita establish a more positive rapport with child welfare, she may learn that there are practitioners and services that are culturally competent and supportive. She may find others like herself who are similarly isolated and struggling to imagine their family's future.

Choosing not to contact child welfare at this time carries some potential positive and negative consequences. On the one hand, it gives Ariba some time to build a rapport with Wanita, thereby gaining her trust and potentially convincing her of the importance of Eli's education and rehabilitation. Given that they come from similar cultural backgrounds, Ariba may feel like this is a real possibility. Because Ariba has assessed Wanita as truly 'caring' for her son, it may also be possible that she can convince her that engaging him in school and therapeutic supports is another way of caring. On the other hand, not calling child welfare may only perpetuate the isolation and potential neglect to which Eli has been subjected. Furthermore, should Eli be further harmed, Ariba could be subject to discipline by her college, as she is a social work professional and is obligated to report all incidents of abuse and neglect, irrespective of the consequences.[4] Exploring the consequences of either reporting or not reporting Wanita allows Ariba to begin a process of reasoning through the best course of action, but does not yet lead her to know the course of action that represents the 'right' decision.

---

4   The crucial question remains whether there is abuse or neglect here.

Legal context

The key legislation informing this case and the ethical dilemma comes from legislation that protects children. In Canada, every province has its own child welfare legislation; in other jurisdictions, the legislation will either be federal or regional. For example, in Ontario, Canada, the Child and Family Services Act[5] (CFSA) sets the minimum standards of care for children. Ontario legislation requires that any person who has reasonable grounds to believe that a child has been abused, or is at risk of abuse, report it to the child welfare authority. More importantly, any professional who becomes aware of abuse or neglect in the course of their duties must immediately report their suspicions. Failure of those who perform professional or official duties with children to report such suspicion is punishable by a fine and may result in a charge of liability under the Criminal Code.[6] Each country is guided by Articles 9, 19, 23 and 24 of the United Nations Convention on the Rights of the Child (United Nations 1989), all of which direct address Eli's rights, as well as the obligations of his legal guardian and the state. Given this legislation, Ariba is obligated to report her concerns about Wanita to child welfare, as Eli may be a child in need of protection. The Children's Aid Society, and not Ariba, must assess whether this is the case.

Research

Social workers are increasingly encouraged to draw on research to inform their practice (Drisko 2014). Although evidence-informed practice models draw on more than just empirical studies, knowledge of observational and intervention-based research plays a key role in understanding and critically reflecting on the ethical dilemma in this case as well as the context within which the ethical dilemma takes place.

First, Wanita is a single parent whose ethnocultural background is non-Western and she is raising two children, one of whom has been diagnosed with autism and epilepsy. The information provided suggests that her son has significant behavioral problems. The epidemiologic literature suggests that up to 70% of children with ASD have at least one other comorbid psychiatric condition such as attention deficit hyperactivity disorder (ADHD) or social anxiety (Siminoff et al. 2008). Similarly, behavioral dysregulation is prevalent in up to 40% of children with epilepsy (Austin et al. 2001). Eli's behavioral problems may therefore be seen to occur in a context that has been documented among children with ASD and epilepsy, and any inferences of a causal relationship between 'bad' parenting and behavior problems should be critically appraised within this complex context. Moreover, there is a paucity of research about how members of different ethnocultural groups view ASD or epilepsy. Even if such data existed, it would

---

5   Child and Family Services Act, R.S.O. 1990, c.C.11.
6   R.S.C. 1985, c.C-46, ss. 218–219.

be difficult (and perhaps unethical) to extrapolate how such findings would relate to how Wanita parents her son.

Given this, it would be important to understand more clearly how Wanita experiences her son's behavior, what her beliefs are about the origins of his behavior and the factors that influence it, and what she thinks is needed to help him to integrate and participate in society. For this reason, Ariba may want more time to explore these questions with Wanita and therefore would not call children welfare authorities, at least not yet. However, the research findings also suggest that seeking support for managing challenging behaviors is as important as medical treatment to improve Eli's social communication and restricted or repetitive pattern of behavior, interests or activities. This type of support may be accessed through the child welfare system, suggesting that Wanita might also benefit from their involvement.

We can also turn to the literature on the efficacy/effectiveness of treatments and best practices recommended for children with ASD in order to clarify whether the treatment approaches that Wanita refuses to use are preventing her son from achieving optimal development. A number of systematic reviews of key approaches have evaluated evidence for Intensive Behavioural Intervention (IBI; Eldevik et al. 2009), Treatment and Education of Autistic and Related Communication Handicapped Children (TEACCH; Virues-Ortega et al. 2013) and Pivotal Response Treatment (PRT; Verschuur et al. 2014). Individual randomized control trials of approaches such as Developmental, Individual-Difference, Relationship-Based (DIR)/Floortime™ (Pajareya & Nopmaneejumruslers 2011) may also provide some guidance regarding how important it is to ensure that Eli has access to treatment. Unfortunately, no single approach comes out as unequivocally superior, and the state of the science is such that no-one can predict precisely which approach works better for which child (Birnbaum et al. 2016). Nevertheless, the research suggests that there are evidence-based rehabilitation approaches from which Eli could benefit, and supports the view that Wanita's refusal to give Eli access to them is a form of neglect that must be addressed immediately. This would increase the urgency for Ariba to make the report.

Self

Reflection on the role that one's personal and sociopolitical self plays in arriving at a way forward in an ethical dilemma is absolutely critical (D'Cruz et al. 2007). Personal history as well as social location contribute to the construction of one's professional identity and may lead Ariba to make assumptions. On the one hand, Ariba may better understand and perhaps even identify with aspects of Wanita's situation (such as the importance of having a first-born son who can grow up to look after his mother), or the stigma and shame in the community associated with having a child with a neurodevelopmental condition (Kediye et al. 2009). Arriving at any kind of cultural understanding of impairment and disability, be it one of shame, blame, exclusion or giftedness, is impossible, as there is a risk of attributing to a specific individual a taken-for-granted cultural assumption that may not reflect their actual belief. Ho (1995) coined the term 'internalized culture', which implies that individuals differentially internalize aspects of their culture and that these should become a source of curiosity and enquiry by practitioners, rather than an assumption. Not everyone from a particular culture will subscribe to the same belief. Ariba should therefore consider what her assumptions are about ASD and what her assumptions are about Wanita's culture. Doing so allows her to separate out her own assumptions from what may or may not be Wanita's assumptions. In this way, she could engage Wanita in a conversation about how she perceives ASD in Eli without imposing preconceived notions onto her culture. Doing so requires more time and so would support the decision to not report immediately. The decision to report or not would therefore be contingent on what she learned from Wanita.

Sharing a similar cultural background may contribute to the building of a strong alliance. Wanita may welcome this as an opportunity to develop a relationship with a professional whom she perceives as having an understanding of and respect for her cultural background and beliefs; at the same time, she may be concerned about the fact that Ariba is from the same community and either withhold or generate a false representation of who she is in order to protect herself and her children. The former would support a decision to not report at this time, while the latter supports a decision to report, as waiting would not yield additional information. Ariba's strong identification with Wanita's cultural background may cause her to over-identify or to be 'blind' to the risks. In her desire to connect with Wanita and develop a trusting alliance, Ariba may not give the same weight to risk factors that are clearly evident in this case. This suggests that she should report, to allow someone with more distance to evaluate the risk.

Epilogue

We have purposefully not arrived at a specific conclusion or 'answer' on how to proceed in this chapter. Instead, we have provided a framework or set of tools to add to a decision-making toolbox that we hope helps readers reflect critically on how to proceed. Critical reflection is an essential aspect of social work practice (Fook & Gardiner 2013). Drawing on the various sources of knowledge identified in this chapter, we begin to have an appreciation for the complexity of decision-making when faced with ethical questions and dilemmas.

The critical reflection approach adopted in this chapter is not unique to social work and has implications for other health and social care disciplines. In any discipline, minimizing the complexity of decision-making in such circumstances reduces practice to its most technocratic components. From a practical perspective, the social worker must arrive at a decision; however, the social worker must also be able to defend their decision. They, as well as other health professionals, can draw on values embedded in their respective codes of ethics, principles and theories that serve as the lens through which their daily practice is guided, the legislative context of practice, research and self-reflection. This will ensure that they can account for the very difficult decisions that are made in practice and can defend those decisions to themselves, their clients/patients, colleagues and institutions, and if needed, in the court of law.

Themes for discussion

- The thinking and deliberations reported in this chapter take time and sophistication. What are the consequences – for the child, the parent(s), the professionals, the community – of simply 'following the rules'? What are the downsides – for the same people – of simply 'following the rules'?

- The approach to the analysis of this story presents an 'on the one hand/on the other hand' back-and-forth set of considerations. Is there ever a 'good answer' in a 'difficult' situation? And for whom is the best answer 'good' or 'bad'?

- What resources are available to professionals when confronted with complicated situations like the ones described here? Are we comfortable to share our own uncertainties and vulnerabilities when we are distressed?

References

Austin JK, Harezlak J, Dunn DW, Huster GA, Rose DF, Ambrosius WT (2001) Behavior problems in children before first recognized seizures. *Pediatrics* 107: 115–122.

Beauchamp T, Childress J (2013) *Principles of biomedical ethics* 7th edn. New York, NY: Oxford University Press.

Birnbaum R, Lach L, Saposnek D (2016). Co-parenting children with a neurodevelopmental disorder. In: Drozd L, Kuehnle K, Saini M, Oleson N, editors. *Parenting plan evaluations: Applied research for the family court* 2nd edn, pp. 205–243. New York, NY: Oxford University Press.

D'Cruz H, Gillingham P, Melendez S (2007). Reflexivity, its meanings and relevance for social work: A critical review of the literature. *Br J Social Work* 37: 73–90.

Drisko J (2014). Research evidence and social work practice: The place of evidence-based practice. *Clin Social Work J* 42: 123–133.

Eldevik S, Hastings RP, Hughes JC, Jahr E, Eikeseth S, Cross S (2009) Meta-analysis of early intensive behavioral intervention for children with autism. *J Clin Child Adolesc Psychol* 38: 439–450.

Fook J, Gardiner F, editors. (2013) *Critical reflection in context.* London: Routledge.

Gilligan C (1982) *In a different voice: Psychological theory and women's development.* Cambridge, MA: Harvard University Press.

Ho DYF (1995) Internalized culture, culturocentrism, and transcendence. *Counsel Psychol* 23: 2–24.

Kediye F, Valeo A, Berman RC (2009) Somali–Canadian mothers' experience in parenting a child with autism. *J Assoc Res Mother* 11: 211–223.

Nash M, Mumford R, O'Donoghue K (2005) *Social work theories in action.* London: Jessica Kingsley.

Pajareya K, Nopmaneejumruslers K (2011) A pilot randomized controlled trial of DIR/Floortime™ parent training intervention for pre-school children with autism spectrum disorder. *Autism* 15: 563–577.

Saleeby D (2002) *The strengths perspective in social work practice.* White Plains, NY: Longman.

Siminoff E, Pickles A, Charman T, Chandler S, Loucas T, Baird G (2008) Psychiatric disorders in children with autism spectrum disorder: Prevalence, comorbidity, and associated factors in a population-derived sample. *J Am Acad Child Adolesc Psychiatr* 47: 921–929.

United Nations (1989) United Nations Convention on the Rights of the Child; http://www.ohchr.org/EN/ProfessionalInterest/Pages/CRC.aspx (accessed 9 March 2015).

Verschuur R, Didden R, Lang R, Sigafoos J, Huskens B (2014) Pivotal response treatment for children with autism spectrum disorders: A systematic review. *Rev J Autism Dev Disord* 1: 34–61.

Virues-Ortega J, Julio F, Pastor R (2013) The TEACCH program for children and adults with autism: A meta-analysis of intervention studies. *Clin Psychol Rev* 33: 940–953.

West HR (2004) *An introduction to Mills' utilitarian ethics.* New York, NY: Cambridge University Press.

Chapter 19

The dilemmas for siblings of children with disabilities: personal reflections on ethical challenges

Peter Blasco

Prologue

Brothers and sisters are bonded in special ways, ways that are not really comparable to other (even special) relationships. Siblings reciprocally shape each other's lives. To what extent this occurs is uncertain – perhaps not as much as parents, but surely more than casual friendships. It seems logical that if one sibling is compromised in some way – neurodevelopmentally impaired, chronically ill or emotionally disturbed – the situation might raise a number of special issues for both of them, but perhaps especially for the well one, the sibling who is not impaired (see also Chapter 20).

It is hard to deny that the siblings of children with disabilities may get short-changed (some would say neglected). Good reviews of the subject are available (Coleby 1995; Lobato 1990), although the literature is conflicting. Influences vary over time, as siblings get older. An older sibling influences their younger sibling (and parents) in ways different from the effects of the younger one on their brother or sister. Factors related to adjustment include sex, age and age spacing, severity of disability, diagnosis, birth order and other family factors like maternal stress. Adolescents and young adults raised with a disabled sibling describe numerous positive and negative effects. Some studies show increased problems, some show benefits to the siblings, and many report that the impact changes over time. The fairly extensive literature on these influences from

Table 19.1   Effects of the child with a disability or chronic illness on healthy siblings

Potential positive effects	Potential negative effects
Maturity	Feelings of parental neglect
Responsibility	Feelings of resentment
Altruism	Perceived parental demands and expectations for achievement
Tolerance	Embarrassment
Humanitarian concerns and careers	Guilt about own health
Sense of closeness in the family	Extra responsibility in the home
Self-confidence and independence	Restrictions in social activity
	Sense of distance in the family

older studies is nicely summarized by Lobato (1990) and for more recent literature by Emerson & Giallo (2014) (Table 19.1).[1]

The following vignette illustrates several basic issues I encountered in a routine clinic follow-up visit.

Clinical scenario

Emanuel (Manny) G is a young patient with cerebral palsy who is having a terrible time with oral feeding. He gains a little weight, he loses a little, he stagnates; it takes his parents 30 minutes or more to feed him; he sounds raspy all the time. He is in need of a feeding gastrostomy tube and the parents want nothing to do with the G-tube. As he moves toward malnutrition, I cannot ignore what is obvious. There is a genuine ethical imperative involved here. The conflict between parental wishes and patient health is dangerous. I am ethically obliged to do something in the best interests of my patient.

Manny gets an enormous amount of attention from his loving parents. He has 6-year-old twin siblings. Jose is in clinic today with the children's mother and I always check in on how the siblings are doing. In the clinic exam room Jose sits engrossed with a hand-held videogame and does not respond to my greeting. He never looks up, never makes eye contact. Mrs G reprimands him: 'Say hello to Dr Blasco, Jose.' No response. He finally mutters at one point complaining about how 'Manny gets what he wants all the time.' His mother apologizes and later reports

---

1   The editors strongly recommend reading David B's emotional graphic-format autobiography *Epileptic*, about growing up with an 'epileptic brother', including getting disheartened at his brother for abandoning his role as the older sibling.

that Jose's behavior has become a problem in school this year after he did well in kindergarten. He has been disrespectful to his teacher, having been sent to the principal's office twice in the past 2 weeks. He is increasingly argumentative at home and he hit his twin sister, Margarita, the previous evening as they were squabbling over the TV remote.

Mr G works a long, hard day. Mrs G tried to go back to work after Manny's birth but had to quit in order to care for him at home because of his many needs.

What is my role in this scenario? As I see it there are two clear issues. The first (Manny's feeding and nutrition issues) is pretty straightforward and it is clinically imperative to address it. I need to spend a considerable amount of time going over Manny's interval history, therapies, equipment, multiple medications and so on, and examine him carefully. I then need to address my conflict with the parents over their unwillingness to accept a gastrostomy tube. But surveying the room, the most needy person at the moment is Jose, and his parents are at as much of a loss about what to do for him as they are about Manny.

I feel uncomfortable about several issues. And I know I do not have time to address them all. With that thought comes a wave of guilt: *ethically* I need to step in on the first issue (Manny's poor nutrition) and I *ought* to step in on the second matter (Jose's deteriorating behavior). Manny does get the lion's share of attention. Jose sees it, experiences it. He cannot really articulate it very well. In the clinic his sullen behavior reflects his anger. In school he acts out. For whatever reason, Margarita seems to roll with things a little better. She is pretty much her usual self except when Jose targets her. In this scenario some would suggest that Jose's behavior is a reflection of his being seriously neglected. From that viewpoint, an ethical (or at least legal) responsibility to intervene arises.

The entire scenario causes me to pause and feel very uncomfortable – with the impaired child's situation, the family's struggles, the sibling's behavior and my own issues of time demand and guilt! The issue with Jose's behavior and his mother's distress and shame over it, although highly charged in the moment, would never get to an ethics board! The 'ethical' challenge here is more of a personal nature. It resides with my willingness to ferret out the problem in the first place and then to confront it. The situation represents a dilemma to be sure, but in my thinking, real *ethical* issues have a more substantive, imperative character to them. In this scenario Manny's inadequate nutrition represents a true ethical imperative. The conflict between parents' wishes and patient health potentially poses a dangerous clinical situation. I am ethically obliged to do something in the best interests of my patient.

Ethics or best practice?

With the sibling scenarios, there are certainly problems – future care, acting out behavior because of feeling neglected, feelings of guilt, feelings of resentment and so on (Table 19.2). Much of the time, sibling issues will not be brought forth in a clinic

Table 19.2 The eight issues affecting siblings of a child with a disability

(1) Over-identification
(2) Embarrassment
(3) Guilt
(4) Isolation
(5) Future
(6) Resentment
(7) Caregiving
(8) Pressure to achieve

visit and there is nothing truly life-threatening going on. It would be excellent family-centered care to uncover and address such issues, but I am uncertain if there is a true ethical imperative to do so. Rather it seems to be more about best clinical practice. As good clinicians, our approach should be to identify these less clear but possibly ethical (certainly often complex) issues. When, for example, a family puts the expectation on a sibling to provide care for the impaired child/ adolescent, does that make us uncomfortable? Are we ethically obliged to discuss this and intervene with the family? The impetus to address things ourselves is not as compelling as in the life-threatening situations with which we deal. But if one views ethical dilemmas as conflicts between competing interests, then these lesser dilemmas may legitimately fall under a personal 'ethical' umbrella. As providers in a family-centered system we should routinely inquire about the well-being of siblings. When problems are uncovered, the clinician should initiate addressing them and help the family find the resources to follow through on the resolution of dilemmas. Depending on availability in one's practice setting, a social worker, the child life specialist and/or a family navigator can be ideally suited to investigate and intervene.

As individuals who know the family and who can be more objective about the problems than the parents or the siblings themselves, we are ideal facilitators for starting the process. We want to avoid paternalism – doctor knows what's best for patients and tells them what to do. I believe professionals *need* (ethically) to seek out and engage these sibling issues. What makes us so important to the task? There are three things to consider:

• To get the facts right – straight and accurate to start with – and then to translate them so they are understandable for the parents (taking into account education, culture and other issues) and for the siblings (age-appropriately).

- To provide sound advice – families look up to us and usually listen. Most crave guidance, even if they may not be overtly asking for it.

- Good care is a two-way street – this is good for us in terms of personal growth, integrity and doing a hard job well. Personal pride in what we do is an important outcome.

The eight sibling dilemmas: advice on how to respond

This letter from a 10-year-old boy illustrates more of the issues faced by siblings of children with complex medical problems.

Dear Mom,

Tonight Dad was telling me how hard it was when Trudy was in the hospital. He doesn't think it was hard for me at all. I missed you. I saw her get all these presents. I saw everyone visiting her and babying her, and there was nothing I could do about it. Sometimes I feel so alone and left out and even unloved. I know I'm overreacting, and I know that some people have so much less than me, but it's not my fault I don't have any medical problems. I wish I did!

Love, Jeffrey
(Quoted from *AAP News* March 2002)

Some of the negative impacts on siblings of being raised with a child with a chronic condition follow logically from the alterations to normal family functioning necessitated by the special requirements of a child who has impairments. Assisting parents in identifying the conflicts underlying sibling problems is a valuable support activity. Physicians and other care providers can have a positive influence on siblings simply by validating their concerns, fears and other issues related to the child with impairments. Based on my personal experience and on discussions with adolescent and adult siblings, corroborated by literature reporting common sibling concerns (Coleby 1995; Emerson & Giallo 2014; Lobato 1990; Scheiber 1989), eight distinct themes emerge from the issues raised. Some simple suggestions to restructure the concern in a positive direction follow below. It is most important to acknowledge the problem or concern first, let the child expand on it or just reflect for a few minutes, and then gently move into redirection. Addressing these issues is largely about 'spin'. What I am referring to is recognizing the dilemma and identifying the complementary positive characteristic (or virtue) that goes with it. Then one can emphasize or promote the positive aspects of the child's negative feelings:

1. *Over-identification* – worrying that they, too, have or will acquire an impairment. Think of this as a close kin to empathy. Providing an age-appropriate explanation for the

cause of the index child's disability and providing the sibling with reassurance that this is not in his or her history or make-up, is a way to defuse it. Identifying with one's brother or sister is good, but it does not mean you are or have the same thing. The clinician is in an authoritative position to help with this explanation.

2. *Embarrassment* – at the brother's or sister's appearance or behavior. Over time this can strengthen a child by prompting in personal and concrete terms the realization that not everyone must be the same. By modeling acceptance of and concern for the child with impairments, the physician can powerfully influence the sibling. In turn, the sibling becomes a good model for peers (and often for adults as well). The virtues of tolerance and understanding the needs of others are fostered. Tolerance and its application to other contexts can be explained and discussed.

3. *Guilt* – because they can live a normal life and their brother or sister cannot. Because of their egocentric perspective, younger children may imagine themselves to be at fault for the impairment. This is primarily a developmental phenomenon of the pre-operational child. It requires reassurance and over time also represents a stimulus for providing information. Accurate, age-appropriate information about the condition is a prerequisite for the development of healthy sibling relationships. In older children, based on the sibling's evolving understanding of the nature and underlying cause of their sibling's disability, guilt may produce added incentive to not waste one's abilities or gifts.

4. *Isolation* – wanting to tell friends but being afraid of the reaction. This can be addressed via special activities – sibling groups, workshops, camp experiences – from which enduring relationships and many insights may evolve. It can be converted from a threat against, to an incentive for, open communication, particularly with relatives and special friends. Simply by modeling open communication with parents and including the sibling in any way, the clinic visit experience can help foster an appreciation for openness.

5. *Fears about the future* – about their brother's or sister's future as well as their own. Who will provide care? Will financial resources be adequate? This can become a stimulus for teaching the concepts of goal setting and advance planning. Reassurance that it is okay to feel worried or concerned and that the index child at his or her level of understanding may want their own independence – as much as possible – is important. Just stating that this is a goal to work toward is reassuring.

6. *Resentment* – of the reduced amount of parents' time and family financial resources. Frustration may be translated into direct rebellion against parents, teachers or other authority figures. This is the reality of 'perceived unfairness'. Adjusting to it (see below) is an important aspect of personal growth.

7. *Caregiving* – Siblings are normally the best equipped and most convenient babysitters. Such caregiving can foster responsibility. However, if caregiving demands are

excessive, siblings may be (or believe they are) deprived of time to themselves and if the demands are made too early, the sibling may be robbed of his or her own 'child-hood'. This really falls to the parents – to be mindful of and to have strategies for assuring that excess demands do not happen. It is the same as setting aside special time, special attention for each sibling. This can be brought up in clinic regardless of whether the sibling is in attendance or not.

8. *Pressure to achieve.* Parental sense of loss experienced when one child has an impairment can lead to (perhaps unrealistically) high expectations for the remaining siblings. Similarly, self-induced pressure to 'please' or ease the burden on parents can heighten anxiety and inhibit communication. If realistic, such pressure can produce direction and motivation. The key is to help the parents and the sibling see the positive aspect of the desire to help and to keep it reined in to an appropriate level.

Although many specific issues come up, as outlined above, the most frequent is that of *perceived unfairness.* When one child's needs demand so much more attention, time, patience and financial resources, the other sibling is easily short-changed (Scheiber 1989). The pediatrician's role in helping the parents and siblings come to grips with this reality revolves around helping each child feel important and positive about him or herself. Siblings need both the opportunity to express their feelings and a supportive atmosphere that allows such a process to be productive. Clinicians might include siblings in interpretive counseling sessions and thereby model for the family the value of open communication and honesty.

Clinical practice

I feel we can strive to do two things well. One is to provide good, accurate information and concrete advice. The eight dilemmas address that challenge. The second is to model good behaviors – always talking to/with the child with the impairment, and always acknowledging, recognizing and seeking the assistance of the sibling. I make sure I have the names of the siblings written down (or I ask directly) so I can bring things up with them by name in clinic. I always say something nice about the sibling who is present and, when finishing up, always thank them for coming along to the visit. These are little things that I believe matter a lot.

There are many factors found in the literature that play into sibling adjustment – sex, age and age spacing, severity of disability, specific diagnosis, birth order and so on – that do not really matter much in the immediate scenario. One would still address each situation in the same way regardless of those details. Additional outside resources should be kept in mind. The goal is to weave advocacy for the whole family into the clinic experience (Blasco et al. 2008). Sibling discussion-group strategies (sibshops, workshops, camps, etc.) are valuable (Tudor & Lerner 2015). Parent involvement with support organizations, such as United Cerebral Palsy Association groups in the USA, various autism societies and so on, can be a great external support. Involvement with those supports can be helpful for the parents and good for the siblings as well.

Themes for discussion

- In this chapter Blasco discusses issues of discomfort regarding his role with the sibling behaviors he observes and hears about. Is it helpful, or even realistic, to describe and define the interface between 'good clinical practice' and 'ethical' practice. For whom does this situation potentially pose an ethical dilemma? Why and how? What are possible ways to manage a dilemma one might perceive?

- There are time and monetary considerations in being concerned about the siblings. How can these realities be considered and refracted through an 'ethics' lens? (In other words – discuss these issues as potential causes of ethical challenges.)

- When we see a situation that is problematic – and potentially within the realm of possibility for us to become involved – we may face an ethical challenge, whatever we do. Has this ever happened to you, and how has it been thought about and considered?

References

Blasco PA, Johnson CP, Palomo-Gonzalez SA (2008) Supports for families of children with disabilities. In: Accardo PJ, editor. *Capute and Accardo's neurodevelopmental disabilities in infancy and childhood* 3rd edn, pp. 775–801. Baltimore, MD: Brookes Publishing.

Coleby M (1995) The school-aged siblings of children with disabilities. *DMCN* 37: 415–426.

David B (2005) *Epileptic.* New York, NY: Pantheon Books.

Emerson E, Giallo R (2014) The wellbeing of siblings of children with disabilities. *Res Dev Disabil* 35: 2085–2092.

Lobato DJ (1990) *Brothers, sisters, and special needs*, pp. 30–61. Baltimore, MD: Brookes Publishing.

Scheiber K (1989) Developmentally delayed children: Effects on the normal sibling. *Pediatr Nurs* 15: 42–47.

Tudor M, Lerner M (2015) Intervention and support for siblings of youth with developmental disabilities: A systematic review. *Clin Child Fam Psychol Rev* 18: 1–23.

Chapter 20

Paying attention to parental mental health: is this our responsibility?

Dinah S. Reddihough and Elise Davis

Prologue

Research indicates that carers (usually parents) of children and adolescents with an impairment currently have substantial unmet mental health needs (Miodrag & Hodapp 2010). Both mothers and fathers of children with an impairment report greater parenting stress and depressive symptoms compared to mothers and fathers of typically developing children (Abbeduto et al. 2004; Oelofsen & Richardson 2006; Singer & Floyd 2006; Smith et al. 2008). A review of 42 studies of the mental health of mothers of children with an impairment demonstrated that mothers consistently report higher rates of depressive symptoms than other mothers, with depression rates ranging from 6 to 49% (Bailey et al. 2007). There is extensive variability in these rates, because the studies involve diverse populations, varying ages and different depression instruments. Computation of a weighted average of reported rates of individuals who passed a screening threshold for depression resulted in an estimated rate of 23.6%.

These mental health problems may in turn influence parental caregiving of children with impairments and limit parental participation in and contribution to social and economic life. Specifically, parental mental health problems have the potential to reduce the quality of care and treatment provided by mothers of children with impairments and their siblings (Stein et al. 2008). Depressed parents are less sensitive and responsive to their children than non-depressed parents (Murray 2009). The last resort for families – relinquishment of their child – is associated with negative consequences for the child, their family and service providers, and is likely to be related to poor carer mental health (Nankervis et al. 2011).

Clinical scenario

Tom is a 12-year-old boy with spastic quadriplegic cerebral palsy (Gross Motor Function Classification System [GMFCS] Level V) secondary to hypoxic-ischemic injury at birth. Although he smiles, he does not have any reliable means of communication (Communication Function Classification System [CFCS] Level V) and seems to enjoy the company of both adults and children. He has an intellectual impairment of uncertain degree. For many years, Tom has been fed by gastrostomy tube (Eating and Drinking Ability Classification System [EDACS] Level V). He has epilepsy that has always been difficult to control and for which multiple antiseizure medications have been prescribed. Tom has also had several interventions for severe spasticity and he has had orthopedic procedures for hip subluxation. Despite this, he still has a dislocated hip.

Jenny, his mother, has attended outpatient appointments regularly. Concerns presented at appointments have usually centered around seizure control or her perceived need for Tom to have more therapy with the aim of optimizing his progress. She has also reported that Tom is often unsettled at night and does not sleep well, which she believes is due to significant pain. She has informed clinicians that she gets up on about four occasions during the night to turn him and make him more comfortable. Despite this significant demand and inevitable sleep disruption, Jenny has not expressed any particular concern about this challenging aspect of his care. The hospital team believes that it provides family-centered care. Jenny's manner has always seemed calm and she presents as an intelligent competent individual, and thus the team has not pursued the family situation further or obtained a detailed psychosocial history. Jenny has always advocated for Tom and, in particular, has been quite successful in obtaining various pieces of equipment for him.

Tom has a prolonged seizure lasting more than 30 minutes and is admitted to hospital. After 2 days he is ready for discharge with a revised antiseizure regimen. It is noted that Jenny does not visit him whilst he is an inpatient. Neither does his father, Michael, although this is not surprising given he never attends the outpatient appointments.

When he is due for discharge, the nursing staff make telephone contact. Jenny states that she and Michael are unable to take him home, as they are at breaking point and they can no longer care for him. She tells the nurse that they have not had a full night's sleep in years and that this in turn is causing substantial conflict. She fears that her marriage will break down if Tom comes home. Jenny states that she is going to leave him in hospital until an alternate place is found for him.

The nursing staff are devastated. How could a parent leave a child in hospital? Particularly a child who cannot communicate well and that is so dependent for every aspect of his care? The medical team is shocked and surprised. It had never realized that this particular mother was not coping well. She had always seemed so competent. They are also extremely angry with Jenny, sharing the same view as the nursing team, that it is heartless to leave such a child unsupported in a strange and alien environment.

Ethical challenges: what this may mean for the individuals involved

The child

Tom is in an unfamiliar and frightening environment. He is being cared for by nursing staff who do not know him and cannot communicate with him. Suddenly, for the first time in his life, Jenny is no longer at his side, looking after him, attending to his day-to-day care and turning him at night. He is unlikely to comprehend why this has happened.

In addition, Tom has a number of physical conditions that may be causing pain and be impacting on his quality of life, including his dislocated hip and his severe movement disorder. His lack of a reliable communication system means that he cannot convey any information to help clarify the source of his pain, nor can he express his distress, anger and disappointment to have been left in hospital. Why had his lack of a communication system not been addressed in the past? It is inevitable that Tom will have been aware of escalating issues at home prior to his admission to hospital. Despite the severity of his impairment, he will at some level be cognizant of parental well-being and will inevitably have been able to detect conflict and unhappiness in his parents. Children with even severe or profound intellectual impairments may be capable of detecting signs of conflict such as raised voices, angry tones or heated conversations. He may have been quite distressed by his home situation yet unable to share his unhappiness because of his lack of a reliable communication system.

Challenges

How can this difficult situation best be managed? It will be important to address his physical issues but also even more important to consider how best to manage his psychological distress. Tom has the right to live in a supportive family and have his care needs met. This is embedded in Article 9 and Article 18 of the Convention of the Rights of the Child, which declares that every child has the right to know and grow up with the support of their family (United Nations 1989). Parents have an obligation to provide for their children's physical and emotional needs. For most parents providing this care is innate, but what if the parents say they can no longer cater for his needs? The United

Nations Convention on the Rights of Persons with Disabilities states that children with disabilities should be able to enjoy all human rights and fundamental freedoms on an equal basis with other children. Importantly, the Convention also states that the best interests of the child should be a primary consideration. Article 23 states that a child should not be separated from his or her parents against their will but it also states that where the immediate family is unable to care for the child, every effort should be made to provide alternate care within the wider family and, failing that, within the community in a family setting (United Nations 2006).

Establishing the best way forward is challenging. Doing the very best for Tom is the primary consideration – his needs are paramount. Time is also an issue. Determining whether this family can be reunited with appropriate supports is likely to be a lengthy process. On the other hand, moving as quickly as possible is important for Tom, to find alternatives if there is no hope of him returning home. For how long should one persist in trying to restore the family situation? Time is also needed for staff to reflect on why this situation has reached crisis point.

In the meantime, providing constant nursing staff may help a little. Exploring the possibility of a member of the extended family becoming more closely involved may also assist this difficult situation. Encouraging the parents to come in to see him as a first step would be useful provided they can be relaxed and responsive to his needs. Is this also the right time to attempt to address his physical issues and to determine whether an appropriate communication system can be put in place?

The parents and the extended family

After several days, Jenny agrees to come to the hospital. Further assessment by the team social worker reveals that she is significantly depressed. She cannot recall being happy in a long time and has little time to reflect on her feelings and ability to cope. Jenny has busied herself with the care of Tom, organizing household matters and persevering with applications for equipment that might make Tom more comfortable. She reports that she has never been able to share her feelings given that in her family, it was considered 'weak' to seek help. She reports that Michael works long hours and has little time to contribute to Tom's care. When he is at home, he tends to drink too much alcohol, which causes significant parental conflict. At times, he becomes violent after periods of drinking.

Challenges

Is it our clinical or ethical responsibility as child health professionals to detect and investigate these family problems at an early stage? Should we have known sooner that Jenny was not coping, was stressed and extremely unhappy, or that there were major family issues? If family-centered practice is key to the way clinicians work, why did the team not assess and respond to the family situation? Healthcare providers have been 'trapped' in the net of attending to this boy's many health and impairment-related needs but overlooked what was the most important factor for Tom – having stable and happy parents caring for him.

What appeared on the surface to be a calm and competent individual was, in retrospect, a façade that was maintained at professional encounters. Is it appropriate or ethical that this boy has received several orthopedic operations and yet staff did not detect the considerable parental distress? Should mental health and psychological issues of the parents be prioritized over physical issues or at least valued equally? Will the parents feel comfortable to disclose their mental health struggles to a health professional who works with their child? How far can we probe into a family's life? Jenny clearly did not want to tell us about how things were for her and her family prior to the situation reaching crisis point. In particular, she has never reported about Michael's behavior and his lack of involvement in caring for Tom.

However, were there more subtle signs that were not picked up in appointments? Could clinicians have delved a bit deeper when asking her how she was feeling? Could it be assumed that maintaining good mental health is challenging given the years of broken sleep and the day-to-day care of Tom? Did anyone ask about her and her husband and whether they were getting some time on their own? Did clinicians check to ensure that Jenny was connected with cerebral palsy specific associations and parent support groups that could provide Jenny and the family with more support?

"Ethically, do clinicians and the program of services have a responsibility to ask about the well-being of the whole family?"

Michael never comes to outpatient appointments. How can we bring him 'to the table' when he attends outpatient appointments so infrequently? Is he using alcohol in an effort to deal with his own depression and anxiety? Should there be mechanisms to identify when parents are not coping well, but also to implement strategies to prevent them and to promote family resilience? If time and resources prevent clinicians from taking the detailed psychosocial history that is required, who else will identify these families? Ethically, do clinicians and the program of services have a responsibility to ask about the well-being of the whole family? Was that done in this situation?

The clinicians directly involved in the story

Up to this time, clinicians have been preoccupied with this boy's many medical needs, including adjusting medications and ensuring appropriate referrals are made to specialists such as gastroenterologists (for gastrostomy care) and orthopedic surgeons (for hip problems). Those working closely with Tom were profoundly upset by the situation and frustrated that they had not detected the issues that were surfacing. They felt guilty that the situation escalated and at that point seemed irreparable.

Challenges

From this scenario, it seems that little attention was paid to the needs of the family, or to the mother's mental health. The clinicians accepted that Jenny was coping, without delving further into the background. Attempts to discuss how the family was getting along were side-tracked into the need for more therapy and better control of the seizures. Mental health issues were overlooked until the time of crisis.

Assessing and managing parental well-being takes significant time and expertise. There needs to be a trusting relationship between the clinician and parent if parents are to disclose mental health issues. Outpatient schedules are always tight and yet this is not an excuse for overlooking a serious situation. That said, if clinicians are going to bring up parental mental health in appointments, there needs to be enough time to ensure that they can listen meaningfully and respond and refer appropriately. Physicians involved in Tom's medical management may not have been well trained in discussing or evaluating mental health issues in parents and carers or had the time or rapport to explore parental mental health.

What ethical responsibility do clinicians have to explore these issues even when they feel they may not have the time or abilities to assess them adequately? Is it ethical to turn a 'blind eye' and trust that someone else will detect and deal with these problems? With whom does the responsibility lie to see, hear, listen and act? Often there are many providers for these children and their families. Should this responsibility rest with a particular health professional, for example, a social worker? What is our responsibility to consider the needs of siblings who may be significantly distressed in this situation? (See also Chapter 19 by Peter Blasco.) Research suggests that very few disability and health professionals enquire about the emotional health of parents, focusing on the child as the unit of care (Wodehouse & McGill 2009). How do we ensure that clinicians gain the expertise that is required? In turn, how do we protect the well-being of clinicians who may be taking on this additional role without feeling adequately equipped?

Even if a problem with parental mental health is detected it may be challenging to find the right services to address the complex needs faced by parents who have a child with severe impairments.

The healthcare system and society at large

A long and challenging hospitalization is an unsatisfactory and expensive way to address the problems faced by this family. Early detection of parental mental health issues and early intervention are both essential for supporting family well-being. It is the role and responsibility of the service system to ensure that mental health is addressed. Clear guidelines need to be developed so that all those involved in the care of children with disabilities are made aware of the importance of this area and that mental health issues cannot be neglected.

Supporting mental well-being

Much emphasis is required to build well-being into our endeavors to reduce mental health problems in carers. We can do this by enquiring whether carers are having some time for themselves, have supportive relationships, and are able to ask for help. Although parents may feel guilty in taking time out for themselves, it is important to highlight the strong relationship between parental well-being and child well-being.

Although a focus on a family well-being approach is consistent with family-centered practice, which has been strongly advocated in childhood disability services, the reality is that services are still set up to provide direct biomedical support to the child and to a lesser extent, to support their parents.

Developing a surveillance system to support family well-being

Regular screening for mental health problems for both parents and siblings is key to early identification of problems and referral for appropriate services. Although there are many tools to choose from, the Kessler 10 (Kessler et al. 2002) is a psychometrically well-developed tool that could be useful to assess psychological distress. For siblings aged 3–18 years, the Strengths and Difficulties Questionnaire (Goodman 1994, 1997) may be useful to assess emotional and behavioral problems. Screening at transition times, such as at the time of diagnosis, school entry and transition to postschool options, is particularly important. Screening may be challenging because of lack of time, lack of comfort and skills to manage mental health effectively, lack of clarity on whose role it is to discuss family mental health and well-being, unclear referral pathways and long waiting lists. For example, a qualitative study of pediatricians in Greece demonstrated that fear of stigmatization was a key barrier to commencing discussions about the possibility of maternal depression (Agapidaki et al. 2014). Additionally, parental perspectives on screening within the child healthcare system require further investigation. However a lack of information about mental health has profound effects for the child and must be prioritized.

Finding appropriate resources

There is a need for resources (e.g. brochures, websites, apps) to support parents to reflect regularly on their health and well-being and increase their understanding about mental health. Although some parents may be able to work through these resources with limited support, others may require more extensive help from health professionals. These resources may be useful for opening up discussions between clinicians and parents. Local resources need to be developed, and knowledge of these resources needs to become widespread with opportunity for more in-depth counseling and psychological and psychiatric help when required.

Resolution

Jenny began to visit Tom. There were many meetings with her, and eventually Michael also came to the hospital. The nursing staff in particular found it difficult to interact with Jenny as they still felt upset over her behavior. Time was set aside so that staff could debrief and also discuss how such a situation could be prevented in the future. Jenny began to have treatment for her depression and she reported that she was feeling better. Tom's stay in hospital was protracted. However, the time was used to investigate the source of his pain and to institute appropriate medical treatment for his proven gastro-esophageal reflux. In addition, the speech pathologist devoted considerable time to assessing his communication skills and was eventually able to provide an electronic communication device. Once a communication system was in place, a child psychiatrist became involved and commenced some individual work with Tom. Tom's rights to have an appropriate means of communication and to enjoy better health were addressed.

Despite these changes in Tom's situation, the parents remained resolved in their decision not to take him home. Finding out-of-home placement was difficult given his complex needs, but suitable foster parents were eventually trained and he could be discharged to their care. The hospital team advocated for and was successful in obtaining increased social worker input for their families and additionally had a number of in-service sessions focusing on parental well-being and ways to promote awareness of mental health issues.

Themes for discussion

- The WHO's International Classification of Functioning, Disability and Health (ICF) is a modern framework for health and many people argue that it should be the organizing principle around which services are provided for children like Tom and his family. In what ways and to what extent, does the ICF framework obligate professionals to engage with families? What are your own thoughts about this?

- Although 'family-centered service' (FCS) is often considered a modern standard approach to the way in which professionals should work with families like Tom's, many people have doubts and concerns about FCS. What are some of the myths and concerns – and how might these be addressed?

- In your program/center/community, how might the issues experienced by Tom's parents and family be approached and managed? Are there opportunities for improvement in whatever is currently available?

References

Abbeduto L, Seltzer MM, Shattuck P, Krauss MW, Orsmond G, Murphy MM (2004) Psychological well-being and coping in mothers of youths with autism, Down syndrome, or fragile X syndrome. *Am J Mental Retard* 109: 237–254.

Agapidaki E, Souliotis K, Jackson SF et al. 2014. Pediatricians' and health visitors' views towards detection and management of maternal depression in the context of a weak primary health care system: a qualitative study. *BMC Psychiatr* 14: 108.

Bailey DB, Golden RN, Roberts J, Ford A (2007) Maternal depression and developmental disability: Research critique. *Mental Retard Dev Disab Res Rev* 13: 321–329.

Goodman R (1994) A modified version of the Rutter Parent Questionnaire including extra items on children's strengths: A research note. *J Child Psychol Psychiatr* 35: 1483–1494.

Goodman R (1997) The strengths and difficulties questionnaire: A research note. *J Child Psychol Psychiatr* 38: 581–586.

Kessler RC, Andrews G, Colpe LJ et al. (2002) Short screening scales to monitor population prevalences and trends in non-specific psychological distress. *Psychol Med* 32: 959–976.

Miodrag N, Hodapp RM (2010) Chronic stress and health among parents of children with intellectual and developmental disabilities. *Curr Opin Psychiatr* 23: 407–411.

Murray L (2009) The development of children of postnatally depressed mothers: Evidence from the Cambridge longitudinal study. *Psychoanal Psychother* 23: 185–199.

Nankervis KL, Rosewarne AC, Vassos MV (2011) Respite and parental relinquishment of care: A comprehensive review of the available literature. *J Policy Pract Intell Disab* 8: 150–162.

Oelofsen N, Richardson P (2006) Sense of coherence and parenting stress in mothers and fathers of preschool children with developmental disability. *J Intell Dev Disab* 31: 1–12.

Singer GH, Floyd F (2006) Meta-analysis of comparative studies of depression in mothers of children with and without developmental disabilities. *Am J Mental Retard* 111: 155–169.

Smith LE, Seltzer MM, Tager-Flusberg H, Greenberg JS, Carter AS (2008) A comparative analysis of well-being and coping among mothers of toddlers and mothers of adolescents with ASD. *J Autism Dev Disord* 38: 876–889.

Stein A, Ramchandani P, Murray L (2008) Impact of parental psychiatric disorder and physical illness. In: Rutter M, Bishop DVM, Pine DS et al., editors. *Rutter's child and adolescent psychiatry*, 5th edn, pp. 407–420. Oxford: Blackwell Publishing.

United Nations (1989) Convention on the rights of the child [Online]; http://www.ohchr.org/en/professionalinterest/pages/crc.aspx.

United Nations (2006) Convention on the rights of persons with disabilities [Online]; www.un.org/disabilities/default.asp?id=150 (accessed 12 January 2015).

Wodehouse G, McGill P (2009) Support for family carers of children and young people with developmental disabilities and challenging behaviour: What stops it being helpful? *J Intell Disab Res* 53: 644–653.

Chapter 21

Tensions regarding the processes associated with decision-making about intervention

Lora Woo, Eunice Shen and Elizabeth Russel

Prologue

In the day-to-day practice of providing occupational and physical therapy services to children with orthopedic and neurological conditions, ethical practice issues arise at many levels. Children with neurodevelopmental impairments require not only therapy services but also case management and coordination among multiple care providers, including parents, physicians, therapists and community services such as schools. Different perspectives, values and priorities may affect parent–clinician, clinician–clinician and clinician–organization interactions in delivering needed therapy services to this population.

The professional organizations for occupational and physical therapy assert that therapists should uphold core values of altruism, equality, integrity, dignity, justice and excellence (American Occupational Therapy Association 2010; American Physical Therapy Association n.d.). However, the complexities of daily practice can create challenging encounters that are difficult to navigate and resolve. Therapists, children and their parents manage their daily needs and responsibilities, ranging from getting to school or work on time to meeting productivity standards or other performance expectations. All involved in the care of children with special needs should have the best interests of the child at the forefront of their intended efforts;

however, other factors – such as organizational structures and policies, workplace and home demands, or personal philosophies, values and beliefs – may cause unwanted or inadvertent discord. Disagreements can emerge with decision-making about interventions for children with neurodevelopmental impairments and an approach to examine these ethical practice issues can be employed to address and resolve such tensions.

Clinical scenario: a typical day in a therapy clinic

It is always a delight on a Monday to start the week with little Sammy coming into the therapy clinic squealing with enthusiasm and love of life. How can Mondays be bad? At 3 years of age, Sammy has been coming to see the therapists at the clinic for treatment of his spastic diplegic cerebral palsy, Gross Motor Function Classification System (GMFCS) II and Manual Abilities Classification System (MACS) II. Both of his moms have been very pleased with his care and with his transition to preschool. They have been diligent in bringing Sammy in for his therapy sessions, arranging their work schedules and family members to help. Now at his routine evaluation, the therapist notes the progress Sammy has made and is recommending periodic monitoring of his abilities with daily living and mobility skills. The therapist feels Sammy really does not need to come in every week for therapy as he has been since he was a baby. However, Sammy's moms are concerned as they feel he's done so well with therapy, how will he continue to make such gains if therapy services are reduced? How will he progress if he does not receive therapy every week? It stands to reason, the more therapy you get, the better you do.

Next comes Kaeko. She is 10 years old, attends fourth grade in school and has a diagnosis of choreoathetosis. It has been 10 months since she was last seen in this publicly-funded therapy clinic as her parents took her out of therapy, disagreeing with the treatment plan at the time. Her parents wanted her to walk, but back then Kaeko had very little weight-bearing ability and could only walk 5 to 10 feet in a gait trainer. Gait training had been provided for 2 years with limited progress and the therapist had wanted to switch to powered mobility training. With divergent beliefs on the direction of therapy for Kaeko, her parents found a private clinic to provide therapy services for her and specifically to work on gait training. However, funding for services at the private clinic eventually ended and now Kaeko returns to this clinic for services. Kaeko's parents bring her and the loaner walker she has been using in therapy, insisting that gait training be continued and that the therapist provide medical justification for the purchase of a walker using public funds. Current re-evaluation shows Kaeko is still functioning at GMFCS Level IV and MACS Level III. Based on the evaluation results, the therapist concludes that walking is not a functional goal and recommends that therapy should concentrate on preparations for powered mobility.

The clinic day ends with the yearly re-evaluation of Jose who is 17 years old and has spina bifida. As part of the re-evaluation, Jose and his therapist complete the Canadian Occupational

Performance Measure (COPM) (Law et al. 2005) and he identifies the desire to be independent with making a simple meal and using public bus transportation to go to community college next year. Additional evaluation findings of environmental and personal factors include: family moved to their current residence last year; Jose's mother has decided to re-enter the work force now that the children are older; and Jose has a girlfriend. The therapist wants to recommend therapy three times a week as Jose is now interested in these specific areas of household and community tasks. However, knowing how short-staffed the clinic is and the facility's philosophy of prioritizing therapy services for infants, toddlers and elementary school-aged children, the supervisor wants the therapist to propose therapy once per week for Jose. Jose's father works at night but is very invested in obtaining the services Jose needs and would be willing to bring Jose to all the therapy appointments, even if this is every day of the week.

In pediatric rehabilitation, healthcare providers may encounter clinical situations that pose ethical dilemmas. However, certain clinical situations may not represent an ethical dilemma at all but rather a legal issue, a difference in professional opinion, or simply the accepted practices of the organization. An ethical dilemma is one characterized by complexity and involves conflicting moral principles or values. Ethical dilemmas differ from legal dilemmas (as no laws are violated) and from practice dilemmas such as simple disagreements on therapeutic interventions, for example, whether providing jaw control for eating is more effective from the front or from the side of the child's face. Generally, there is no simple solution in a genuine ethical dilemma and resolution often involves collaboration and consensus building while respecting the integrity of the individual's values and beliefs.

In therapy, there are several models or methods for ethical decision-making including the 'Realm-Individual Process-Situation Model of Ethical Decision-Making' (Swisher et al. 2005), the 'Patient-Centered Care Ethics Analysis Model for Rehabilitation' (Hunt & Ells 2013) and the 'Clinical Ethics and Legal Issues Bait All Therapists Equally Method for Analyzing Ethical Dilemmas' (Kornblau & Burkhardt 2012). However, for the purposes of this chapter, we will explore each of these scenarios using an adaptation of Morris's ethical decision-making model (Morris 2003; Slater 2011). This model provides a sequential process by addressing pivotal questions to determine if the situation is actually an ethical dilemma and then analyzing and evaluating a course of action for resolution:

- Am I facing an ethical dilemma here?
  - What are the relevant facts, values and beliefs?
  - Who are the key people involved?
  - What exactly is the dilemma? Is this an ethical issue, involving conflicts of principles or values, or a practice dilemma?

- Analysis
  - What are the possible courses of action?
  - What are the conflicts that can arise from each action?
  - Propose a course of action
- Evaluate proposed course of action
  - Applicable ethical principles/code of ethics

The Occupational Therapy Code of Ethics and Ethics Standards from the American Occupational Therapy Association (2011) and the Code of Ethics for the Physical Therapist from the American Physical Therapy Association (n.d.) will be used to analyze the following ethical dilemmas (see also Appendix 21.1, p. 248).

Sammy and ongoing therapy

Sammy has made nice progress with therapy services three times per week. Now that he is in preschool, the demands on his daily schedule have changed. He loves going to school, playing with his friends and learning new things every day. He has wonderful support with both of his mothers and extended family and friends. His parents want to ensure he receives the best of everything they can possibly provide for him, including advocating for therapy services.

What is the ethical dilemma?
The following are the relevant facts, values and beliefs:

- Providing therapy three times per week would take Sammy away from the natural environment of school and from participating in play activities, thus limiting his social interaction.

- He has made good progress with previous therapy, meeting goals at appropriate levels but has now plateaued.

- His family believes more therapy is better and values therapy services.

- His therapist enjoys working with Sammy and his mothers. Parents are consistently cooperative and enthusiastic, responsive to home program suggestions. On one level, the therapist would like to maintain him as a patient and is not sure that someone else can do as well as she can with facilitating his development. On another level, she feels committed to her clinical judgment that decreasing the frequency of therapy is most appropriate at this time and that integration of learned daily activity skills in a natural environment is best to promote participation.

The key people involved:

- Although Sammy is minimally physically involved, his social-emotional development is that of a typical 3-year-old desiring peer contact and social interaction provided within the preschool setting.

- Mothers are invested in what is best for Sammy, and having seen the rapid progress in the early intervention program, they want this level of progress to continue. They question whether the decreased therapy services can continue this level of progress (provide what Sammy needs at this time) and strongly believe that 'more is better'.

- With an extended family, Sammy has a supportive social network including grandparents, aunts and uncles and cousins. They all want what is best for Sammy and cheer him on with his developmental achievements despite the impairments; they are all willing to do anything to help him participate in his activities (e.g. school, therapy, play dates).

- The school teacher has 15 years of experience in preschool education and feels strongly that education can provide what a child at Sammy's level needs. She wants him fully involved in the classroom program and activities and not pulled out for therapy treatment.

- The therapist has extensive experience in early intervention. She feels that Sammy's rapid progress is a result of intervention, as well as typical central nervous system maturation. What Sammy needs now is to practice developmental skills in the natural environment.

- The director of the facility is satisfied when parents and therapist work together effectively. She encourages collaboration with her staff in order to reduce conflict.

- From a societal viewpoint, the evidence supports the importance of preschool in the development of social skills necessary to become an active member of society.

The dilemma: this is an ethical dilemma for the therapist because of the conflict between her values and those of the parents. Is it permissible for the therapist to provide the amount of therapy services as requested by Sammy's parents despite her professional judgment based on assessment results and evidence to the contrary?

Analysis of the dilemma
There are a number of possible courses of action and consequences or conflicts that can arise with each action:

- Do nothing different/continue to provide therapy three times per week.

  - Avoid conflict between parents and therapist.

- The therapist may feel conflicted over providing therapy services in a clinic setting as requested by the parents, when the practice of skills in the natural environment would best meet Sammy's needs.

- May not be doing what is best for the child – he could be socializing with school friends.

- Discuss progress with the family and rationale for current recommendations with reassurance that the therapist is not abandoning Sammy but will continue to monitor and provide intensive services as needed.

  - The family may still insist on three times per week therapy.

  - Sammy may not continue to progress developmentally without the intensive intervention.

- Work with the teacher to incorporate skills into school activities/environment.

  - The teacher may not be receptive to the therapist's input, may not see this as part of their job.

  - The parents may still not be satisfied with this alternate approach to therapy services.

- Decrease therapy services as recommended.

  - The family may be upset with the therapist for not agreeing with them.

  - The family may complain to the therapist's supervisor.

Proposed course of action: Discuss with the family exactly what goals they wish to accomplish, review the progress Sammy has made, emphasize opportunities for Sammy to use the skills he has developed in the new environment of school, explain evidence indicating the benefits of periods of intense treatment followed by practice in natural environments (e.g. home, school) and offer availability to consult with the school teacher and family.

Applicable professional guidelines
The following ethical principles and code of ethics, from the American Occupational Therapy Association (AOTA) (2011) and the American Physical Therapy Association (APTA) (n.d.), have bearing in this situation with Sammy.

AOTA ethical principles and code of ethics:

- Beneficence

  - Provide appropriate evaluation and plan of intervention specific to needs.

- Re-evaluate child to determine if goals are being achieved and whether intervention plans needs to be revised.
- Use to the extent possible, evaluations, planning and intervention that are evidence-based.
- Autonomy
  - Establish a collaborative relationship with child, family and significant others in setting goals and priorities.

APTA ethical principles and code of ethics:

- Professional duty
  - Provide information necessary to allow family to make informed decisions.
  - Collaborate to empower in decisions about care.
- Excellence
  - Demonstrate professional judgment informed by best evidence, patient values and practitioner's experience.
- Social responsibility
  - Avoid overutilization of therapy service.

In this situation there are conflicting aspects of ethical principles. The therapist's viewpoint is supported by the principle of beneficence (e.g. by providing appropriate and evidence-based intervention), as well as the principle of social responsibility by avoiding overutilization of therapy services. However, the principles of autonomy and professional duty highlight the need to collaborate with the family and allow the family to make informed decisions.

Resolution

Although collaboration with the family is a hallmark of excellence in pediatric therapy, the wishes of the family cannot be the only factor to determine therapy needs. The therapist proceeds with her recommendation to decrease the frequency of services. She meets with the parents and the teacher to explain and reassure them that she is available at any point for consultation. The mothers meet with the facility supervisor to request maintenance of level of services and the supervisor agrees to a compromise of once per week for a semester, with which the therapist concurs.

Kaeko and therapy goals

Kaeko's parents make it clear that they feel the private therapy was better and state that their family pediatrician concurred with this. Despite talking with the parents about the appropriateness of powered mobility for Kaeko at this time, the parents are not persuaded. The therapist is frustrated and finds it hard to hide her anger, sharing with her supervisor and the staff her feelings that some parents can be unrealistic, insisting that children should walk when evidence is available to show that this is highly unlikely.

What is the ethical dilemma?
The following are the relevant facts, values and beliefs:

- The therapist feels offended that the parents went elsewhere for therapy and they were not able to trust the therapist's judgment about mobility.
- The parents value therapy services but believe that private therapy was better (e.g. Kaeko using a walker).
- The clinic therapist and administration value family-centered care in the provision of therapy services.
- The family pediatrician feels Kaeko would be able to walk given sufficient skilled intervention.
- Society generally places great value in the ability of individuals to walk independently.

The key people involved:

- Kaeko enjoyed going to therapy at private clinic.
- The parents liked the private therapy clinic and therapist, and want to continue gait training.
- The family pediatrician sees nothing wrong with continuing gait training.
- The facility management wants no conflicts.
- The clinic therapist desires recognition of her clinical professional judgment regarding the functional outcome of walking.
- The private therapist feels more time spent in gait training is appropriate.
- On a societal level, public funds should be used in a fiscally responsible manner.

The dilemma: Is it permissible for the therapist to recommend the purchase of a walker for gait training despite her clinical professional judgment in favor of powered mobility?

Analysis of the dilemma
There are a number of possible courses of action and consequences or conflicts that can arise with each action:

- The clinic therapist can disparage the private therapist and pediatrician.

  - The private therapist and pediatrician may file a complaint with the clinic therapist's supervisor.

  - The therapist may be reprimanded by the supervisor for unprofessional behavior.

- The clinic therapist can meet with parents and present research evidence to support her conclusion that walking was tried for 2 years with limited success and continuing this approach is not appropriate at this time.

  - The parents may still insist on use of a walker.

  - The parents may enlist support of private therapist and pediatrician for a walker.

- The parents may complain to the management that the therapy being offered is not right for their daughter and threaten to sue.

  - The clinic therapist may be instructed to provide what parents want.

- The clinic therapist can do what parents ask and see Kaeko for gait training with walker.

  - The parents will be happy.

  - The therapist may become angry or frustrated.

  - This may possibly be a poor use of available resources.

- The clinic therapist can contact the private therapist for further information and clarification of her position.

  - The private therapist may provide justification for a walker and gait training, thus not supporting a change to powered mobility training.

Proposed course of action: The clinic therapist gathers all viewpoints by calling the private therapist and pediatrician, explaining her reasoning for not pursuing gait training at this time. She meets with the family to present evidence on walking and continues to recommend powered mobility training.

Applicable professional guidelines
The following ethical principles and code of ethics from AOTA (2010) and APTA (n.d.) have application in the situation with Kaeko.

AOTA ethical principles and code of ethics:

- Beneficence

  - Use, to the extent possible, evaluations, planning and intervention that are evidence-based.

- Fidelity

  - Respect competencies of own and other professions.

  - Use conflict resolution to resolve organizational and interpersonal conflicts.

APTA ethical principles and code of ethics:

- Integrity

  - Recognize personal biases and not discriminate against other practitioners.

- Compassion, professional duty

  - Provide services with compassionate and caring behaviors.

- Integrity

  - Demonstrate professional judgment informed by best evidence.

  - Communicate and collaborate with other health care professionals.

The primary ethical principles revolve around recognizing personal biases and respecting the competencies of others, including a difference in treatment philosophy. Both therapists feel that their professional judgment is informed by the best available evidence. The clinic therapist is also dealing with the issues of providing services with compassion when her professional expertise is being questioned.

Resolution

Despite the therapist's attempts at collaboration with family, physician and private therapist, the parents continue to disagree with the therapist's recommendations and with due process proceed to formal dispute resolution in a fair hearing process. The hearing officer decides in favor of the family and orders the public agency to purchase the walker and provide therapy for gait training.

Jose and frequency of therapy recommendations

Jose has had intensive therapy intermittently over the years. Legally soon to become an adult, Jose is very excited and eager to be more independent and to embark on vocational training. With Jose's motivation and self-identified goals for therapy, parental support and evaluation findings the therapist recommends therapy three times per week; however, the supervisor wants therapy only once a week due to the limited number of staff to provide services. Given Jose's enthusiasm and readiness to learn to function more independently, his family support of his goal attainment and the age-appropriateness of his desired developmental skill acquisition, the therapist struggles with the supervisor's request.

Based on the clinical evaluation, knowledge of his health condition and his contextual factors, the therapist believes Jose would benefit from skilled therapy intervention three times per week. However, the therapist is also aware that this would potentially place an undue burden on the therapy staff and the program to provide therapy services this frequently. The therapist could face resentment or hostility from co-workers and, being a therapist new to this facility, she does not want to cause any trouble so early in her career here. Nonetheless, is it not the therapist's professional obligation to make recommendations based upon the patient's individualized needs? Is this not why she pursued a career as an occupational therapist – to help people develop skills to participate in important and meaningful daily activities and thus be able to participate as a member in society? Yet the therapist is acutely aware of the need to heed her supervisor in order to maintain this new job.

What is the ethical dilemma?
The following are the relevant facts, values and beliefs:

- Jose is ready to progress with community skills.

- Jose values being more independent as he will soon legally become an adult. He would like to be able to get around and interact with his peers without having to rely on his parents for transportation.

- The father is interested in Jose being more independent and participating more with peers.

- The facility is understaffed.

- The therapist does not want to upset colleagues with a possible increase in workload.

- The therapist's supervisor needs to ensure patients are receiving recommended services given available resources (e.g. staffing).

- Society values productive contributing members who are not a burden to others.

The key people involved:

- Jose is now in late adolescence and has come to the realization that he wants to be more independent and wants to do more things with his friends, especially his girlfriend. He now states he is ready to participate actively in therapy.

- The father is very supportive of Jose increasing his independence.

- The therapy supervisor wants to be able to provide services to all patients cost-effectively.

- The facility administrator wants to maintain solvency by maximizing cost-effectiveness strategies.

- The therapist does not want to disobey the supervisor, but wants to be an ethical therapist.

- Disability rights advocacy group wants to advocate for patients and their rights to receive appropriate and needed services.

- Society values individuals who are self-sufficient, but challenges exist with funding for such rehabilitation services.

The dilemma: The therapist made recommendations for the frequency of therapy services based on the results of the evaluation and her professional judgment. Is it permissible for her to comply with her supervisor's order to limit therapy services due to staff shortage?

Analysis of the dilemma
There are a number of possible courses of action and consequences or conflicts that can arise with each action:

- The therapist can discuss the therapy frequency recommendation with the supervisor.
  - The supervisor may still not agree with therapist.
- The therapist recommends therapy once a week.
  - The supervisor may be delighted as this therapy recommendation would be easier to fulfill with existing staff.
  - Other staff may also be content as this would not require more work from them.
  - Jose may not make functional changes as quickly (benefit from therapy services).

- The therapist recommends therapy three times per week.
  - The therapist may incur displeasure from the supervisor.
  - Other staff and, possibly also the supervisor, may become hostile or resentful towards the therapist.
- The therapist informs the father of the disagreement regarding the frequency of therapy recommendations.
  - The father could go to the supervisor and insist on more therapy.
  - The father could involve an advocate to assist with obtaining the needed therapy services.

Proposed course of action: The therapist discusses with the supervisor, Jose and his father the rationale for therapy frequency, include collaborating with others (e.g. school teacher, vocational rehabilitation counselor) to work on community skills, and proposes three times per week with direct treatment and collaboration for 2 months followed by reassessment of needs.

Applicable professional guidelines
The following AOTA (2010) and APTA (n.d.) ethical principles and code of ethics are relevant in this situation with Jose.

AOTA ethical principles and code of ethics:

- Beneficence
  - Provide appropriate evaluation and plan of intervention for all recipients specific to their needs.
- Non-maleficence
  - Avoid compromising client's well-being based on arbitrary administrative directives by exercising professional judgment and critical analysis.
- Autonomy
  - Establish collaborative relationship with recipients of services in setting goals and priorities.
- Social justice
  - Advocate for just and fair treatment for all patients and encourage colleagues to abide by the highest standards of social justice.

APTA ethical principles and code of ethics:

- Professional duty, compassion
  - Provide information necessary to allow patients to make informed decisions.
  - Collaborate with patients to empower them in decisions about their health care.
- Integrity
  - Demonstrate independent and objective professional judgment in patient's best interest.
  - Communicate and collaborate with peers as necessary.
- Accountability
  - Promote practice that supports professional judgment.

The primary ethical issue is to avoid compromising a patient's well-being by failing to act in their best interest. The therapist has the responsibility to advocate for therapy services based on evaluation results and the intervention plan. The facility administration has the responsibility to ensure fair treatment for all patients given the resources available.

Resolution

Ethical practice dictates that the needs of the patient would pre-empt the needs of the organization. The supervisor calls a staff meeting with all involved to discuss adjustments to schedules to allow for the recommended treatment for Jose. Jose is also referred to vocational rehabilitation services for assessment.

Epilogue

Ethical and professional practice involves continual learning and self-reflection. For therapists, situations may arise where there is an ethical concern that requires an immediate response. Resolution to an ethical dilemma in such situations may not always be ideal as these situations may be fraught with emotions. However, reflecting back and analyzing the situation critically, using a model for ethical decision-making, can foster professional growth and development. In this chapter, the authors have utilized an adaptation of an ethical decision-making model offered by Morris (Slater 2011). It is hoped that this chapter provides therapists with guidance in approaching and resolving ethical situations regarding therapy interventions.

Themes for discussion

- In the cases used to illustrate issues in this chapter the authors refer to discipline-specific guidelines that can provide guidance in behaving in an ethical manner. What are the resources available to you? Can you find them? Have you read them? Have you ever had occasion to refer to them?

- As illustrated in these cases, it is almost always true that there are many 'actors' in the 'play' that is enacted in the course of our work? Is there a hierarchy in the 'cast'? Should there be? How can the potential tensions among the 'players' be addressed?

- The recommendations clinicians make about 'therapies' reflect both our views of what is important, and always reflect choices and trade-offs. What do you think might be the impact of hours of therapy to facilitate walking on the child's internal world – and what might the 'cost' of that therapy be?

References

American Occupational Therapy Association, Ethics Commission (2010) Occupational Therapy Code of Ethics and Ethics Standards 2010 edition. *Am J Occup Ther* 64: S17–S26.

American Physical Therapy Association (n.d.) *Code of ethics for the physical therapist* [online]; www.apta.org/uploadedFiles/APTAorg/About_Us/Policies/Ethics/CodeofEthics.pdf#search=%22ethics%22 (accessed 11 February 2012).

Hunt MR, Ells C (2013) A patient-centered care ethics analysis model for rehabilitation. *Am J Phys Med Rehab* 92: 818–827.

Kornblau BL, Burkhardt A (2012) *Ethics in rehabilitation: A clinical perspective* 2nd edn. Thorofare, NJ: Slack.

Law M, Baptiste S, Carswell A, McColl M, Polatajko H, Pollock N (2005). *Canadian occupational performance measure (COPM)* 4th edn. Toronto, ON: CAOT Publications ACE.

Morris JF (2003) Is it possible to be ethical? *OT Practice* 8: 18–23.

Slater DY, editor (2011) *Reference guide to the occupational therapy code of ethics & ethics standards* 2010 edn. Bethesda, MD: AOTA Press.

Swisher LL, Arslanian LE, Davis CM (2005) The Realm-Individual Process-Situation (RIPS) model of ethical decision-making. *Am Phys Ther Assoc, Section on Health Policy & Administration* 5: 1–8.

Appendix 21.1: American Occupational Therapy Association and APTA core values and code of ethics

AOTA	APTA
Core values	
Altruism: placing needs of others before one's own	Altruism
Equality: promoting fairness	Social responsibility
Freedom: personal choice	Integrity
Justice: structures organized so that all can function and flourish	Accountability
Dignity: treating others with respect	Compassion/caring
Truth: providing accurate information	Excellence
Prudence: using reasoning, judgment and reflection to make decisions	Professional duty
Code of ethics	
(1) Beneficence: concern for well-being and safety of others	(1) Respect inherent dignity and rights of all (compassion, integrity)
(2) Non-maleficence: do not cause harm	(2) Trustworthy and compassionate in addressing rights and needs of others (altruism, compassion, professional duty)
(3) Autonomy: right to individual self-determination	(3) Accountable in making sound professional judgments (excellence, integrity)
(4) Social justice: promote fairness and equality	(4) Demonstrate integrity in relationships with others (integrity)
(5) Procedural justice: comply with regulations	(5) Fulfill legal and professional obligations (professional duty, accountability)
(6) Veracity: provide accurate information	(6) Enhance expertise through lifelong learning (excellence)
(7) Fidelity: treat others with respect and fairness	(7) Promote organizational behaviors and business practices benefiting patients and society (integrity, accountability)
	(8) Participate in efforts to meet health needs of all people (social responsibility)

Source: American Occupational Therapy Association (2010) and American Physical Therapy Association (n.d.)

Chapter 22

Can't you just do therapy? When there is disagreement about discharge from therapy

Janey McGeary Farber and Harriet Fain-Tvedt

Prologue

Yvonne W is a 15-year-old girl with cerebral palsy (CP) and a complicated medical history. Like so many of our patients, she presented a challenge to her care team in determining the appropriate frequency, dosing and timing of therapy services. After a pathologic fracture, Yvonne's caregivers were reluctant to continue with her home exercise program and her mother was concerned that Yvonne was having increased pain. During the episode of care focused on modifying the home program and supplying caregivers with strategies to reduce pain, hydrotherapy was trialed. Although Yvonne did not actively participate in activities in the pool, her mother perceived that pain was decreased for a few days after each session. The therapist provided education so that the program could be continued outside of therapy and discharged Yvonne from skilled services. Shortly thereafter, she returned to the clinic with an order from her community physician for pool therapy three times a week.

The ethical dilemmas we discuss in this case scenario revolve around the idea of 'futility', although one may be loath to employ the term so often used in reference to end-of-life issues. Effectiveness, benefits and burdens of treatment must be explored and analyzed in order to make decisions about the optimal course of care. The question of what is meant by physical therapy needs to be addressed, and with that, concepts of distributive justice. The human dimensions of hope and empathy cannot be overlooked.

Yvonne's primary diagnosis is spastic quadriparetic cerebral palsy, Gross Motor Function Classification System (GMFCS) Level V (Palisano et al. 2008), Manual Ability Classification System (MACS) Level IV (Eliasson et al. 2006), Communication Function Classification System (CFCS) Level IV (Hidecker et al. 2011) and Eating and Drinking Ability Classification System (EDACS) Level V (Sellers et al. 2014). She also has medically intractable epilepsy and multiple anomalies of the brain and spinal cord. Yvonne has significant kyphoscoliosis and wears a thoracolumbosacral orthosis (TLSO) when upright, in order to maintain a functional sitting (or standing) posture. Two orthopedic surgeons have recommended against corrective surgery for her spinal deformities: Yvonne has a history of long and complication-filled recoveries from surgery; she has very poor bone density and she tolerates the TLSO well. While wearing the TLSO, she has maintained good pulmonary and gastrointestinal health. She has a ventriculoperitoneal (VP) shunt that has been revised twice since its original placement at 18 months of age and she has a history of multiple pathological fractures including, most recently, a femoral fracture 10 months ago.

Yvonne is dependent for all activities of daily living and receives her nutrition through a feeding tube. She is also totally dependent on her caregivers and family for transfers and all mobility and is not able to participate in stand pivot transfers with any level of assistance. At baseline, she is placed in a stander daily for 25–40 minutes at a time. She is unable to sit or stand without total support, but does demonstrate good head control in these positions. Expressive language is very limited, but Yvonne can use facial expressions and vocalizations to communicate with her family, and her mother is aware of when she is experiencing pain.

Yvonne lives with her 41-year-old mother and her older brother, who serves as her personal care attendant. Her father passed away several months ago from complications following a stroke. Yvonne has 24 hour nursing care. She attends school daily and is in a special education classroom for five out of seven classes.

After her femoral fracture was fully healed, physical therapy services were provided one time a week for 45 minutes for a 6-month period. Caregivers were not completing her stretching exercises because they were fearful about causing a repeat fracture. Her mother was very concerned that Yvonne was experiencing pain a good deal of the time, but was reluctant to increase medications to address pain because of her concerns about side effects such as excessive drowsiness.

The plan of care included modifying the existing home exercise program to help her various caregivers avoid accidental fracture. The primary focus was to return her safely to the level of function she enjoyed before her fracture – that is, participation in her standing program and use of the gait trainer for physiological ambulation without signs of pain. Transcutaneous electric nerve stimulation (TENS) had been tried during a previous episode of care, but Yvonne had a reaction to the adhesive in both types of electrodes that were trialed. Her mother had expressed interest in trying a therapy session or two in the pool and this was supported by the physical therapist as a potential adjunct to a home program.

Attendance was good during the episode of care. All of the goals were achieved and Yvonne's mother reported that she was pleased with the outcomes of the episode of care.

Seven sessions of physical therapy were done in the pool and during these sessions, the therapist attempted to elicit active movement, including walking, reaching for toys in standing and kicking or paddling during supported swimming. When the primary physical therapist was on vacation, a second therapist who knew Yvonne well treated her in the pool. Despite using several different treatment and motivational strategies, the therapists were never able to stimulate active movement; however, Yvonne seemed to very much enjoy being supported in a floating position, with gentle movements side to side.

During the time that pool therapy was being trialed, the therapist spoke often with Yvonne's mother, reporting that she was noting no active participation. The therapist provided information and training to the family as to how to support Yvonne in a floating position and how to gently move her back and forth while floating. On one occasion, Yvonne's mother was able to participate in a pool session and had an opportunity to practice these skills.

On discharge, the physical therapist provided written home exercise program handouts personalized for Yvonne. One set of exercises consisted of passive and active assisted range of motion exercises and the other had activities for the pool, including the activities that her mother had practiced with her. Additionally, a list of community swimming pools was provided.

Three months after physical therapy services had been discontinued, Yvonne returned to the clinic with a prescription from her community physician for physical therapy three times a week, in the pool. During the evaluation, Yvonne's mother told the therapist that Yvonne's pain was decreased when she was in the pool: 'It just makes her feel better.' No other goals were identified. When asked if she had been able to try some of the techniques on her own in community pools, Yvonne's mother explained that the pools close enough to her were not within the family's budget.

The therapist contacted the physician to report on the results of the evaluation and determine if, perhaps, the physician had additional goals for therapy services. No goals were identified and the physician asked the physical therapist, 'Can't you just do therapy?' The therapy team was conflicted about this request because they felt that the benefits Yvonne received from being in water were not skilled therapy services.

The caregiver's perspective

Yvonne's mother knows that after Yvonne gets into the pool, she feels better, at least for a few days. She has never given up hope that Yvonne will someday improve and feels that the therapists are 'giving up on her daughter' when they recommend discharge from therapy or do not recommend ongoing services. Joining a health club or other community pool would place a burden on the family as Yvonne's mother works full-time and struggles financially, so both time and money would be barriers to the recommended approach.

Analysis

Does treatment in the pool help Yvonne feel better? As is often the case with parents of children with severe impairments, only Yvonne's mother is able to understand and interpret her daughter's communication. Even though Yvonne is not able to use verbal language or assistive technology to communicate, she can communicate with people with whom she has spent the majority of her life. Solely in terms of time, the physical therapist has spent 18–20 hours with Yvonne, while even accounting for school and sleep, her mother has been with her for thousands of hours. Simply put, Yvonne's mother should be considered an expert on Yvonne. This is an important foundation in most, if not all, definitions of family-centered care (Bamm & Rosenbaum 2008).

Thus, acknowledgement of the expertise of her mother should allow us to assume that Yvonne's pain is, indeed, positively affected by being in the pool.

By not recommending ongoing direct physical therapy services, is the physical therapist 'giving up' on Yvonne? What is her ethical responsibility in light of this lifelong reality? Lifelong impairments may require lifelong therapeutic intervention, but the level of intervention is titrated based on the need of the patient at that moment in time. Physical therapy includes, along with hands-on direct care, consultation, the development of home programs to continue therapeutic interventions and recommendations for community resources. Ethical practice includes understanding when direct physical therapy services are no longer warranted. Principle 3A, in the Code of Ethics for the Physical Therapist (PT) (APTA n.d.), states that 'PTs shall demonstrate *independent* and *objective* professional judgment in the patient's/client's best interest in all practice settings.' In Yvonne's case, even though the order from the physician is for physical therapy three times per week, the physical therapist is obligated to evaluate objectively the need for physical therapy. A home program has been established that has been shown to be effective in assisting with pain management. Education on implementing this home program has been completed. If this education were effective, there should not be a need for further physical skilled (direct) therapy at this point in time. Yvonne's caregivers should be able to provide her with the interventions that help maintain her current level of function.

Principle 3B enjoins physical therapists to '… demonstrate professional judgment informed by professional standards, evidence (including current literature and established best practice), practitioner experience, and patient/client values'. The best evidence in this case indicates that Yvonne's gross motor capacity will not improve over time. Best efforts were made to elicit increased participation toward progressive goals. Principle 8C guides physical therapists to '… be responsible stewards of healthcare resources and … avoid overutilization or underutilization of physical therapy services'. It is easy to understand that providing unnecessary services for the financial gain of the physical therapist is unethical. Is this ethical responsibility somehow invalidated if it is the patient who asks for services that are not necessary? Additionally, if physical therapy is provided three times per week for Yvonne, this is time that cannot be offered to other patients.

The pediatric physical therapist has the responsibility to support and inform patients and their caregivers, ensuring they have the information and resources necessary to carry out recommendations made for practice in the natural environment. This helps to avoid overutilization of services, while ensuring that children with impairments receive the interventions that help them most. This can be a truly challenging task as the pediatric physical therapist balances empathy with practical concerns.

Skilled physical therapy services are not indicated, but it is important to ensure that education has been effective.

How then to consider the issue of the financial burden that will be placed on Yvonne's mother to join a community pool? In making a case to a third-party payer for physical therapy, a therapist is expected to complete an evaluation that documents in detail the medical necessity for the proposed treatment, together with functional, measurable, achievable and time-limited goals. Functional goals may be defined as '… the individually meaningful activities that a person cannot perform as a result of an injury, illness, or congenital or acquired condition, but wants to be able to accomplish as a result of physical therapy' (Randall & McEwen 2000). During the last episode of care for Yvonne, the physical therapist explored many strategies to determine if therapy in the pool could help to achieve functional goals. Initially, one to two sessions were agreed upon, but in fact seven sessions were completed. The therapist reasoned that patients sometimes require a certain amount of repetition before beginning to respond to novel stimuli and made a recommendation to add a few sessions in order to fully explore the possibilities of this modality. Various techniques were attempted and a different therapist was even used, in case the lack of response was due to interpersonal factors. None of these strategies resulted in

Yvonne's active participation in exercises and activities. Aquatics appears to be a modality to which Yvonne responds positively. Additionally, it provides her family with the perception that someone is 'doing something' for Yvonne. In actuality, it does not meet the clear-cut criteria for medical necessity and continuing to recommend it as a therapy may be unethical. This expectation creates a dilemma for the therapists.

Physical therapy goals must be functional, measurable, achievable and time-limited.

The ordering physician's perspective

If a patient's mother reports that a given intervention, with no adverse effects, is helping her child, the physician may feel compelled to sanction or enable this treatment in the context of family-centered care.

Analysis

Why not 'just do therapy'? Physicians and therapists alike are keenly aware of the placebo and other positive 'side' effects and can often employ these to benefit a patient; whether that benefit is a measurable one can, at times, be a moot point. For example, a caregiver may report that a sensory technique such as compressions helps a child be more attentive. Even if the therapist does not observe any effect in attention with the compressions, they may endorse the continued use, because no harm is expected and the cost (in time and resources) is negligible. Perhaps a caregiver will report the benefits of an herbal remedy to the physician. After researching the remedy, the physician may, similarly, endorse its use if no harm is expected, even if she does not believe it will be helpful.

Physical therapy cannot analogously be employed as an anodyne – the therapist cannot 'just do therapy' – because interventions and treatment strategies are not, on their own, physical therapy. They are only a fraction of an autonomous practice that includes examination, evaluation, physical therapy diagnosis, prognosis, intervention and outcomes (see Guide to Physical Therapy Practice 3.0, http://guidetoptpractice. apta.org/). Physical therapy treatment cannot occur without assessment and development of objective goals.

Physical therapy treatment cannot be provided without a complete examination and evaluation, and subsequent careful documentation of medical need; a physical therapy episode of care includes functional goals, outcome measures and a plan for discharge.

The therapist's perspective on the ethical dilemmas inherent in this story

Physical therapy needs to be goal-directed and medically necessary. Charging for services the therapist feels are not beneficial violates the physical therapy code of ethics and is considered fraud under many systems, including Medicare. In some physical therapy practices, or in organizations that provide care, resources are limited, and providing services not medically necessary for one patient may result in resources not being available for other patients whose conditions meet the criteria for medical necessity. The prognostic power of the GMFCS allows therapists to formulate goals that are reasonable for each patient with cerebral palsy (Rosenbaum et al. 2008). That being said, there is always the child whose functional gains surprise even the most seasoned therapists. Families and therapists alike are not immune to the optimism that these anecdotal successes create.

Analysis

Would ongoing physical therapy three times per week in the pool be goal-directed and medically necessary? Yvonne's mother's stated goal for this episode of care is for her daughter to 'feel better'. She has refused increases or changes in pain medication because of concerns about side effects and TENS has been ruled out as an option. She reports that Yvonne feels good for two to three days after being in the pool and then starts having pain again. She would like therapy to continue for 'as long as it works', but there is, clearly, fundamental disagreement on what constitutes 'physical therapy'.

Although a pediatric physical therapist should be expected to work with a family to develop goals that are both based on the family's desired outcomes and are measurable, functional, achievable and time-limited, this does not seem possible in Yvonne's case. A goal to decrease pain would present difficulties in all four categories. Measurement would be limited to parental report and would be difficult to quantify, given Yvonne's communication impairments. No functional changes are to be expected, based on past performance and on functional ability predicted by Yvonne's age and GMFCS level. Although it is reported that it is possible to decrease Yvonne's pain, the goal is achievable only ephemerally, as there does not appear to be any long-lasting effect through the modalities that physical therapists can offer. Finally, it seems clear that the goal is not time-limited.

Three times weekly is considered an 'intensive' frequency for therapy services; it is recommended that intense episodes of care correspond to a time that a child is able to make rapid gains, or when there is a clear indication that rapid functional losses will occur without therapy (Bailes et al. 2008). Given Yvonne's functional level and her prognosis, a more appropriate model of services would be either periodic or consultative (once a month or less).

Justification of a physical therapy plan of care at a frequency of three times a week and without a plan for discharge cannot ethically be made based on current examination results.

Is there an option to provide these services but not to charge for them? The ethical principle of distributive justice must be considered here. Practically, if the physical therapist were to provide care free of charge, the 135 minutes each week would be time not available to other potential patients. Physical therapists 'must seriously consider their moral responsibility not only to their own patients but also to the many that could benefit from their services if resources were available' (Purtilo 1992).

Providing free services that are not medically necessary may result in de facto *resource shortages.*

Synthesis

It seems that the team is at an impasse. Yvonne has pain that is temporarily relieved by being in the pool. Her mother does not see any affordable options to carry on a program in a community pool. The physical therapist cannot justify skilled services at the frequency recommended by the ordering physician and desired by Yvonne's mother, and providing services free of charge is not a viable option.

Outcome

A team meeting was scheduled with the ordering physician, the physical therapist and Yvonne's mother, as well as a social worker who had previously worked with the family. During this meeting, it became apparent that Yvonne's mother was concerned that she did not possess adequate skills to carry out the recommended activities in the pool (even if she had access) and was worried about how she would train Yvonne's attendants. The decision was made to schedule four additional sessions in the pool, with the goal being to provide training to each of Yvonne's regular caregivers. Additionally, the therapist would teach Yvonne's caregivers some activities meant to facilitate more active participation and specify what responses might indicate that Yvonne was making changes. Yvonne's mother was told that, should she see any of these changes, the therapist would be more than happy to evaluate her again. During the month that these sessions were scheduled, the social worker planned to work with Yvonne's mother to explore alternate funding sources.

The four sessions were completed and handouts were given that included photographs of the recommended activities. A community recreation center near Yvonne's home offered reduced-rate memberships that were within the family's budget.

Themes for discussion

- The notion of 'futility' (though we recommend to use the term 'ineffectiveness') – a word that carries many dire connotations – is introduced at the beginning of this chapter. How is this term – this idea – thought about and what implications does its use have on professionals' behavior? On families' perceptions of their loved one? On their own lives and actions? And what are the ethical implications of using this term?

- As professionals working with young people with complex impairments and their families we are often confronted – as in the case described in this chapter – with issues that defy easy resolution and sometimes draw us in 'over our heads', creating discomfort and ethical challenges. How can we/do we/should we think about and address these issues in an ethically and empathically appropriate manner?

- This case suggested that there may be important gaps between the clinical and life situation realities of some of the people we serve and the rules, regulations and policies of the agencies and professional colleges with which we are affiliated. How might these issues and gaps be addressed to relieve some of the stresses experienced by both patients and professionals?

References

APTA (n.d.) *Code of Ethics for the Physical Therapist. HOD S06-09-07-12 [Amended HOD S06-00-12-23; HOD 06-91-05-05;HOD 06-87-11-17; HOD 06-81-06-18; HOD 06-78-06-08; HOD 06-78-06-07; HOD 06-77-18-30; HOD 06-77-17-27; Initial HOD 06-73-13-24] [Standard]*; http://www.apta.org/uploadedFiles/APTAorg/About_Us/Policies/Ethics/CodeofEthics.pdf.

Bailes AF, Reder R, Burch C (2008) Development of guidelines for determining frequency of services in a pediatric medical setting. *Pediatr Phys Ther* 20: 194–198.

Bamm EL, Rosenbaum P (2008) Family-centered theory: Origins, development, barriers and supports to implementation in rehabilitation medicine. *Arch Phys Med Rehabil* 89: 1618–1624.

Eliasson AC, Krumlinde-Sunholm L, Rosblad B et al. (2006) The Manual Ability Classification System (MACS) for children with cerebral palsy; scale development and evidence of validity and reliability. *Dev Med Child Neurol* 48: 549–554.

Hidecker MJC, Paneth N, Rosenbaum P (2011) Developing and validating the Communication Function Classification System (CFCS) for individuals with cerebral palsy. *Dev Med Child Neurol* 53: 704–710.

Palisano RJ, Rosenbaum P, Bartlett D, Livingston MH (2008) Content validity of the expanded and revised Gross Motor Function Classification System. *Dev Med Child Neurol* 50: 744–750. Purtilo RB (1992) Whom to treat first, and how much is enough? Ethical dilemma. *Int J Technol Assess Health Care* 8: 26–34.

Randall KE, McEwen IR (2000) Writing patient-centered functional goals. *Phys Ther* 80: 1197–1203.

Rosenbaum PL, Palisano RJ, Bartlett DJ, Galuppi BE, Russell DJ (2008) Development of the Gross Motor Classification System (GMFCS) for cerebral palsy. *Dev Med Child Neurol* 50: 249–253.

Sellers D, Mandy A, Pennington L, Hankins M, Morris C (2014). Development and reliability of a system to classify the eating and drinking ability of people with cerebral palsy. *Dev Med Child Neurol* 56: 246–252.

Chapter 23

Concurrent therapy in pediatric neurorehabilitation

Marilyn Wright, Sandra Gaik and Kathleen Dekker

Prologue

Parents want their children to reach their fullest potential. To achieve this goal, some families of children with neurodevelopmental impairments may engage in concurrent therapies, including treatment from more than one therapist of the same profession during the same time period. Such involvement in concurrent therapy can be a positive experience; however, in some situations challenging, complex and multifaceted ethical dilemmas can arise and have the potential to result in moral confusion for all involved. Ideally, professionals enter into collaborative relationships with other service providers, but in some circumstances therapists may find themselves unsure of their roles due to a lack of coordination or even conflicting rehabilitation principles and practices. Clinical ethical issues can be encountered in the care of individual families and organizational ethical inquiries may arise when a facility attempts to act in accordance with regulations and espoused values. In this chapter, several cases are presented to illustrate how one can work through a decision-making framework that can help service providers approach dilemmas like these in a thoughtful and organized way.

Ethical issues pertaining to the provision of concurrent therapies vary greatly, as illustrated in the following scenarios.

Clincal scenarios

- *A family of a child with cerebral palsy functioning at Gross Motor Function Classification System Level IV is receiving therapy for their child from two physiotherapists. One therapist is addressing impairments with the goal of independent walking, while the other is focusing on power mobility, positioning for comfort and efforts to address potentially preventable secondary impairments such as contractures, and participation in community recreational programs for fitness and socialization.*

- *A child is being seen by two occupational therapists for feeding problems. The family questions one therapist about the other therapist's recommendations. The family is advised to contact the other therapist with their questions, as two therapists addressing feeding could lead to safety concerns. Going forward, in order to establish who will be doing what aspect of treatment with the family, the first therapist tries to reach the second; however, the latter therapist does not respond to attempts to communicate.*

- *A publicly funded team of therapists and a team of therapists from a private agency are seeing a child concurrently. The privately funded team suggests approaching a particular charity to pay them for more frequent services such that the funding, which can only be accessed once every five years, would be used up in a short time. When the child needs other expensive equipment, such as an adapted bike or a wheelchair van, funding will not be available.*

- *A speech-language pathologist is working on a young child's functional communication abilities, including both non-verbal and emerging verbal communication skills. The family has been told by another speech-language pathologist that their child should work on blowing through straws and horns to support the development of speech skills and talking. This clinician offers to sell these items to the family. The claims that the private speech-language pathologist is making regarding the outcomes of the blowing activities are not evidence-based.*

- *A family registers their child for treatment at two publicly funded treatment centers in two municipalities using two different addresses.*

Decision-making frameworks can help engage stakeholders in collaborative and rigorous decision-making processes by facilitating the analysis of ethical quandaries and identifying approaches to address situations at organizational or individual levels. One such framework can be captured in the acronym ISSUES (Hamilton Health Sciences 2011).

1. Identify the issue and decision-making process.

2. Study the facts.

3. Select reasonable options.

4. Understand values and duties.

5. Evaluate and justify options.

6. Sustain and review the plan.

As ethical decision-making is not linear, some of these steps may be revisited throughout the process as additional questions arise or new facts emerge. This framework was used to address the issues of concurrent therapy in a pediatric rehabilitation facility, specifically situations when a family receives services from more than one therapist of the same discipline during the same period of time for similar issues.

Identify the issues and decision-making processes

This process involves the following steps:

- Determine the issues most relevant to the scenarios under consideration and identify relevant stakeholders to ensure that all perspectives are considered.
- Select a process to facilitate decision-making.

The most relevant issues were incongruent goals and practices, safety concerns, adherence to therapists' college guidelines and the responsible use of resources. Families, therapists and administrators were identified as the primary stakeholders. A process for decision-making to address the issues was developed and included the following:

- Compilation of further information pertaining to concurrent therapy
- Collection of ongoing, iterative feedback through email and formal and informal meetings to maintain transparency and constructive engagement with stakeholders
- Consultation with clinical and organizational ethics, institutional decision support and risk management
- Translation and exchange of knowledge

Study the facts

In studying the facts, the following should be considered:

- Perspectives of stakeholders
- Contextual features
- Relevant evidence and best practices
- Internal and external directives, legal considerations, human resource and financial implications

When families were asked, they spoke of how they wanted the best opportunities for their children. Parents reported that they seek concurrent therapy to obtain an intensity of therapy that is not available from their publicly funded provider or to access different approaches. They noted they sometimes do not feel adequately skilled to perform certain home program exercises, do not have the time or energy to carry out recommendations, or encounter behavioral issues when working with their own children. In some cases they seek additional resources so they 'can live without regrets'. Some families also noted that they felt uncomfortable admitting they were seeking additional therapy and in some circumstances 'felt like hiding it'.

Issues from the perspectives of pediatric rehabilitation professionals and administrators were explored through a focus group. This process provided a forum in which to reflect on the opportunities and challenges encountered when providing concurrent therapy and to identify specific concerns. A constellation of clinical and organizational ethical issues emerged, as reflected in the scenarios. Professionals found themselves unsure of their roles when working in concurrent therapy situations that were incongruent with their pediatric rehabilitation principles and practices. It was acknowledged that there are finite publicly funded resources, but the use of family or other resources should be legitimate.

A need for the following was identified:

- Clarification of terminology for concurrent therapy, duplicate treatment, dual treatment, complementary therapy and alternative therapy (see Appendix 23.1, p. 270)
- Establishment of clinical and organizational practice guidelines
- Development of family education materials

A review of the literature yielded negligible information. An electronic survey was conducted of practices at similar facilities. Responses varied from not participating in the care of children whose families were receiving therapy from other same discipline service providers due to the risk regarding which party holds responsibility should consumer complaints or any alleged wrong-doing be reported, to working with families to ensure concurrent therapy was provided in an open, safe and collaborative manner.

Contextual features include internal and external directives. In our program, there were no specific internal directives regarding concurrent therapy, but there was a corporate policy for working with patients who were engaged in complementary treatments. External directives included professional regulatory associations (colleges) standards from the colleges of physiotherapy, occupational therapy and speech language pathology. These state that concurrent treatments must be appropriate, compatible and done with consultation and coordination between professionals, and that there should be no unethical duplication of services (College of Audiologists and Speech-Language Pathologists of Ontario n.d.; College of Physiotherapists of Ontario 2007).

Select reasonable options

• Identify the options

Options included (1) being supportive of families pursuing concurrent therapy, specifically duplicate treatment and developing guidelines in accordance with professional regulations, or (2) not providing services for families when they are receiving services that would be considered duplicate.

Understand values and duties

• What values and duties are relevant to the options and scenarios?

• Consider principles and practices that inform ethical decisions or service delivery.

Family-centered service acknowledges that each family is unique and recognizes that parents know their child best. This model of service delivery promotes respectful, supportive and collaborative partnerships between families and service providers and supports the family's role in decision-making about services for their child. This support includes sharing information so families' decisions are informed (Baum & Rosenbaum 2008).

Relationship-centered care recognizes that the formation and maintenance of relationships are central to care and have the potential to be a source of satisfaction and positive experiences for families and practitioners. There are four dimensions: relationships between families and clinicians, and relationships of clinicians with other clinicians, with the community and with themselves (Beach & Inui 2006).

Traditional ethical principles include autonomy, respecting the rights of families to make their own choices; beneficence, doing what is best for the greatest number of people; non-maleficence, doing no or the least harm; and justice, doing what is fair and equitable.

Best practice principles include the following:

• Use of evidence-based practice

• Goal setting within the framework of the International Classification of Functioning, Disability and Health (World Health Organization 2001)

• Setting realistic goals and expectations based on prognosis

• Holistic and lifespan approaches

• Consideration of quality of life

• Recognition of the importance of transitions and provision of extra support through times of change

- Respect for the confidentiality of families and professionals

- Inter-professional service delivery and communication

- Promotion of ownership of one's health

- Moral and responsible use of family and institutional finances and time

Evaluate and justify options

- Choose the option with the best consequences and alignment of duties, principles and values.

- What are the possible harms and benefits to various stakeholders of various options?

Parents can make decisions about their child's therapy services. Being supportive of families who choose to receive services from more than one provider of the same discipline is consistent with the philosophy of family-centered care and the ethical principle of autonomy. However, if concurrent therapy is to be in the best interests of a child it must be practiced appropriately – in a safe manner, consistent with the regulatory guidelines of the professional associations and ideally in a collaborative manner that reflects the previously mentioned values and best practice principles.

Education/informed decision-making

Although parents can make decisions regarding services, they should be enabled and supported to make informed decisions. Parents may believe that increased amounts of therapy are beneficial or that functional abilities are a direct result of the amount of therapy procured since diagnosis (Beveridge et al. 2014). Professionals should answer questions and guide families with the best available evidence, another tenet of family-centered care. There is an ever-increasing number of high-quality research studies to support professionals in this role, and in many cases evidence about efficacy or effectiveness (or lack thereof) can be shared with confidence. However, providing advice can be complicated when research evidence does not provide definitive answers to questions such as 'which therapy approach, at what intensity and for how long?' There is often little evidence to answer these questions or demonstrate the superiority of one approach or intensity over another (Gibson et al. 2009).

Evidence-based practice involves the integration of the best available evidence from systematic research with clinical expertise and values. However, combining research with clinical expertise and values can be challenging as there will be great variation in clinical practice based on one's experience, passion, method of compensation and restrictions on service provision due to resources. Attitudes can also be impacted by local community dynamics or advocacy groups.

Parents can be confused when faced with complicated decisions. They may be uninformed or misinformed by testimonials or misleading claims. Even when presented with best evidence for effectiveness or safety they can be persuaded to follow non-evidence-based approaches – they may have 'knowledge in their heads but hope in their hearts'.[1]

Providing information regarding prognosis can be particularly challenging. For some families it can be difficult to find a balance – to not dispel hope but to work towards achievable goals.

Communication and collaboration

The basis of managing positive and appropriate concurrent therapy is open and honest communication. Families have a responsibility to disclose any involvement with concurrent therapies. Professionals should create an atmosphere in which families feel comfortable doing this. Service providers will also need to reflect on why families pursue certain service pathways and accept that some families may seek additional services.

Transparent collaboration among all involved in concurrent care is paramount to safe practice and is a requirement according to regulatory guidelines (College of Audiologists and Speech-Language Pathologists of Ontario n.d.; College of Physiotherapists of Ontario 2007).

Although concurrent practice can sometimes reflect questionable ethical elements, there are many situations where clinicians can be allies with the potential to appreciate the importance of a shared mission, be open to alternate ideas, have mutual respect and trust, learn from each other and engage in reflective practice. Working together in an open and collaborative manner can result in satisfying and trustworthy relationships between professionals as well as with families.

Appropriate concurrent therapy requires clarity about goals, roles and approaches. There needs to be consensus around overall therapy goals. However, there may be situations when a combination of specific goals or approaches could be beneficial. Rather than debating the importance of differing short-term goals or superiority of particular approaches, it may be possible that a child could benefit from a combination of foci or approaches (Gibson et al. 2009). This can be best determined through collaborative discussion between the family and the respective professionals.

---

1   Comment from a parent.

There are clearly benefits to respecting and accepting differing views, but there may be situations when the other professional providing intervention has completely different care objectives or a conflicting approach to treatment that could result in an overall detrimental effect for the child or the family. In such circumstances or when a professional cannot determine the nature of the other intervention, they must consider whether there is a reasonable risk of harm and advise the family accordingly. Some situations may involve safety concerns or blatant evidence contradicting another approach. In some cases, if there is unethical, incompetent or unsafe practice by another practitioner, a professional may be obligated to seek advice from a regulatory college (e.g. in the authors' setting these would include the College of Physiotherapy of Ontario and the College of Audiologists and Speech and Language Pathologists of Ontario).

There are, however, situations with more subtle or gray zone harm issues, for example when there are questions such as 'How much is enough and is there such a thing as too much?' All therapists need to be cognizant of unintentional harms inflicted by burdening families with feelings of inadequacy if they are unable to follow through with program suggestions because of competing responsibilities, fatigue associated with regular parenting or parenting a child with neurodevelopmental needs, impact on the parent–child relationship, or the risk of neglecting other children, a spouse or extended family. There can also be feelings of disappointment, both for children and parents, associated with working hard towards a goal that may not be achieved or even be achievable. Social and psychological harms imparted to children through the time and effort devoted to therapy that might otherwise be spent on participation in more satisfying and typical childhood pursuits must also be considered (Gibson et al. 2009). The importance of ongoing communication between the family and professionals offering the services is key in monitoring issues such as these, the effects of therapy and outcomes.

Sustain and review the plan

- Determine how best to document, implement, communicate and reflect on the decision and the process.

Practice guidelines were developed and are described below. Processes are summarized in an algorithm (Fig 23.1).

Overall guiding principle: Families who seek concurrent therapy are supported in their efforts if the interventions are considered to be appropriate based on practice guidelines.

Processes are initiated by ascertaining whether families are involved with other professionals when first assessed and on an ongoing basis. If they are seeing another professional of the same discipline, they are informed of the reasons for initiating and maintaining communication between therapists and consent for ongoing communication is requested. Written educational materials are provided. This allows professionals to consult with

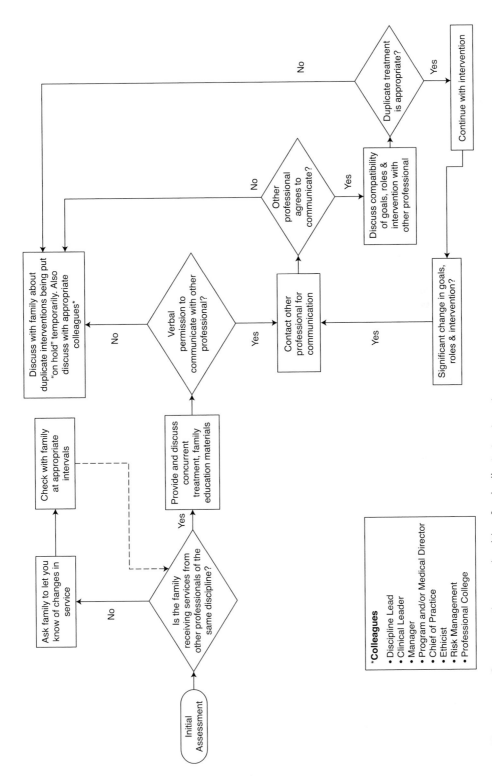

Figure 23.1 Concurrent therapy: algorithm for duplicate treatment.

each other and determine whether concurrent therapy is appropriate. Concurrent therapy would be considered appropriate if the treatment goals were complementary or enhance each other, if professional roles were defined and if interventions were coordinated.

Concurrent therapy would be considered questionable if the goals, roles or interventions of the concurrently treating professionals were conflicting in philosophy or approach, or were thought to pose safety risks; if there were no communication between practitioners; or if services represented an unethical or inefficient duplication of publicly funded health services.

If concurrent therapy is questionable, the situation must be discussed with the family. Consultation, as appropriate, with colleagues, administrators, ethicists, risk management specialists or professional college advisors can facilitate and inform the development of a plan. Treatment may have to be put on hold temporarily until appropriate practices are in place. All actions regarding concurrent therapy intervention must be documented according to institutional and professional association guidelines.

The guidelines were vetted by a parent representative, the institutional ethics committee and policy specialists, and incorporated into practice. Knowledge translation and exchange were promoted through the development of family education materials, presentations at conferences and incorporation into academic programs.

Concurrent therapy, practiced in an ethical manner, involves regard for values and duties, communication and collaboration as described in the following scenario.

Clinical scenario

John, a 6-year-old boy with cerebral palsy functioning at Gross Motor Function Classification System Level II, has received concurrent physiotherapy services through publicly funded children's treatment centers and a private agency since infancy. Results of brain imaging during his neonatal period suggested he would have cerebral palsy; however a formal diagnosis was not given. The children's center in the family's region would not provide therapy until a diagnosis was made, therefore the family engaged in private therapy. The private therapist has provided a source of consistent services when there were staffing changes within the children's treatment center and also when the family moved and services were transferred to another children's treatment center. The private services provide the family with a frequency of treatment that is not possible at the children's treatment center where resources are finite and the service delivery model relies on home programs in which caregivers participate. The concurrently treating therapists communicate regularly via email and phone to ensure services are coordinated and everyone is working towards the same goals. Collaboration around issues such as timing of botulinum toxin injections and serial casting as well as exercise programs support working towards the achievement of optimal outcomes. This model of care requires significant family coordination and resources, which are not available to many children.

Themes for discussion

- In the scenarios described in this chapter, families told the service providers in the community-based programs that they were using additional outside therapists. What is an appropriate response when families do not disclose the use of other services and we learn about them from other sources?

- What are the policies, in the programs in which you work, regarding families receiving what might be competing services from more than one program or professional? Have these policies been arrived at with an 'ethical' lens to guide their development?

- It can sometimes feel like a slap in the face when families seek additional or alternative services. In these circumstances is it ethical for us to discharge the family from our program? If not, what are alternative ways to 'deal with' (or support and accommodate) such families?

References

Baum EL, Rosenbaum P (2008) Family-centred theory: Origins, development, barriers, and supports to implementation in rehabilitation medicine. *Arch Phys Med Rehabil* 89: 1618–1624.

Beach MC, Inui T, Relationship-Centred Care Research Network (2006) Relationship-centred care – a constructive reframing. *J Gen Intern Med* 21: S3–S8.

Beveridge B, Feltracco D, Struyf J et al. (2014) 'You got try it all': Parents' experiences with robotic gait training for their children with cerebral palsy. *Phys Occup Ther Pediatr* 35: 327–341.

College of Audiologists and Speech-Language Pathologists of Ontario (n.d.) See http://www.caslpo.com/Portals/0/positionstatements/mpsintervention.pdf.

College of Physiotherapists of Ontario (2007) See http://www.collegept.org/Assets/registrants'guideenglish/standards_framework/standards_practice_guides/StandardConcurrentTreatmentOfPatient.pdf.

Gibson BE, Darrah J, Cameron D et al. (2009) Revisiting therapy assumptions in children's rehabilitation: Clinical and research implications. *Dis Rehabil* 31: 1446–1453.

Hamilton Health Sciences. Hamilton Health Sciences Ethics Framework. Andrea Frolic and the HHS Clinical Ethics Committee (2011) See http://corpweb.hhsc.ca/workfiles/CLINICAL_ETHICS/OrganizationalEthicsWorkSheetHHSEthicsFramework.pdf.

World Health Organization (2001) *International classification of functioning, disability and health.* Geneva: WHO Press.

Appendix 23.1: Definitions

Concurrent treatment occurs when a client/family receives service for the same condition/issues in more than one setting. There are different types of concurrent treatment in the context of pediatric rehabilitation. For this chapter, the following definitions were used:

- Alternative treatments are not, or not yet, widely accepted as 'mainstream' interventions. They may be practiced in non-traditional clinical settings. They are not currently considered evidence-based or best practice within similar children's treatment centers. Examples are hyperbaric oxygen and craniosacral massage.

- Complementary treatments may be considered 'mainstream', but are not practiced traditionally within similar children's treatment centers. Examples are acupuncture and massage therapy.

- Dual treatment occurs when a client receives interventions from a therapist of the same profession in another setting for issues beyond the scope of those provided by the children's treatment center. An example would be a school health support services program.

- Duplicate treatment occurs when a client receives intervention from a therapist of the same profession in another setting for the same symptoms or issues and towards the same goals. This would occur when a child receives privately funded therapy in addition to publicly funded therapy.

Chapter 24

Ethical considerations regarding surgical treatment of severe scoliosis in children with cerebral palsy

M. Wade Shrader

Prologue

As healthcare providers, we try to weigh and consider the benefits and risks – the pros and cons – of every intervention we recommend to our patients and their families. We draw on our training, experience and medical literature to inform everyone involved of possible future outcomes for each individual patient. In this process, we also consider the psychological impact of medical decisions. When faced with difficult decisions due to significant risks, the decision-making process can be as important as the decision itself. This chapter discusses some of the ethical considerations that may arise when making treatment decisions about severe, progressive scoliosis in patients with CP.

Clinical scenario

Mark is a 15-year-old who presents to the pediatric orthopedic surgery clinic with his mother with concerns over poor posture and increasing difficulty sitting in his wheelchair. He has bilateral spastic cerebral palsy, Gross Motor Function Classification System (GMFCS) Level V. He has a moderate intellectual impairment and is in a special education classroom at his local school. Mark lives with his mother and father, along with two younger siblings. His mother is his primary caregiver and takes time off from her job at a local supermarket to bring him to his medical appointments.

Mark was born preterm at 28 weeks' gestation and had an 8-week neonatal intensive-care unit (NICU) stay complicated by seizures. He was enrolled in an early intervention program and participated in community physical, occupational and speech therapy services. When Mark was 18 months old, his neurologist explained the diagnosis of cerebral palsy (CP) to his parents and described developmental impairments in this context. He referred Mark to a pediatric orthopedic surgeon, who followed him regularly every 6 months. Between the ages of 2 and 5 years, he had several surgical procedures to correct his strabismus. He used a wheelchair from the age of 5. At the age of 6 years, increasing spasticity and pain were ascribed to deterioration of bilateral hip dislocation. He underwent bilateral hip reconstructions, which was emotionally very traumatic to Mark and the family due to severe postoperative pain. After that episode, the family followed up with orthopedics only every 2 to 3 years to get prescriptions for new orthotics and a new wheelchair.

Over the years, Mark has had significant feeding issues, requiring gastrostomy and a Nissen fundoplication. He is followed by pediatric nutrition and gastroenterology services, but despite close follow-up, he is extremely small and under-nourished. He has developed a progressive restrictive lung disease and has been followed recently by a pediatric pulmonologist. He has had four respiratory illnesses in the past 12 months, two of them requiring hospital admission and antibiotic therapy. A sleep study showed repeated obstructive apneic episodes and the family has been counseled about the possible need for oxygen and non-invasive ventilation support (Bi-pap).

On musculoskeletal examination, Mark has severe spasticity with contractures of all four limbs. He also has a significant spinal deformity with a large pelvic obliquity and skin at risk under his ischial tuberosity, and a skin crease where his ribs are impinging on his pelvis. His spine radiographs show a 120-degree, long, sweeping scoliosis curve. The pediatric orthopedic surgeon explains about it and the fact that adapted seating has not succeeded in preventing the scoliosis. When he discusses the possibility of performing a posterior spinal fusion to correct or improve the spinal deformity, ameliorate respiratory health and perhaps reduce pain, Mark's mother becomes noticeably emotional and has difficulty completing the visit.

Scoliosis is common in CP, especially in children and adolescents with GMFCS Levels IV and V. The spinal deformity often progresses over several years and can lead to significant negative impacts on functioning and quality of life (QoL), including increased pain, poor seating tolerance, decubitus skin issues, rib–pelvis impingement, restrictive lung disease and a possible shortened life span (McCarthy et al. 2006).

Primary and secondary preventive measures typically focus on postural hygiene and adapted seating and possibly on bracing. Beyond those measures, surgical posterior spinal fusion (PSF) can be proposed for progressive curves greater than 50 degrees in order to improve spinal alignment and halt the curve progression. PSF leads to significant improvements in functioning and improved handling by caregivers in a large proportion of patients (Bohtz et al. 2011; Watanabe et al. 2009). These studies were based on patient/proxy reports – so, although they have not been studied in conventional ways, this is the kind of information parents are likely to want to know from other parents. In our experience, patients who have undergone this procedure typically experience substantial improvements in seating, decreased occurrence of pressure ulcers, and the halting of the progression of their lung disease. However, PSF in children with CP carries a significant risk of complications, including worsened respiratory insufficiency, occasionally precluding postoperative extubation in patients who did not have a tracheostomy preoperatively. Reported complication rates in the literature range from 20 to 58%, including infection in 10–35% and perioperative mortality in 1% (Mohamad et al. 2007; Sharma et al. 2013; Tsirikos et al. 2008).

Without surgical treatment, the risk of progressive deterioration in the child's functioning is substantial (McCarthy et al. 2006). That progressive curve may make it difficult for the patient to sit upright, may be associated with significant pain, can lead to the development of significant skin issues and may contribute to severe, potentially fatal pulmonary disease.

For these reasons, families and healthcare providers have a significant dilemma when faced with severe scoliosis in a patient with CP. Should they agree on a treatment that aims at improving their functioning and QoL, while accepting the risk of not achieving this and of peri- and postoperative complications including death? Or should they decide against surgical treatment, knowing that the disease process will continue to progress and function will decrease, possibly leading to worsened QoL and a shorter life span? The ethical dimensions of this dilemma are multifaceted.

Ethical issues

Patient
When patients are capable of expressing their own perspectives, it is very important to respect patient autonomy (Deatrick et al. 2003). If the child or adolescent has the capacity to participate in the process, they should be encouraged to do so. If the patient is considered legally competent to make healthcare decisions, then they may be able to make an independent choice. Alternately, the patient who is legally a minor may be allowed to give a formalized assent, and many children's hospitals have such an assent process. In most ways, if the patient is capable of decision-making (with or without the assistance of their family and healthcare providers), there is much less potential for ethical conflicts. If the patient can communicate effectively, they may be able to describe

clearly how much pain they are experiencing. They may be able to discuss the social and interpersonal consequences of having poor sitting balance and posture. Patients may be able to say openly and directly that they are willing to face the significant risks of PSF rather than continue to live with their current spinal deformity.

However, many young people with CP have concurrent intellectual impairments. In severe cases, they typically are not able to participate in the informed consent and decision-making processes. In this situation, the parents or legal guardians bear the responsibility of making the decision.

Family
As the legal guardians of their child, parents of a child with communication and intellectual impairments have the right to make informed decisions about their child's healthcare. It is imperative that the family is supported through this process. The family may need several sources of assistance during this time, including help from compassionate healthcare providers, social workers, friends and family, and special needs support groups.

Families in this situation may have substantial feelings of guilt relating to the evolution of the condition, fear of making the wrong decisions and despair. These children have often had many medical procedures, and the thought of undergoing a large surgery like PSF, with its potential risks, is something that they cannot easily consider. Throughout the decision-making process, it is essential that healthcare professionals work with families to help them identify and articulate their concerns and dilemmas in order to try to ensure that all these issues can be considered and factored into the eventual decision about PSF for their child (Boudreaux & Tilden 2002; Watanabe et al. 2009).

Prior experiences may impact how families view PSF. Previous surgical procedures may have been significantly painful for the child, and the parents may assume that a spinal surgery will be more painful than these earlier surgical experiences. The child may have had a life-threatening illness in the past, requiring an extended ICU and hospital stay. Memories of those experiences may significantly influence the perception of this approaching surgery.

Some families may feel that they need to be proactive in the care of their child (see also Chapter 7 by Noritz), wanting to do as much as possible to prevent disease progression. Those families may be keen to proceed with PSF, to the point that they ignore or underestimate some of the substantial risks. Other families may feel that they could accept a significant complication or perioperative death knowing that they had 'done everything that they could to help their child'.

Depression and fatigue are common in families raising children with special healthcare needs (Majnemer et al. 2012; Raina et al. 2005) (see also Chapter 20 by Reddihough & Davis). Those psychological issues must be identified because of the impacts they may make on the parents' ability to decide whether to proceed with PSF. Families may feel that they are 'at the end of their rope' and may not currently have the appropriate resources to care optimally for their impaired child, which may result in a decision rooted in their own despair rather than in their child's best interests. These feelings of hopelessness should be recognized by the healthcare team and should be fully discussed, allowing the family to share their thoughts and doubts. Family counseling should be offered when appropriate.

Healthcare provider
Healthcare providers should have, or should acquire, a solid understanding of the medical evidence regarding outcomes of PSF. This includes awareness of the limitations of the literature so that a complete picture of the potential outcomes can be presented to the family to assist them in the decision-making process. Although complication rates and the improvements in functioning and QoL have been described in several studies (Bohtz et al. 2011; Watanabe et al. 2009), the current level of evidence in the medical literature is still limited, as most of it is based on retrospective series (Corona et al. 2013). The difficulties and the limitations in the literature lie in the identification of patients who are most at risk. Risk stratification is important in all areas of healthcare, but is vitally important in the decision process for PSF for those with CP.

In many settings, the care for children with CP is primarily under the medical responsibility of the pediatric orthopedic surgeon. Families often identify the orthopedist as their child's 'main doctor', notwithstanding their relationship with their primary care physician (Lindseth 2000). Many of the factors affecting a decision about scoliosis surgery in the setting of CP are multidisciplinary rather than pure surgical issues. Therefore, coordinated care for these children with special healthcare needs is vital good practice. Such coordination is often organized by special primary care physicians with expertise in care for adolescents with special needs, special needs clinics, or specific nursing care coordinators. Specialists from other areas ought to be involved as well, including those from gastroenterology, pulmonology, orthopedics, neurology, physiatry and possibly neurosurgery. When all stakeholders can communicate effectively, both among themselves and with the family, everyone can make a better-informed decision about whether and when to proceed with scoliosis surgery.

Palliative care consultations should be considered for many families in this situation. It must be ensured that the family and patient understand the alternatives to the proposed surgical treatment. Palliative care physicians who are involved with the patient care conference can add a different and important perspective, providing the family with much needed information about treatment and comfort alternatives.

Unfortunately, there are times when a family is perceived as being 'demanding' (see also Chapter 7 by Noritz) in desiring spine surgery for their child with CP. This situation can occur when the pediatric orthopedic surgeon is hesitant to proceed because of substantial surgical risks, yet the family wants the procedure done. A common scenario involves a child with poor nutrition and a significant curve, usually greater than120 degrees. When the spine deformity reaches such an advanced stage, the family is now faced with the very difficult task of caring for that child, who is probably in considerable discomfort.

There are several reasons why a parent may strongly desire the surgery for their child. Parents may feel reluctant to start on an approach referred to as palliative care as they may understand this as an end-of-life process. Some parents might be willing to take any chance to improve their child's life. In this situation the ethical conflict between the physician and the family can be one of patient/family autonomy versus one of medical ineffectiveness. If the healthcare team regards that the surgical risks are too high for this particular patient, then they may feel uncomfortable proceeding with the operation, despite insistence from the parents.

Even after extensive discussion, care planning and counseling, families and physicians may continue to disagree about the appropriateness of spine fusion surgery. In those rare instances, if a care conference truly does not resolve the differences, then a formal ethics consult may be necessary.

Shared decision-making

The family should be supported throughout the process of making a surgical decision. The parents should be allowed to share their fears and concerns openly with the healthcare team. Likewise, the patient and any siblings should be able to voice any concerns they have and should be encouraged to ask questions during the process leading up to the possible surgery date. Also, the family has the expectation and right to receive from the healthcare team all the pertinent medical facts to assist with their decision-making (Hoffman et al. 2014).

Institutions may use a formal process to facilitate this shared decision-making process between family, patient and the care provider team. Decision aids may also be useful to help facilitate a meaningful discussion and to provide evidence-based information about the risks and benefits of the treatment options for neuromuscular scoliosis (Shirley et al. 2014). In addition, implementing regular care conferences can be an effective mechanism to give the family the freedom and environment necessary for them to feel comfortable with whatever decision they make. Regardless of whether a formal tool or process is utilized, the importance of shared decision-making cannot be overstated; it should envelop the entire preoperative evaluation period.

Resolution

Initially, Mark's mother was adamant about not proceeding with surgery. She was terrified that her son might not survive the perioperative period and she was afraid of the need for tracheostomy and long-term ventilation. The team provided the mother with support and proposed a comprehensive team approach to help with the decision-making process, including calling for a complex care team discussion. The surgeon suggested several consults, including from the gastroenterology, pulmonology and palliative care services. The gastroenterologist advised calorie supplementation prior to surgery. The pulmonologist suggested preoperative non-invasive Bi-PaP. The palliative care consultation was beneficial to the mother and father, who better understood the non-operative alternatives. After a care conference with the mother, father, other family members and all providers, the parents consented to proceed with the surgery and all the suggested treatments. Posterior spinal fusion was performed uneventfully. Mark's pulmonary situation did not improve significantly but did not deteriorate any further. His nutritional status improved and pain stopped being an issue.

Themes for discussion

- It is suggested that when families and clinicians are faced with difficult decisions 'we try to weigh and consider the benefits and risks, pros and cons, of every intervention we recommend to our patients and their families'. Does your program have a formal process by which this is done – and if not, should we have such an approach?

- How do we – how can we – help families and each other when we are involved with difficult clinical challenges for which there are no 'good' answers and where every possible course of action can be considered risky and less than perfect?

- Modern clinical decision-making is meant to be 'evidence-based'; unfortunately, there is often a paucity of good evidence. However, even when there is solid evidence about an issue (such as the benefits of scoliosis surgery to address a problem such as that described in this case), what additional 'evidence' and information need to be added to the decision-making process?

References

Bohtz C, Meyer-Heim A, Min K (2011) Changes in health-related quality of life after spinal fusion and scoliosis correction in patients with cerebral palsy. *J Pediatr Orthop* 31: 668–678.

Boudreaux AM, Tilden SJ (2002) Ethical dilemmas for pediatric surgical patients. *Anesthesiol Clin North Am* 20: 227–240.

Corona J, Miller DJ, Downs J et al. (2013) Evaluating the extent of clinical uncertainty among treatment options for patients with early-onset scoliosis. *J Bone Joint Surg Am* 95: e67.

Deatrick JA, Dickey SB, Wright R et al. (2003) Correlates of children's competence to make health-care decision. *J Clin Ethics* 14: 152–163.

Hoffman TC, Legare F, Simmons MB et al. (2014) Shared decision making: What do clinicians need to know and why should they bother? *Med J Aust* 201: 35–39.

Lindseth RE (2000) Ethical issues in pediatric orthopaedics. *Clin Orthop Relat Res* Sep(378): 61–65.

Majnemer A, Shevell M, Law M, Poulin C, Rosenbaum P (2012) Indicators of distress in families of children with cerebral palsy. *Disab Rehabil* 34: 1202–1207.

McCarthy J, D'Andrea LP, Betz RR et al. (2006) Scoliosis in the child with cerebral palsy. *J Am Acad Orthop Surg* 14: 367–375.

Mohamad F, Parent S, Pawelek J et al. (2007) Perioperative complications after surgical correction in neuromuscular scoliosis. *J Pediatr Orthop* 27: 392–397.

Raina P, O'Donnell M, Rosenbaum P et al. (2005) The health and well-being of caregivers of children with cerebral palsy. *Pediatrics* 115: e626–e636.

Sharma S, Wu C, Andersen T et al. (2013) Prevalence of complications in neuromuscular scoliosis surgery: A literature meta-analysis from the past 15 years. *Eur Spine J* 22: 1230–1249.

Shirley E, Bejarano C, Clay C, Fuzzell L, Leonard S, Wysocki T (2014) Helping families make difficult choices: Creation and implementation of a decision aid for neuromuscular scoliosis surgery. *J Pediatr Orthop* 35: 831–837.

Tsirikos AI, Lipton G, Chang W-N et al. (2008) Surgical correction of scoliosis in pediatric patients with cerebral palsy using the unit rod instrumentation. *Spine* 33: 1133–1140.

Watanabe K, Lenke LG, Daubs MD et al. (2009) Is spine deformity surgery in patients with spastic cerebral palsy truly beneficial? A patient /parent evaluation. *Spine* 34: 2222–2232.

Chapter 25

Considering best interest, quality of life, autonomy and personhood in the intensive care unit

Michael A. Clarke

Clinical scenario

Charlie M is 13 years old. He experienced a chronic partial intrapartum asphyxial insult. He now has spastic quadriparetic cerebral palsy (CP) (Gross Motor Function Classification System [GMFCS] Level V, Manual Ability Classification System [MACS] Level V) with severe scoliosis, significant learning difficulties, limited communication (Communication Function Classification System [CFCS] Level V), visual impairment and epilepsy with daily convulsive seizures. He has been gastrostomy-fed since the age of three (Eating and Drinking Ability Classification System [EDACS] Level V) and has severe gastro-esophageal reflux. Charlie's parents describe his brother Ben, aged 6 years, as 'boisterous and naughty'. Charlie loves it when Ben is around. Charlie's dad (Mike) is his full-time carer and his mum (Sarah) works as an administrator.

Charlie has always had recurrent acute respiratory symptoms. In the past year there have been four admissions to the pediatric intensive-care unit (PICU) for assisted ventilation (intermittent positive pressure ventilation, IPPV) and it is becoming increasingly difficult to wean him from the ventilator.

Intensivists discussed Charlie's worsening respiratory difficulties with Mike and Sarah and reported that Charlie's medical condition had deteriorated. They indicated that that would continue and that Charlie would have increasingly frequent episodes of acute respiratory failure. As a consequence it would become increasingly difficult to wean Charlie from IPPV and eventually he would develop progressive lung disease, leading to chronic respiratory failure and a much-shortened life expectancy. Charlie's parents were aware of this reality, though no one had ever been clear about the possible degree of shortened life expectation.

The doctors said that repeated PICU admissions were distressing for Charlie and were not achieving anything positive for him. They believed that Charlie's worsening medical problems meant that his quality of life (QoL) was deteriorating. Mike and Sarah felt that the doctors were implying that Charlie should no longer be admitted to PICU and objected to doctors making assumptions about Charlie's QoL. They would not countenance any suggestion that limitations be placed on Charlie's treatment. They were angry, especially when an intensivist implied that resources used to provide care for Charlie could be better used.

Communication between the medical team and parents became difficult. Mike and Sarah spoke with an experienced PICU nursing sister (Jo) whom they trusted. Jo said the nurses were distressed that Charlie was suffering and not getting better, and that they (the nurses) were not sure that all the treatment Charlie was having would benefit him in the long run. Mike and Sarah agreed to a discussion about what was the right thing to do for Charlie. At the same time they felt that some of the doctors only seemed to see Charlie as a problem, while they saw him as their 'little boy'.

Team meeting with Mike and Sarah

The clinical team and the parents agreed that there were decisions to be made about Charlie's medical management; that what was decided had to be the right course of action for Charlie; and that this involved trying to answer ethical questions raised by Charlie's situation.

Despite this common ground there was no agreement as to what the ethical issues were. For the nurses, the right thing to do was to prevent suffering; for the doctors, intensive care did not bring Charlie overall benefit; and for the parents the question was whether the doctors had the right to question their wishes that 'everything should be done'. The manager's ethical question (expressed to professional staff outside the meeting with parents) was whether it is morally right to continue to use scarce resources for Charlie's medical care with little evident benefit.

Jo chaired the meeting and said, 'Everyone wanted what was best for Charlie'. Eventually, everyone (professionals and family) agreed that it was acceptable to ask the question 'Is it in Charlie's best interests to continue to provide IPPV for episodes of respiratory failure?' There was also agreement that not answering the question was not an option. Mike and Sarah remained suspicious that the doctors were 'fed up' with treating Charlie and that there was a financial pressure on the hospital not to give full treatment to children like Charlie.

The discussion centered on delineating Charlie's medical problems, available medical options, and what was likely to be achieved. The doctors said repeated IPPV would not alter the natural history of Charlie's respiratory difficulties. Mike and Sarah said doctors had been wrong previously. Charlie's PICU nurse Lisa said Charlie was distressed and frightened. She said that Charlie suffered, especially when he was extubated; at those times he had struggled a lot, barely maintained adequate saturations, and had needed to be re-intubated, only to repeat the cycle of ventilation and weaning.

Nothing was agreed. Mike and Sarah understood the medical issues more clearly, but they just couldn't think about being without Charlie.

What is meant by 'best interests' and 'quality of life' (QoL)?

The UN Conventions on the Rights of People with Disabilities (Article 7) and the Rights of the Child (Article 3) state 'In all actions concerning children/children with disabilities the best interests of the child shall be the primary consideration'. Impaired or well, children lack the capacity to make informed choices, and decisions are made in their best interests by others. However, the United Nations Convention on the Rights of the Child (UNCRC) emphasizes that, where possible, due weight must be given to the child's views when his best interests are being determined.

When a decision is made for someone else it has to be the best one for that person, with all possible options considered. The decision should bring the greatest benefit with the least possible restriction on the person's rights and future options.

In judging Charlie's best interests, we have to satisfy his right not to be subjected to medical treatments (i.e. medical interventions) that are of doubtful medical benefit, and also his right to respect for private and family life (Articles 3 and 8, European Convention on Human Rights). Decisions about best interests evolve over time and with changes in a child's clinical condition. Coming to a decision requires gathering views from both family and professionals, including professionals external to the specific clinical care of this child.

Best interest judgments may involve the following considerations (adapted from Larcher et al. 2015):

- Does the proposed management plan meet the child's medical needs in the most clinically beneficial way?

- Do the proposed medical interventions provide greater benefit than burden?

- Do the proposed actions relieve suffering?

- Does our proposal maximize the child's autonomy and ability to choose?

- Are we acting in conformity with the legal rights of the child?

- Will our proposal maximize the child's QoL and possibly quantity of life?

- Does our proposed course of action meet the child's social, family, cultural and spiritual needs?

- Will our proposed plan result in the least possible pain and distress?

- Will our plan enhance the child's social participation?

When considering best interests we are drawing up a balance sheet, weighing the advantages of continuing a treatment/intervention against the advantages of withdrawing it. Not all factors will be seen as having equal weight. For example, avoiding what some would consider to be an 'intolerable life' by withdrawing treatment may be judged of greater importance than the possible benefits that result from continued medical treatment. In addition to weighing advantages and disadvantage, we might also consider perspective. For example, when considering withdrawal of life-sustaining treatment, our goal may not be to determine if it is in a person's best interests to die, but rather whether it is in a person's best interest for their life to be prolonged.

Interests can be understood as factors that influence a person's QoL; that is, what is of value to this person in his life. Every person involved in a story like that of Charlie and his family will have individual value systems (and biases) and therefore may have different value judgments when considering 'best interests'. Individuals may also have varied understanding of the relevant facts. It is crucial to establish the parents' understanding of the current medical situation.

When assessing medical interventions one increasingly common consideration is QoL. In the World Health Organization's terms, QoL refers to '… an individual's perception of his position in life in the context of the culture and value systems in which he lives, and in relation to his goals, expectations, standards and concerns' (WHOQOL Group 1993). An individual's perception of their 'health-related' QoL includes their perceptions of mental and physical health and of the social–environmental impact of their impairment (Davis et al. 2006). For children whose profound impairments compromise cognitive or communicative capacity, QoL is commonly obtained as a proxy measure derived from information from the primary caregiver. Of course the primary caregiver's perception of their impaired child's QoL will be influenced by their own health, personality, coping, resilience and self-esteem. It is recognized that parental distress is negatively correlated with parent proxy-reported QoL for children with neurodevelopmental impairment such as cerebral palsy (Davis et al. 2012). In addition, a doctor's rating of an impaired child's QoL influences decisions made about treatment (Morrow et al. 2012). On the other hand, it should be remembered that QoL that is viewed as intolerable to an able-bodied person may not be intolerable to someone who is born with impairment – an idea referred to as the 'disability paradox' (Albrecht & Devlieger 2009; Larcher et al. 2015).

Healthcare teams may judge this impaired child's QoL as poor. Professionals can confuse the value and meaning of life with the QoL. Hospital doctors may not have seen profoundly impaired children at home with their families when they are well and happy. Doctors should make judgments about impaired children's QoL (especially the more subjective components) with caution. An important factor that affects QoL is the quality of care and support that is provided for children with impairments and their families – and of course the quality of care and support provided to families by the community services to which they turn. What gets parents down more than anything else, and often causes more distress and anger than their child's neurodisability, are issues like having to repeat the history again and again, difficulty with access to services, quality of services, buck-passing, professional arrogance, not being listened to, superficial judgments being made about their child, and their need for recognition that they themselves (as parents) are experts about both their own child and their values (Kirk & Glendinning 2002).

Clinical team meeting

The clinical team met, but Mike and Sarah were not present. Jo reported back that Mike and Sarah could see what the nurses were saying about Charlie's suffering. They were shocked about how limited Charlie's life expectancy was thought to be. Sarah and Mike thought some of the doctors did not 'value' Charlie as much as unimpaired children, that the doctors implied that medical treatment was not doing Charlie much good, that Charlie would never be able to express his wishes or lead a full life, and would always need lots of care. He would never have any independence and his QoL was and would remain poor.

There were differences of opinion about Charlie's best interests. What lay 'beneath' these differences was not so much about specific issues of medical management as about the issues that Charlie's parents had picked up on. These issues included bioethical principles of personal autonomy and personhood.

Autonomy and personhood

Beauchamp and Childress (2009) write '… common morality contains moral norms that are basic for biomedical ethics'. These principles are respect for autonomy, non-maleficence, beneficence and justice.

Beauchamp and Childress hold that these moral principles function as an analytical framework and '… are a suitable starting point for biomedical ethics'. Beauchamp and Childress write '… it is usually a mistake in bioethics

"… it is usually a mistake in bioethics to give an overriding status to one principle over another doing so can be seriously misleading"

to frame issues as giving an overriding status to one principle over another' – and that doing so 'can be seriously misleading' (Beauchamp & Childress 2009 p. 13).

Autonomy has two components: independence from controlling influences and the capacity for intentional action. An autonomous person has capacity for self-governance; that is, has understanding, reasoning and an ability to deliberate, and can choose independently. An autonomous person also has the capacity for intentional action. Beauchamp and Childress emphasize autonomous choice and note that there are persons who are generally incapable of autonomous decision-making; that is, they lack capacity but can (at times) make autonomous choices (e.g. people with intellectual impairment). Personal autonomy is on a continuum and a person can have diminished autonomy. This is not a simple matter of there being a 'cut-off' point above which autonomy is present and below which it is absent. These same authors write that '... autonomy stretches from being fully present to being wholly absent' (Beauchamp & Childress 2009 p. 101). Lariviere-Bastien and Racine (2011) emphasize the importance of 'empowering autonomy' – facilitating a young person's autonomy when, due to impairment, they have diminished autonomy. The danger is that clinicians, while having respect for personal autonomy as a bioethical principle, may judge that certain 'types' of people (e.g. those who are severely cognitively impaired) or those who do not have and who will never have personal autonomy, cannot have their personal autonomy respected. Beauchamp and Childress (2009 p. 105) write 'Our obligations to respect autonomy do not extend to persons who cannot act in a sufficiently autonomous manner ...'.

Considering these principles as they apply to ourselves, we may realize that we are rarely, if ever, fully autonomous. It may also be the case that people who are severely cognitively impaired, though having much diminished autonomy, may not completely lack personal autonomy. For example, in Charlie's case he is obviously happy when Ben is around being noisy and creating mayhem. This observation shows that Charlie's behavior is unlikely to be purely reflexive or instinctive and therefore may indicate his preference for social interactions. In other words, even a significantly cognitively impaired person may be able to make some (perhaps limited) choices (a key component of autonomy); for example, they may show that they want to do this or that, demonstrating that the capacity for choice-making is there even if the person cannot do all of what they want to do alone. Charlie cannot, by his own acts, create the conditions for Ben to be noisy and cause mayhem, but he may well have a degree of decisional autonomy even without having executional autonomy (i.e. he cannot do what he may want to do on his own).

In sum, therefore, personal autonomy is not an all-or-nothing issue for the individual, and should not be considered as such when bioethical issues are being considered regarding an individual.

Autonomy is intimately related to individual freedom. For many people, personal autonomy has become the highest moral principle, despite the admonition of Beauchamp and Childress (see earlier) not to prioritize one principle over another. This potentially puts people who do not have the capacity to make autonomous decisions, and who will never have that capacity, at risk of being treated and cared for in ways that are different (and less favorable) when compared to people who are judged to have full personal autonomy and therefore have the right to have this respected by others.

When the rights of the person, such as respect for personal autonomy, become conflated with inherent human dignity (i.e. what a person is), a person with intellectual impairments who does not have personal autonomy, or in whom it is diminished, is at a disadvantage. What can result is that clinicians (and others) may believe that a life with diminished autonomy (perhaps because of the indignities that can result) is a life less 'worth living'.

What is at stake here is the question of whether a severely impaired person without autonomy is due the same personal respect, and respect for their rights, as the unimpaired person with autonomy.

What a 'person' is has always been a central issue in philosophy. Singer (2011) defines a person as a rational self-conscious being. He writes. '… the profoundly disabled child is indisputably a member of the species homo sapiens, but is not self-aware, does not have a sense his future, or capacity to relate to others'. In Singer's view, the profoundly impaired human being does not have personhood, and thus the inevitable implication for him is that being a member of the human species does not necessarily mean they have a life that is worth living. Profoundly impaired humans therefore do not have the individual rights that are the privilege of people having personhood. Singer also says that only a person who can grasp the difference between dying and continuing to live can autonomously choose to live. Individuals with severe impairments are thus placed at a profound disadvantage if a certain level of functioning and behavior defines personhood. If this profoundly impaired child does not have personhood, what moral status do they have?

Each of us has to answer the question 'Do I believe that there is no intrinsic difference between myself and this profoundly impaired child; we have personhood, does he?' Philosophically, what is at issue here concerns what is the manner of being. This is not the same as how this being acts, or what he can and cannot do. The concept 'being' is stable, unchanging and the deepest core of what a person is. How a being acts, or how they are functioning (what they can and cannot do), can never alter their manner of being (i.e. what they are).

This is where the concept of personhood fails, insofar as it says the converse, that is, that functioning defines the manner of being. This idea creates a huge disadvantage for people with impairments, particularly cognitive limitations. This is functionalism, and is the principle on which Singer's conceptualization of personhood is based. One could argue that Singer is confusing what a being *does* with what a being *is*, and does not tell us what they are – that is, their essence is at the deepest core of their being.

Many would regard Singer's views as extreme, but the issue of what a person is is very important. Is a person defined by his physical or psychological attributes (as Singer would suggest)? The German philosopher Kant distinguished between things, which only have extrinsic value, and persons, who must always be regarded as having objective, absolute, intrinsic worth. This is the Judeo-Christian view of the person; each individual person is created by God and therefore has unalterable intrinsic worth. The Judeo-Christian stance is that each person matters and no human life is ever redundant.

Another conceptualization of personhood includes the idea that a unique capacity of human beings (as distinct from other species) is that persons have the ability to reflect on their actions. By reflection, a person is able to derive a set of principles to guide choices. The relationship of the concept of the reflective person to a person having individual autonomy is evident.

Finally, another view of personhood is that personhood depends on the standing or status that is bestowed on a human being by others in the context of relationship as a social being. Each person has a context (based on relationship with others) in which personhood is manifested (McCormack & McCance 2010). People with severe cognitive impairment are perhaps not self-reflective, but they do have relationships with others and these are often intense, as can be seen in the relationship between Charlie and his parents. One might say, however, that such a relationship is one-way only – from Mike and Sarah to Charlie. Most parents of impaired children would strongly argue that the relationship is in fact reciprocal. In my experience, many parents will go further and will say that their impaired child's need for help and his response to them gives them something that is very powerful, very human and brings out their best.

The principles of autonomy and personhood can therefore act to the impaired person's disadvantage. However, we have to ask ourselves 'What is a person?' and at least consider the conclusion that this 'impaired' individual has the same intrinsic worth as an unimpaired individual. An individual should be respected as a person for their intrinsic worth (manner of being) and because of their relationships with others, independent of their attributes or capacity for reflection.

Further meeting of the clinical team

This was an informal meeting when a trainee in pediatric intensive care said she was at a loss as to what should be done in this all-too-frequent situation. The doctors acknowledged that their attempt to limit Charlie's treatment could be (and probably was being) interpreted by Charlie's parents as the doctors holding that Charlie was 'less of a person' than other patients without such profound impairments and therefore may have less right to treatment.

The intensivists were concerned by the way in which PICU practice had evolved. A senior intensivist related how, when he had started as a consultant, practice had involved the delivery of life-saving interventions to acutely and dangerously ill children. PICU practice had changed and was now about managing the medical complications of chronic (often neurological) childhood disorders. He said, and his colleagues agreed, that they felt pressurized into attempting to alter the natural history of chronic impairments where this was not possible, and that expensive PICU resources were often not delivering benefits for the severely impaired child or for society; and making judgments about how resources were used did not necessarily mean that a 'value' was being put on individual patients. Wanting proper use of resources did not of itself lead to disadvantage for some (impaired) children though they recognized that talking about the greatest benefit to the greatest number creates difficulties for respecting individual's rights.

Further meeting with Mike and Sarah

Jo chaired the meeting. Mike and Sarah had reflected on the discussion about best interests and could see the sense of this. Sarah said Charlie was a 'miracle child' and should be given another chance. She said 'It just seems you want Charlie to die and the sooner the better. You say you are acting in Charlie's best interests but you are not, you just want to get it over and done with.'

There was a break in the meeting.

Jo had a discussion alone with Charlie's family and then with the clinical team. She said that Charlie's family felt that Charlie was being discriminated against and there was a negative attitude towards Charlie, and some of the discussions about quality of life or questioning the purpose of medical treatment were, to them, predicated on the fact that Charlie was so impaired.

The family understood that Charlie's respiratory difficulties would worsen; they had seen this for themselves. They agreed to further discussion about Charlie's best interests in respect to respiratory management. What they couldn't abide were their feelings that some of the clinical staff seemed to them to see Charlie as somehow a different kind of person with different rights compared to children who did not have severe impairments.

The clinicians feared they would be forced to continue interventions that caused suffering without benefit. Some clinicians noted that this was another example where treatment was continued long beyond what was best medically or in the child's best interests.

Jo suggested to the doctors that an impasse was inevitable if the parents continued to perceive that Charlie was being treated less favorably than an unimpaired child. Jo said it would be best to concentrate on Charlie's medical needs and options for meeting these needs. The doctors should discuss quality of life when considering options but they must acknowledge that the best judges of Charlie's quality of life were Charlie's parents. She stressed that the doctors needed to say directly that the discussion with them as Charlie's parents would be the same as the discussion with the parents of a child who did not have neurological impairments, but who had *progressive respiratory failure and for whom it was thought repeated PICU admission was not appropriate. Jo said it was possible to have this discussion focusing on medical needs without communicating either explicitly or implicitly that Charlie's capacity, his autonomy, his moral status as a person, or his ability to choose were issues in determining the advice that was given. The message had to be got across that Charlie was not being judged, as a person, in a less favorable way to other unimpaired children.*

Final meeting with the family

Five days later, Charlie had been successfully extubated and transferred to the neurosciences ward. The discussion focused on medical needs, but the doctors emphasized that Charlie was not being viewed as someone with lesser rights than an unimpaired child. The parents said they were glad that the issue of Charlie's rights was discussed openly.

As regards IPPV it was agreed that Charlie would have each episode of acute respiratory symptoms evaluated and that he would receive IPPV for acute episodes until it became clear – either on the basis of clinical course or the results of investigations – that he had progressive rather than acute respiratory failure. They said they now had a better understanding of the medical issues and that it was the medical issues that were the most important to them in deciding what to do. They still felt that they and other parents in a similar situation had to advocate for their children to ensure each child was fairly treated.

Outcome

Charlie was not admitted for the next 9 months, when he had a short period of IPPV. He had been less distressed on a day-to-day basis, and his parents thought this was because he was in less pain.

He was found dead in bed 6 months later, his death being ascribed to sudden unexpected death in epilepsy (SUDEP). (See also Chapter 27.)

Summary and conclusions

- Cognitively impaired children often do not have age-appropriate capacity and may never develop that kind of capacity. Decisions have to be made on the basis of their best interests.

- Having (or lacking) personal autonomy is not an all-or-none attribute.

- Personhood is a complex concept and, if based mainly on an individual's attributes, will result in those with cognitive impairments receiving less favorable treatment.

- Clinical professionals need to be helped to be aware of the possibility that they may place an often not-expressed lesser 'value' on impaired children, and then may resist seeing an individual impaired child as anything more than their diagnosis or list of impairments.

- It is best to focus on medical needs, but also to make clear by our (professional) behavior and by what is said that each child is unique and each child has equal moral status as a person, whatever the severity of impairments.

Themes for discussion

- Thinking of a complex case or scenario in which you or your colleagues have been involved, were any of the issues presented in this chapter by Clarke raised and discussed? If not, should they have been – and might a fuller discussion of these issues possibly have changed whatever decisions were reached?

- There is frequent reference in this chapter to the issues and challenges associated with assigning 'value' to a human life. Whose perspectives are important in addressing this complex issue – and where might clashes arise? Is there anything that can be done either to prevent such clashes, or to address them thoughtfully?

- There is often a *conceptual* argument made about the need to use specialized resources like pediatric intensive care units as judiciously as possible. Have you ever been in an *actual* situation where there was competition for a bed or resources between a typically developing child and one with significant neurodisabilities? Is this argument a fair and honest one – or one that reflects bias and a negative view of 'the disabled'?

References

Albrecht GL, Devlieger PJ (2009) The disability paradox: High quality life against all odds. *Soc Sci Med* 48: 977–988.

Convention on the Rights of People with Disabilities (2006) United Nations; http://www.un.org/disabilities/convention/conventionfull.shtml.ii

Convention on the Rights of the Child (1989) UNICEF; www.unicef.org/crc/files/Rights_overview.pdf.

Beauchamp T, Childress J (2009) *Principles of biomedical ethics* 6th edn. Oxford: Oxford University Press.

Davis E, Mackinnon A, Reddihough D, Graham HK, Mehmet-Radji O, Boyd R (2006) Paediatric quality of life instruments: A review of the impact of the conceptual framework on outcomes. *Dev Med Child Neurol* 48: 311–318.

Davis E, Mackinnon A, Waters E (2012) Parent proxy-reported quality of life for children with cerebral palsy: Is it related to parental psychosocial distress? *Child Care Health Dev* 38: 553–560.

Kirk H, Glendinning C (2002) Supporting 'expert' parents and professional support and families caring for a child with complex health care needs in the community. *Int J Nurs Studies* 39: 625–635.

Larcher V, Craig F, Bhogal K, Wilkinson D, Brierley J (2015) Making decisions to limit treatment in life-limiting and life-threatening conditions in children: A framework for practice. *Arch Dis Childhood Educ Pract* 100(Suppl. 2): S1–S23.

Lariviere-Bastien D, Racine E (2011) Ethics in health care services for young persons with neurodevelopmental disabilities: A focus on cerebral palsy. *J Child Neurol* 26: 1221–1229.

McCormack B, McCance T (2010) *Person-centred nursing: Theory and practice.* Chicester: Wiley Blackwell.

Morrow AM, Hayen A, Quine S, Scheinberg A, Craig J (2012) A comparison of doctors', parents' and children's reports of health states and health-related quality of life in children with chronic conditions. *Child Care Health Dev* 28: 186–195.

Singer P (2011) Taking life: Humans. In: *Practical ethics* 3rd edn, Ch 7. New York, NY: Cambridge University Press.

WHOQOL Group (1993) Study protocol for the World Health Organization project to develop a Quality of Life assessment instrument (the WHOQOL). *Qual Life Res* 2: 153.

Chapter 26

How much is too much care? Interventions and life support in children with profound impairments and life-threatening conditions

Christopher J. Newman and Eric B. Zurbrugg

Clinical scenario 1[1]

Mary was a 7-year-old girl with a rare neurometabolic disease, who had been followed in a tertiary center at least twice a year from the age of 6 months. She had profound developmental impairment and interacted minimally with people around her (CFCS Level V); she was non-mobile, had spastic quadriplegia (GMFCS Level V) and had always been dependent on her caregivers for all activities of daily life (MACS Level V), including feeding by a gastrostomy tube from the age of 1 year. Over her first few years of life she developed severe scoliosis, despite bracing, accompanied by a progressive restrictive lung disorder. From the age of 5 years she presented with more and more frequent episodes of pneumonia, possibly related to aspiration, sometimes with major respiratory distress, but from which she recovered, usually in hospital with intravenous antibiotics, respiratory physiotherapy and oxygen. Pressure sores became an issue from age 6 years. Throughout these years, because her condition was objectively worsening, several attempts were made to discuss end-of-life planning with her parents, encouraging them to adopt a care plan primarily oriented towards Mary's comfort. The parents were adamant

---

1   The cases reflect situations in which the authors were directly implicated. Identities, timelines and elements of the children's personal history have been modified in the scenarios in order to strictly ensure their anonymity.

that complete cardio-pulmonary resuscitation (CPR) and maximal life support measures be provided for their child whose 'rights are the same as any other child' and 'who loves life, is communicative and knows exactly what she wants'.

A few days before her seventh birthday Mary was admitted to the center's intermediate care unit with a new episode of pneumonia and rapidly worsening respiratory distress. The medical and nursing team on rotation concluded that cardiopulmonary resuscitation (CPR) would be futile and communicated this opinion to the parents, who strongly opposed any such suggestion. Mary recovered from this episode following a week of antibiotics and non-invasive ventilation, although her neurological condition deteriorated even further, leaving her with no apparent interaction with her surroundings or signs of awareness. New discussions took place, involving the parents, hospitalists, neurological and physiatry specialists, as well as the primary care pediatrician, to decide what should be done in the event of a new episode. The participants all agreed on maintaining an open and non-judgmental atmosphere. The medical team, including the specialists who had followed the child regularly from early childhood, held to their suggestion of a palliative care plan whose primary objective was to ensure Mary's comfort, associated with a 'do not resuscitate' (DNR) recommendation in order to avoid invasive medical treatment aimed at prolonging her life. The parents responded that the team 'wanted to kill their child' and insisted that 'everything be done' if this were to happen again. In any case they said their family 'would not survive Mary's death'. Mary passed away 4 months later at home in her sleep, with no forewarning infectious or respiratory symptoms.

A few months after Mary passed away, the parents were seen by one of her long-time consultants, within a follow-up program offered to bereaved parents. The parents and the physician were respectfully and openly able to exchange their memories and experiences surrounding Mary's life and death. Even as the parents were grateful for the care that had been offered throughout Mary's lifetime, the evocation of the DNR discussions remained very painful for them. They were resentful toward the medical team who had managed Mary's last life-threatening situation and remained unable to understand or accept the DNR approach that had been recommended.

Clinical scenario 2

Trey was a 10-year-old boy who had periventricular leukomalacia as well as periventricular hemorrhagic infarctions associated with maternal cocaine abuse and extreme prematurity. Abandoned by his biological mother, he was a ward of the State Department of Children and Family Services and had been in the court-appointed care of an elderly, distant cousin. As such, and although non-ambulatory with spastic quadriplegia (GMFCS Level V), no verbal abilities (CFCS Level V), profound intellectual disability and cortical blindness, he had infrequent emergency room encounters and only rare hospitalizations, as his cousin had mastered the arts of hydration, nutrition and medication administration via gastrostomy tube (EDACS Level IV).

Then his caretaker had a stroke. She was discovered a few days later dehydrated, with hemiplegia and aphasia. Trey had persistent seizures. He was admitted to the pediatric intensive care unit (ICU) where he was intubated, ventilated and monitored with continuous electroencephalogram (EEG) for his intractable status epilepticus.

A new child neurologist came on service at day 5 of admission and found growing dissatisfaction with the neurology team among ICU staff as attempts to wean intravenous anti-seizure medication and move toward extubation were met with re-emergence of clinical seizure activity. The neurologist sought colleagues' advice on alternative anti-seizure treatment options, without success, as most standard and novel strategies had already been tried. There was severe census pressure in the ICU at the time, leading the health team to ask 'What are we doing here with this child?' The neurologist became aware of individual discussions among the ICU staff debating upon the quality of Trey's life – past, present and future – expressing their frustration about the current situation, and promoting the desirability of an expedited tracheostomy and transfer to a step-down unit to free up a bed in the PICU. Withdrawing life support never came up openly as an alternative in team discussions.

A court-appointed guardian ad litem *is customary in such cases. Trey's guardian had only recently graduated from law school. In her first job, it was clear to the neurologist that she was taking her role as advocate for Trey very seriously. She appeared devoted to the ideal of maximum care for all regardless of disability. During their first discussion the neurologist found her to be perturbed by the discussion of the proposed tracheostomy, asking 'Isn't this a bit extreme?' The neurologist in turn felt inadequate because of his inability to communicate the reality of the clinical situation to the young attorney. These feelings were additive to his inability to control Trey's seizures and meet the ICU staff's expectations. The guardian learned quickly what the ICU staff was saying about the clinical options for Trey and relented on the issue of tracheostomy. The neurologist never felt that the guardian was interested in a collaborative relationship with clinical staff as opposed to her self-interest in avoiding being criticized for making the wrong decision.*

Trey's previous caretaker survived and was in a rehabilitation facility, permanently unable to resume her caretaker role. The process had begun, with no firm timeline, to find another person to care for Trey when discharged from the ICU with a tracheostomy.

Discussion

Progress in medical technology during the second half of the 20th century, with improvements in resuscitation and intensive care, has offered medical teams recent possibilities to sustain and prolong life beyond what was previously its natural course. Life-threatening situations in children with profound neurological impairments epitomize the moral dilemmas that arise in modern medicine by putting into play questions such as 'What is a valuable life, and how is this judged?' and 'Who can judge which human life has meaning?'

In answering the question 'How much is too much care?', a starting point is to identify the parties with a stake in the outcome. In general order of importance these are as follows: (1) the child, whose interests should be paramount and protected from others' agendas; (2) the child's family, whose wishes are traditionally considered and protected; (3) the medical and nursing staff assigned to the child and providing their care, who have investments in time, emotion and perhaps the lost opportunity to care for others with potential for a better outcome; and (4) society at large, which pays for medical care through insurance premiums and taxes and which demands that its values be respected, and thus codifies many of these values in laws and policies.

The child

As healthcare providers, our mission is to place our patients' well-being and interests first. Our opinions regarding life support measures in children with profound impairments usually weigh the benefits (in terms of quality of life, including aspects such as happiness, relational capabilities and awareness) that can be expected from, for example, complete CPR, against the constraints linked to these treatments (in terms of pain, discomfort and potential additional functional limitations). From a child's point of view, and irrespective of the severity of their impairment, the recognition of their inherent dignity, which is the basis of human rights, is paramount (International Covenant on Civil and Political Rights, preamble 'Recognizing that these rights derive from the inherent dignity of the human person'; UN General Assembly 1966). Human dignity is one of the central parameters in this type of situation, because prolonging life by any and all medical means may lead to what certain people may judge to be an 'undignified' existence or to an artificial prolongation of the dying process.

What makes Mary's and Trey's lives valuable? Should one consider a universally intrinsic value of human life itself, in which case their lives could be deemed equally valuable and therefore as deserving of prolongation as any other, or is the value of life also determined by components of living that are instrumental to a 'good' quality of life? Most Western philosophers, starting with Aristotle and culminating with utilitarianism and its refinements, adopt the second position, arguing that there is variation in the value, meaning and quality of individual lives (Bickenbach & Wassermann 2006). On the other hand the approach that prioritizes the intrinsic

"Every human being has the inherent right to life. This right shall be protected by law."

value of life is strongly engrained in Judeo-Christian tradition, emphasizing the sanctity of life, with the correlate that one should neither intentionally kill nor intentionally allow someone to die. This moral heritage has inspired Western and international policies (International Covenant on Civil and Political Rights, Article 6.1: Every human being has the inherent right to life. This right shall be protected by law. No one shall be arbitrarily deprived of his life; UN General Assembly 1966), and most nations have enacted laws that aim to protect and preserve life. Yet emerging legislation on assisted dying (e.g. in the Netherlands, Belgium and Switzerland) and 'futile'[2] care (e.g. the Texas Advance Directives Act), illustrates the adoption in law of the notion that life has an instrumental value (Jox et al. 2013).

One of the main challenges when trying to assess the quality of life of children with profound impairments is our difficulty to access or comprehend their own experience of life, because we, and they, lack a means of communication. In medical practice, two notions seem to emerge as determinant factors when judging a profoundly impaired child's quality of life. These can be defined both in terms of experience and the lack thereof. The experience of chronic pain and suffering by a profoundly impaired child – or at least of what is perceived as such by external observers – frequently enters the equation when discussing life-prolonging decisions. However, these aspects often only intervene secondarily in relation to profoundly impaired children's potential lack of experience in terms of awareness and autonomy.

In Western thinking, the locus of what makes the person a person is strongly situated in the mind, symbolized by Descartes' famous dictum 'I think therefore I am'. When awareness is apparently absent or very limited (most often interpreted as a lack of thought processes, especially when supported by diagnostic tools such as electroencephalography or structural/functional brain imaging) people may devalue the profoundly impaired child as a person (see Chapter 25 by Clarke). The notion that the essence of the personhood is in the mind – an idea that most of us take for granted and as absolute – is a cultural construct based on Western scientific rationalism. Other cultures, for example in Eastern Asia, do not locate a person's identity exclusively in the brain (Bowman & Richard 2003). This is important to recognize, not only when discussing issues with families from diverse cultural backgrounds, but also when comprehending our own set of values and beliefs.

"Autonomy, the human capacity to will actions and to be independent moral agents, is at the heart of our ethical thinking in clinical situations"

Autonomy, the human capacity to will actions and to be independent moral agents, is at the heart of our ethical thinking in clinical situations. It is the pillar of values such as respect for the individual and individual freedom and was viewed by Kant as the source of human dignity. Autonomy is supported in international law by the Universal Declaration of Human Rights and the Convention on the Rights of Persons with Disabilities. Children progressively evolve from dependent non-autonomous beings to independent and free-willed adults, and as such are represented and protected by

---

2   As discussed further in this chapter, the editors recommend to use alternative terms, such as ineffectual, to replace the term 'futility'.

their parents or guardians in medical decision-making until they become capable of discernment. Children with profound neurological impairments are strongly limited in their autonomy, with, in most cases, no prospect of improving this capacity. Again, the value we place on autonomy can devalue the way these children are viewed as persons, even if our respect for them is based not solely on respect for their autonomy, but also on our obligations to other human beings. To Mary and Trey our questions should be 'What are your best interests?' and 'Could we harm you with our medical technology?' Given their lack of awareness and autonomy we had to rely on their family or guardian, as well as our own medical and moral judgments, in order to elucidate these questions.

The child, the family, the team

In Mary's situation the medical team judged further CPR and intensive care to be 'futile', with respect to their judgment of a very poor quality of life, with no chance of functional improvement given the nature of her condition, and increasingly painful and distressing complications. This view was completely opposed to her parents' assessment of Mary's quality of life, which they judged as excellent within a loving and caring family, and reading in their child's eyes and expressions the pleasure and interest she had in living (although at the end of her life the child was, to an external observer, without facial expression). This of course made the medical team's opinion all the more difficult to accept and contributed to the parents' distress during discussions, even as the physicians strove to remain empathetic and non-judgmental. Faced with a non-communicative and non-interactive child, both professionals' and family members' judgments are based not only on observation but also on interpretations, personal experience, feelings and beliefs.

The medical team faced a situation in which the child's interests and those of the parents seemed opposed. They struggled with this issue of 'who to put first'. Insisting or even unilaterally deciding to withhold life support in the face of a new life-threatening event (the latter decision was legally not possible) would certainly have created great suffering, sadness and anger for the parents. On the other hand, having to perform what was considered by some to be 'futile treatment' would in the team's opinion have gone against the child's dignity and interests and would have created, at the least, an important unease among the professionals who would have had to apply the life-prolonging measures (Kompanje et al. 2013).

For Trey, despite – or maybe because of – the absence of a family member or strongly determined guardian, the decision-making process seemed no easier. In this case, even though the notion of futility was voiced within discussions, reluctance around openly considering the interruption of life support seemed to prevail in team meetings, most probably due to regional medical culture as well as legal constraints. Also, symbolically *removing* life support might prove a more morally complex act than *withholding* life-saving measures (although both are identical from the legal perspective), because in the first case the child dies by an action of a professional (turning off the machine), whereas in the second case he dies by an inaction (Sulmasy & Sugarman 1994).

In Mary's case, the medical team considered that repeating life-saving measures in the event of a new life-threatening situation would be pointless. In Trey's situation the usefulness of maintaining ongoing life support and treatment was debated. The concepts of 'medical futility' have waxed and waned in the medical literature during recent decades (Helft et al. 2000). Certain authors distinguish the two notions of quantitative and qualitative 'futility', whereas others postulate that the term 'futility' should only apply to physiologic futility (Racine & Shevell 2009). Quantitative, physiological futility is defined by the very low statistical probability (traditionally <1%) of an intervention proving successful (e.g. initiating CPR after 15 minutes of cardiac arrest), and is rarely an issue in the type of situation described above. Qualitative futility has been known by various definitions, of which most include the provision of treatments that either preserve permanent unconsciousness or fail to end a patient's total dependence (Goh & Mok 2001). 'Qualitative medical futility' is an essentially subjective and inherently value-laden judgment generally emitted by medical teams, and mirrors our assessments of quality of life. A number of authors have cautioned against this acceptance of futility (Lo 2009; Racine & Shevell 2009; Wilson 1996), because it *de facto* constitutes a judgment about quality of life, with the consequence of being used to qualify parental demands that are considered unreasonable (i.e. 'futile' requests from parents). This controversy has persisted for over two decades, and a broadly accepted definition of 'futility' may ultimately prove unachievable (which may be a good reason to avoid using it).

In a majority of life-threatening situations involving children with profound neurological disabilities, parents and medical teams seem to reach an explicit agreement on withholding or withdrawing life support (Launes et al. 2011), with parents' greatest concern being that the child might suffer. The decision-making process per se has seldom been described. Recently it has been shown that despite several retrospective studies demonstrating that parents wish to be involved actively in the process, in practice only a minority of parents are explicitly asked to share in the decision-making (de Vos et al. 2015). The authors of this research make a strong case that opening the possibility to parents to share in end-of-life decisions (in effect 'giving them permission' to consider it) is a more important duty for physicians than protecting them from guilt or doubt.

The death of a child, severely impaired or not, is fundamentally and emotionally unacceptable for any parent, and a heartbreaking moment of their existence. In a minority of situations a consensual decision cannot be achieved within the team, within the family, or between the family and team. Certain disagreements find their roots in strong family beliefs that may be religious or cultural, or concern the origins of their child's impairment. In the latter situation families may, for example, attribute a child's impairment to an adverse, supposedly iatrogenic, neonatal adverse event, whereas the child objectively presents a genetic disease. This may lead to a deleterious 'them and us' situation where our medical knowledge is pitched against their families' beliefs, with both parties acting defensively. In other cases the disagreement may stem from the popular, but also to a certain extent medical, belief that physicians are ultimately equipped to stave off death. In this respect, death is considered as a failure of modern medicine, even more so when a child is concerned. Associated with third-party coverage of medical costs and a strong shift towards patient autonomy that has superseded physician paternalism since the 1960s, this has 'led to the perception that the patient can demand, and the physician must provide, whatever the patient or family requests' (Paris 2010). Recent literature on patient autonomy in end-of-life situations usefully reminds us that this notion entails the personal right to refuse treatment, but in no case a right to be provided with any requested intervention (Billings & Krakauer 2011). Service provision is of course not only a matter of interaction between providers and recipients of care, but is to a large extent determined at a societal level.

The child and the society

For society 'How much is too much care?' opens the further questions of equity and the appropriate use of costly medical resources, and of its mirror notion, rationing. Our ICUs are regularly under strain and pushed to their maximum capacity, and putting Mary or Trey under life support could ultimately have deprived another child, with a better long-term prognosis, of optimal care (e.g. by having to transfer that child to another hospital with the entailed risks in a vital situation). Also, pushing the first scenario to its opposite conclusion – that is, had Mary required further resuscitation – it is likely that she would have ended up on long-term or even definitive invasive ventilation with a tracheotomy to prolong her life. This is a scenario that the medical team had envisioned, and had the situation evolved in that direction they had considered resorting to the available legal measures to withhold life support. Not only did the team consider tracheostomy ventilation to be excessively invasive and ethically questionable, they also considered it to be an extremely costly measure in order to maintain an unconscious and totally dependent life. Practices vary between countries and cultures in this respect; they are probably determined by societal views on impairment and disability and on the acceptability of 'natural' or sometimes even expedited death in children with severe and incurable chronic disorders, and of course also by the laws enforced in each country that regulate end-of-life decisions. (In addition, of course, resources determine possible courses of action, as discussed poignantly in Chapter 15.)

The right to life is enshrined in Article 3 of the United Nations Universal Declaration of Human Rights: 'Everyone has the right to life, liberty and security of person'. In theory, and morally, a year of human life is priceless. Does this imply that society should mobilize all and any available resource if a profoundly impaired child, with a predicted poor outcome, requires these resources to stay alive? In reality, governments and insurance agencies, whose assets are not limitless, are increasingly resorting to the use of cost–effectiveness analysis in determining coverage of medical procedures. Health economics markers such as 'quality adjusted life years' (QALY) place the cost of an additional year of life of good quality (i.e. without disability) anywhere between US$50 000 and 200 000 in developed countries (Neumann et al. 2014). Does this type of information have any place when taking decisions on life-prolonging measures in children who are and would remain profoundly impaired? There is most certainly a taboo in many Western countries to even consider the issue of cost when discussing the provision of care for children with impairments, when the quality of a society is also judged by its ability to protect its most vulnerable members. Recent history marked by early 20th-century eugenics, which ultimately led to the mass extermination of hundreds of thousands of children and adults with physical and mental impairments, has certainly made us all the more wary of discussing issues of life and death based primarily on notions of 'social cost' (Ronen et al. 2009). Ultimately, the factor of financial cost may not prove to be a determinant in our decision-making, noting that this possibility prevails only in well-off developed economies (see also Chapter 15 by Esmaili & Ntizimira). However, with transparency and equity in mind, we believe that there is nothing inappropriate in envisioning the potentially very high cost (financially and in human resources) of, for example, long-term life support in situations where survival will most likely be associated with a poor quality of life.

Disagreement and negotiation

In Mary's situation thoughts were shared and discussions took place with the family, medical and nursing colleagues, therapists, teachers, the institutional ethics board and the departmental and hospital managements. While these exchanges helped the medical team to advance in its reflections and attain consensus on its recommendation, this sadly did not relieve any of the distress on the family's side and only to a certain extent did it help with the distress of the professionals who directly cared for Mary. With a family, the physician and care team are well advised to listen to all members, seen and often unseen, empathetically and compassionately, thoroughly acknowledging their concerns and rights, and documenting every conversation completely. For Trey, with the state as the legal guardian, the physician and care team may or may not have experienced less ambiguity in the direction of care because of existing laws and policy.

The most effective way to address life and death issues is through open and balanced communication. The reality of decision-making, especially in situations of disagreement, is probably best conceptualized as a negotiation. It is simplistic to describe medical teams as bringing knowledge and evidence to the negotiating table while families bring their values. Physicians are persons with values; these will inevitably and often positively transpire into discussions and even decisions. Families are often well informed of the possibilities of modern medicine and have developed their own expertise in the care of their child. For children at risk, discussions about implementing or withholding life-sustaining technologies should ideally take place in a timely fashion, ahead of life-threatening events. Personal resuscitation plans for children with impairments and life-threatening conditions have been shown to be useful and empowering for families, as well as medical and nursing staff (Wolff et al. 2011). A strong respect for the cultural background and religious beliefs of each family is essential, aiming to understand and take into account how these may affect their views on themes such as the role of physicians and medicine, life and death, independence and interdependence.

In the rare cases of irreconcilable positions between family and medical teams, most large medical institutions apply codified processes, typically including mediation, consulting an ethics committee, seeking second opinions and/or transferring to another institution before ultimately resorting to law and a court order. The latter step is often experienced as a failure of communication by medical teams. We would contend that a minority of disagreements and conflicts simply cannot be successfully negotiated and resolved and that our personal and medical ethics do on rare occasions frontally and durably oppose us with families. In these cases, resorting to justice is no more than appealing to the official body mandated by most democratic societies to determine what is just, what is right or wrong.

Epilogue

Until very recent history, medicine's limited capacity to modify life's course set a limit on what could or should be done to preserve life. Our societies have barely half a century of experiencing the ethical dilemmas that go with the possibility of prolonging life technologically, and we are still in the process of developing the collective wisdom necessary to face and resolve these issues. The particular questions raised by life support in children with profound impairments are emblematic in that they test to their limits the four principles of modern medical ethics (beneficence, non-maleficence, justice and autonomy – Beauchamp & Childress 2008). They illustrate to what extent these principle-driven standards on which we strongly rely in our decision-making can be conditioned by personal morals, beliefs, politics, laws and culture. Feminist philosophers have argued that the Western tradition in ethics strongly reflects a male discourse, and that the embodied ethical caring that women are more likely to follow may provide a more concrete set of ethical rules, especially in healthcare services (Fotaki 2015). The ethics of care can prove complementary to principlism, particularly in seemingly inextricable situations, by displacing the focus of our ethical thinking from the constraints of supposed impartiality towards the quality of our responses, and by emphasizing the essential ethical components of care – attentiveness, responsibility, competence and responsiveness (Tronto 2001).

Our deep respect for human life does not dictate that we choose life always. Preserving dignity and providing relief and comfort may take the upper hand over artificially prolonging life. There should be no such thing as discontinuity of care, and in a majority of situations, such as those discussed in this chapter, families and professionals consensually decide on individual care plans. The motto 'First, do no harm' has been used as a guiding principle for physicians since Hippocrates. Another might be 'Cure occasionally, relieve often, care always'.

"Cure occasionally, relieve often, care always"

Themes for discussion

- As noted elsewhere in this book, much of modern clinical training focuses on evidence-based care, but rarely are the ethical aspects of an issue as clearly expressed. How might we go about introducing 'ethical' perspectives and frameworks into a case discussion in which there were dilemmas or conflicts?

- Decision-making in complex cases is usually seen to be the responsibility of senior medical staff and families. What is/should be the role of 'allied health professionals' – and whatever our answer, why do we answer that way?

- Many of the issues discussed in this book – and certainly in this chapter – concern young people whose impairments may make their lives appear to have a lower 'value' than others' lives. What are the forces and influences in the development and lives of professionals that might contribute to these perceptions – and what can be done to address these apparent gaps in perception?

- Terminology and empathy are important components of communication with families in similar situations. List terms that would be useful to connect with parents and those that would potentially antagonize families.

References

Beauchamp TL, Childress JF (2008) *Principles of biomedical ethics* 6th edn. Oxford: Oxford University Press.

Billings JA, Krakauer EL (2011) On patient autonomy and physician responsibility in end-of-life care. *Arch Intern Med* 171: 849–853.

Bickenbach JE, Wassermann D (2006) The good life and the quality of life. In: Bickenbach J, Mitchell DT, Schalick III WO, Snyder SL, editors. *Encyclopedia of disability*. Thousand Oaks, CA: Sage Publications.

Bowman KW, Richard SA (2003) Culture, brain death, and transplantation. *Prog Transplant* 13: 211–215, quiz 216–217.

De Vos MA, Bos AP, Plotz FB et al. (2015) Talking with parents about end-of-life decisions for their children. *Pediatrics* 135: e465–76.

Fotaki M (2015) Why and how is compassion necessary to provide good quality healthcare? *Int J Health Policy Manag* 4: 199–201.

Goh AY, Mok Q (2001) Identifying futility in a paediatric critical care setting: A prospective observational study. *Arch Dis Child* 84: 265–268.

Helft PR, Siegler M, Lantos J (2000) The rise and fall of the futility movement. *N Engl J Med* 343: 293–296.

Jox RJ, Horn RJ, Huxtable R (2013) European perspectives on ethics and law in end-of-life care. *Handb Clin Neurol* 118: 155–165.

Kompanje EJ, Piers RD, Benoit DD (2013) Causes and consequences of disproportionate care in intensive care medicine. *Curr Opin Crit Care* 19 : 630–635.

Launes C, Cambra FJ, Jordan I, Palomeque A (2011) Withholding or withdrawing life-sustaining treatments: An 8-yr retrospective review in a Spanish pediatric intensive care unit. *Pediatr Crit Care Med* 12: e383–e385.

Lo B (2009) *Futile interventions. Resolving ethical dilemmas, a guide for clinicians* 4th edn. Philadelphia, PA: Lippincott Williams & Wilkins.

Neumann PJ, Cohen JT, Weinstein MC (2014) Updating cost-effectiveness – the curious resilience of the $50,000-per-QALY threshold. *N Engl J Med* 371: 796–797.

Paris JJ (2010) Autonomy does not confer sovereignty on the patient: A commentary on the Golubchuk case. *Am J Bioeth* 10: 54–56.

Racine E, Shevell MI (2009) Ethics in neonatal neurology: When is enough, enough? *Pediatr Neurol* 40: 147–155.

Ronen GM, Meaney B, Dan B, Zimprich F, Stogmann W, Neugebauer W (2009) From eugenic euthanasia to habilitation of 'disabled' children: Andreas Rett's contribution. *J Child Neurol* 24: 115–127.

Sulmasy DP, Sugarman J (1994) Are withholding and withdrawing therapy always morally equivalent? *J Med Ethics* 20: 218–222, discussion 223–224.

Tronto JC (2001) An ethic of care. In: Holstein MB, Mitzen PB, editors. *Ethics in community-based elder care.* New York, NY: Springer.

UN General Assembly (1966) *International Covenant on Civil and Political Rights.* United Nations Treaty Series 999: 171.

Wilson BE (1996) Futility and the obligations of physicians. *Bioethics* 10: 43–55.

Wolff A, Browne J, Whitehouse WP (2011) Personal resuscitation plans and end of life planning for children with disability and life-limiting/life-threatening conditions. *Arch Dis Child Educ Pract Ed* 96: 42–48.

Chapter 27

Discussing sudden unexpected death in newly diagnosed epilepsy

James J. Reese Jr. and Phillip L. Pearl

Clinical scenario

Carter, a previously healthy and developmentally normal 8-year-old boy, is evaluated following two separate and unprovoked generalized tonic-clonic seizures 6 months apart. Neurological examination, electroencephalogram (EEG) and brain magnetic resonance imaging (MRI) are normal. He and his family are being seen for their first visit with a child neurologist following referral by their pediatrician. The family has many questions about diagnosis and prognosis. They ask 'Do children die from epilepsy?'

This common scenario is laden with emotional and ethical considerations. When counseling a family about the diagnosis of epilepsy, the neurologist must decide whether, when and how to disclose information about dying from seizures, including sudden unexpected death in epilepsy (SUDEP). SUDEP is used to describe the syndrome in which a person with epilepsy dies unexpectedly and suddenly without clear etiology, including trauma, drowning and status epilepticus. The pathophysiology is currently unknown, with debates over possible cardiac or respiratory dysregulation. The ethical conflict arises because of the difficulty of balancing how best to inform families without causing undue distress. Neurologists are left with the challenge of providing such sensitive information in the proper context versus considering whether sharing the information at a particular time is relevant, helpful or potentially so distressing to the family that the discussion is postponed or avoided.

Case and clinical context

Mortality in epilepsy may be related to status epilepticus, seizure-related accidents, suicide and complications of underlying systemic or Neurological disease, but SUDEP has emerged as a leading phenomenon associated with patient fatalities. There is some ability to stratify risk, as the incidence of SUDEP is 1:10 000 person-years in newly diagnosed patients, but as high as 1:100 person-years in patients with medically intractable epilepsy who are being evaluated for epilepsy surgery (Tomson et al. 2008). Although SUDEP predominantly affects young adults, other risk factors include the presence of increasingly active generalized tonic-clonic seizures, early life onset of epilepsy, duration of epilepsy and presence of post-ictal generalized suppression on EEG (Lhatoo et al. 2010; Nilsson et al. 1999; Thurman et al. 2014). SUDEP has been observed to have a strong association with particular genetic disorders, such as Dravet syndrome (Kalume 2013; Skluzacek et al. 2011).

The risk in the patient described in the scenario above is small but not zero. Whether it is higher than the death rate in the general population is debatable, and uncertain. In an analysis of four pediatric cohorts of over 2200 patients followed for more than 30 000 person-years from epilepsy onset, the death rate from SUDEP was only 9 per 100 000 person-years in those with uncomplicated epilepsy (versus 98 per 100 000 person-years in complicated epilepsy) (Berg et al. 2013). The overall death rate in persons with uncomplicated epilepsy (i.e. without associated neurodevelopmental impairments) was not significantly different from that of the general population, and the death rate from SUDEP was comparable to accidents, the leading cause of death in the pediatric age group.

The SUDEP conversation, however, is not an easy one. To date, the experience of SUDEP disclosure appears to reflect this. In an online survey of 1200 American and Canadian neurologists, fewer than 7% reported discussing SUDEP with nearly all epilepsy patients and 12% reported never discussing it (Friedman et al. 2014). The majority responded that distress and anxiety on the part of patients and families were a common response to the disclosure. In contrast, appreciation and relief were expressed far less often. Physicians are thus faced with balancing information of extraordinarily high emotional valence, with low likelihood of occurrence, with a wish not to alarm or unnecessarily distress patients and families with anxiety or grief.

Framing of the problem

The possibility that a family could give informed consent for a SUDEP discussion is arguable but illogical. An informed decision by patients and families concerning whether or not they would like to hear about SUDEP cannot possibly be completed because the neurologist would first have to explain or discuss the concept in order to ask them in a truly informed manner if they would like to discuss it. In these circumstances, the neurologist must therefore balance beneficence and non-maleficence to determine how to balance the benefit and harm of disclosure of information. It may be possible to circumvent the details of the topic and ask patients something along the lines of 'Would you like to discuss rare but severe potential complications associated with epilepsy?' However, a lack of details in asking the family questions would limit the family's ability to provide truly informed consent to answer. Consequently, neurologists must balance their own perceptions and assumptions about how the patient and family would exercise their autonomy in this situation.

Navigating the conundrum

An ethical analysis presents several potential approaches to SUDEP disclosure. There could be arguments for each of the following:

• Withhold discussion of SUDEP with all families

• Proceed with SUDEP disclosure selectively

• Discuss SUDEP with all epilepsy patients and families

The argument to withhold discussion of SUDEP

Barriers that prevent SUDEP disclosure include the notions that certain patients are at minimal or no greater risk than the general population, that there is no proven way to prevent it, and that the information itself could adversely affect the patient's and family's quality of life or mood (Friedman et al. 2014). Other reasons expressed by neurologists are the rarity of the event, so that the risks of discussion outweigh the potential benefits, lack of time for this discussion, lack of resources for a proper discussion, and lack of an opportunity to form a trusting relationship with the family at that point of the clinical interface.

Some of these reasons have overlapping rationales. The idea that the patient is at minimal or almost no risk may align with the suggestion that the frequency of SUDEP is so low that the risks of discussion outweigh the potential benefits. Other barriers mentioned are very real yet more logistically based. The logistics of the conversation are a real challenge. Clinics are increasingly busy as neurologists are faced with greater pressure to see patients more efficiently. Spending appropriate time to counsel a family about SUDEP may not fit with administrative pressures and may detract from the time required to address pressing issues of even more relevance if not immediacy to that patient.

Overall, a lack of evidence, to date, that SUDEP is preventable leaves some neurologists wondering why or how the patient or family may benefit from knowing about SUDEP.

The argument to discuss SUDEP selectively
Neurologists may choose to discuss SUDEP with selective populations known to be at higher risk. Alternately, other neurologists may invoke SUDEP when a patient is showing poor compliance, perhaps in an effort to provide motivation to improve medication adherence. In the latter scenario, initial potential psychological harm of creating fear of death would potentially be superseded by more potential long-term benefit. A neurologist may analyze all patients on a case-by-case basis and decide that some combination of patient/parental questions, risk factors and the clinical situation indicate that the patient and family are more likely to benefit than be harmed by the conversation.

In the case of a child with newly diagnosed childhood absence epilepsy, for example, it would seem essentially irrelevant to raise the prospect of SUDEP. How productive can that discussion be for the patient and family? One could argue that SUDEP is *diagnosed* rarely enough (which is different from *occurring* rarely enough, because it may be under-diagnosed) that a neurologist is more likely to effect positive change in the child's life by spending time discussing seat belt use, pedestrian safety, the importance of avoiding smoking or even healthy dietary habits than by discussing SUDEP. The counterargument could be made, however, that these children are also at risk for generalized tonic-clonic seizures. In that case, it would seem more appropriate to raise the SUDEP discussion if and when convulsive seizures appear in that patient's clinical course. There is also the slippery slope problem that excluding SUDEP from discussion in certain patients with epilepsy could be extended to syndromes that are typically felt to be 'benign' and unas-sociated with early mortality in epilepsy, whereas it is unknown whether *any* epilepsy patients are actually immune from SUDEP.

The argument to discuss SUDEP with all patients and families with epilepsy
Some neurologists make an extra effort to discuss SUDEP with the majority or entirety of their epilepsy patients. Patient survey data appear to suggest that parents of both high-risk and low-risk children are glad to have had the discussion, even though it may increase initial anxiety (RamachandranNair et al. 2013). Neurologists may be projecting their own opinions on families when deciding that it would create too much harm for families to have this discussion.

A qualitative study of young adults with epilepsy who were recently told about SUDEP reported that 81% supported uniform disclosure (Tonberg et al. 2015). Some of these patients also admitted to improving their compliance or changing behavior based on their discussion of SUDEP.

The discussion of SUDEP can vary in terms of content and depth based on the interest expressed by the patient and parents/caregivers as well as the patient's level of risk. For example, for a patient with childhood absence epilepsy, the neurologist may let the family know that SUDEP exists and that children with childhood absence epilepsy are at extremely low – probably imperceptibly low – risk for it. Acknowledging that SUDEP exists and placing this in context represent the couching of information that allows for the palatable disclosure that is an intrinsic component of clinical medicine.

Analysis

Principles

Several ethical principles are applicable to this scenario. Autonomy is the principle by which patients and families should have the right to make decisions in their own best interests. Beneficence is the principle by which physicians act in the best interests of the patient. Non-maleficence is the principle by which doctors avoid doing harm to patients.

In this scenario, the patient lacks the appropriate ethical maturity and legal status to make independent decisions as to his own best interests, and his parents act as his surrogate decision-makers. The physician must use humility, honesty and compassion to balance and contrast the autonomy of the patient – or the parents as surrogate decision-makers – to make decisions about applying their own ethical values, compared to the possible paternalism of the neurologist deciding whether disclosure is in the patient's and family's best interest. Although it may seem paternalistic to make the unilateral decision to avoid disclosure and discussion of SUDEP to 'protect' families, there are many other items that are not disclosed to patients. It is logistically impossible to cover every possible diagnostic, therapeutic and outcome scenario in every clinical setting. For example, busy clinicians may decide that they lack sufficient time to manage a thorough and sensitive discussion of all rare events, including rare side effects from medication or SUDEP. Other clinicians may fear that their patient ratings, which have become increasingly ubiquitous due to proliferating patient satisfaction surveys, may decrease by discussing an unexpected and emotionally laden topic. A certain level of risk must exist to warrant any such discussion in a clinical setting. Autonomy can be difficult to exercise in this case because of the neurologist making the decision about the disclosure and discussion of SUDEP.

The principle of non-maleficence could suggest that neurologists should not discuss SUDEP because of the discomfort, anxiety or fear it could produce in patients and families. Yet there is the matter of whether there are indeed actionable items that patients and families could undertake to mitigate their own level of risk. SUDEP has been observed most commonly in persons with a prone sleep position, and thus behavioral modifications, such as a change in sleep position, or the use of devices such as a lattice pillow or seizure detection device, may serve to reduce risk (Liebenthal et al. 2014). Furthermore, it seems at least plausible that achieving improved seizure control, whether with increased adherence to treatment programs or even use of epilepsy surgery where applicable, could reduce the risk of SUDEP and serve as a rationale for making these healthcare choices.

Promoting autonomy of patients and families in this case can present unique challenges. They cannot easily be given sufficient information to decide if they would like to have their neurologist disclose and discuss SUDEP. Several studies have been performed to examine this question and appear to support disclosure. A qualitative analysis performed in Canada used focus groups and detailed interviews to explore parents' views of learning about SUDEP (RamachandranNair et al. 2013). The authors found that parents report a desire for pediatric neurologists to discuss SUDEP face to face, most commonly at the time of epilepsy diagnosis, and that the parents should decide whether the child is present during the discussion. These factors were listed despite the emotions of being overwhelmed and anxious following the discussion.

Families who have actually experienced SUDEP have compellingly argued that it is better to have known of this as a possibility as opposed to first learning about it in the aftermath of a devastating event (Gayatri et al. 2010; Stevenson & Stanton 2014). Until more studies can provide more detailed factors to help neurologists predict which patients and families may not want to discuss SUDEP, information so far suggests that neurologists may underestimate the numbers of patients and families who want to participate in this discussion.

Reconciling the different arguments
The decision about whether to disclose SUDEP universally in the practice of epilepsy care brings several viewpoints (Brodie & Holmes 2008). A variety of opinions exist and, at least in Australian law, neurologists are not found negligent for avoiding a discussion of SUDEP (Beran 2015). Yet the ethical dilemma is in a state of flux as new information becomes available about risk factors, potential interventions to reduce risk and family reactions to undergoing SUDEP's devastating consequences without previously having been aware of this possibility. There may be situations where the discussion could lead to more harm than benefit, but it must be recognized that patients have ready access to information on SUDEP, and discovering its existence on sources such as the Internet would seem less preferable than participating in a guided discussion about it. Additionally, patients and families may sense some damage to the relationship with their neurologist if they find out about this topic they perceive to be incredibly important and suspect that their neurologist was potentially avoiding disclosure. Even in cases where families would welcome the discussion, they are less likely than the physician to initiate it during a clinical encounter. There is an increasing call for physicians to inform and educate patients about risks in low-incidence adverse outcomes (Palmboom et al. 2007).

In the case discussion at hand, the parents are motivated and desirous of counseling. This would be most appropriate in a calm, rational discussion of risk factors and placing them in context. In this particular case of uncomplicated epilepsy, the risk of SUDEP does not appear to be significantly higher than other causes of death, but the existence of SUDEP as an entity requires acknowledgement and an opportunity to frame the wide spectrum of epilepsy and its complications in perspective.

With regards to a more general approach, limited studies suggest that many patients and families would exercise their autonomy by choosing to participate in a discussion of SUDEP. Furthermore, patients and families may benefit from the discussion if this provides sufficient motivation to improve some modifiable risk factors for SUDEP, including medication compliance. Non-maleficence should be considered in how the discussion occurs so that honesty and compassion help guide the discussion with an appropriate setting and timing to help address all applicable concerns from the patient and family.

Many of the barriers to conducting an appropriate discussion of SUDEP with a patient or family can be overcome, although investment of resources will be needed to ensure that neurologists have adequate knowledge of SUDEP and its risk factors. Key knowledge gaps include delineation of risk factors and whether interventions actually reduce risk and prevent its occurrence, the effects of the discussion on patients and families, and the optimal methods of disclosure.

Themes for discussion

- The authors suggest that selective discussion of SUDEP be based on clinicians' sensitivity to a family's (or indeed child's) apparent awareness of this possibility. What 'hints' might a family drop, and what questions can professionals ask, that could be used as indications of a family's readiness to have 'the conversation'?

- This chapter discusses the challenges associated with a conversation about a relatively rare but hugely important possible outcome for a young person with epilepsy. What can professionals do to learn and practice how to start such a conversation? (See also Chapter 8 by Novak et al.)

- The clinical challenge of the 'SUDEP conversation' is probably familiar to many readers of this chapter. Have you ever had a discussion with colleagues about this issue as an ethical dilemma? If you were to start such a conversation, how would your colleagues respond, and why do you think they would respond that way?

- The authors point to a number of possible reasons for not having the 'SUDEP conversation'. Some of these are patient-and-family related issues, but some sound like defensive 'excuses' by professionals to avoid an unpleasant encounter. How do these several 'reasons' resonate with your clinic? Is there an opportunity for your team to have an open and honest discussion about these, or even practice how to discuss SUDEP with your colleagues?

References

Beran RG (2015) SUDEP revisited – a decade on: Have circumstances changed? *Seizure* 27: 47–50.

Berg AT, Nickels K, Wirrell EC et al. (2013) Mortality risks in new-onset childhood epilepsy. *Pediatric* 132: 124–131.

Brodie MJ, Holmes GL (2008) Should all patients be told about sudden unexpected death in epilepsy (SUDEP)? Pros and cons. *Epilepsia* 49: 99–101.

Committee on Injury, Violence and Poison Prevention (2010) Policy statement – prevention of choking among children. *Pediatrics* 125: 601–607.

Friedman D, Donner EJ, Stephens D, Wright C, Devinsky O (2014) Sudden unexpected death in epilepsy: Knowledge and experience among U.S. and Canadian neurologists. *Epilepsy Behav* 35: 13–18.

Gayatri NA, Morrall MC, Jain V et al. (2010) Parental and physician beliefs regarding the provision and content of written sudden unexpected death in epilepsy (SUDEP) information. *Epilepsia* 51: 777–782.

Kalume F (2013) Sudden unexpected death in Dravet syndrome: Respiratory and other physiological dysfunctions. *Respir Physiol Neurobiol* 189: 324–328.

Lhatoo SD, Faulkner HJ, Dembny K, Thippick K, Johnson C, Bird JM (2010) An electroclinical case-control study of sudden unexpected death in epilepsy. *Ann Neurol* 68: 787–796.

Liebenthal JA, Wu S, Rose S, Ebersole JS, Tao JX (2014) Association of prone position with sudden unexpected death in epilepsy. *Neurology* 84: 703–709.

Nilsson L, Farahmond BY, Persson PG, Thiblin I, Tomson T (1999) Risk factors for sudden unexpected death in epilepsy: A case control study. *Lancet* 353: 888–893.

Palmboom GG, Willems DL, Janssen NBAT, de Haes CJCM (2007) Doctor's views on disclosing or withholding information on low risks of complication. *J Med Ethics* 33: 67–70.

RamachandranNair R, Jack SM, Meaney BF, Ronen GM (2013) SUDEP: What do parents want to know? *Epilepsy Behav* 29: 560–564.

Skluzacek JV, Watts KP, Parsy O, Wical B, Camfield P (2011) Dravet syndrome and parent associations: The IDEA League experience with comorbid conditions, mortality, management, adaptation and grief. *Epilepsia* 52(Suppl. 2): 95–101.

Stevenson MJ, Stanton TF (2014) Knowing the risk of SUDEP: Two family's perspectives and The Danny Did Foundation. *Epilepsia* 55: 1495–1500.

Thurman DJ, Hesdorffer DC, French JA (2014) Sudden unexpected death in epilepsy: Assessing the public health burden. *Epilepsia* 55: 1479–1485.

Tomson T, Nashef L, Ryvlin P (2008) Sudden unexpected death in epilepsy: Current knowledge and future directions. *Lancet Neurol* 7: 1021–1031.

Tonberg A, Harden J, McLellan A, Chin RFM, Duncan S (2015) A qualitative study of the reactions of young adults with epilepsy to SUDEP disclosure, perceptions of risk, views on the timing of disclosure and behavioural change. *Epilepsy Behav* 42: 98–106.

Chapter 28

Ethical challenges of diagnosing fetal alcohol spectrum disorder: when diagnosis has socio-political consequences

Ilona Autti-Rämö

Prologue

Knowledge of the long-term effects of prenatal alcohol exposure has increased in recent years. It is acknowledged that there is no safe quantity of alcohol to drink during pregnancy, yet drinking among women of reproductive age has increased multifold during the last decades. The risk of the teratogenic effects of alcohol has simultaneously increased, but the etiology-specific diagnosis – fetal alcohol spectrum disorder (FASD) – is still seldom used in clinical practice. This chapter discusses the ethical challenges of diagnosing FASD, which are relevant worldwide.

Clinical scenario

Ann is 7 years old. She was sent to the neuropediatric department for diagnostic evaluation and developmental intervention. She had been in home care until the age of 6. Her developmental difficulties were identified at preschool and became more evident at school. Ann's mother has confirmed that, prior to recognizing she was pregnant, she drank one to two bottles of wine every weekend and sometimes one to two glasses of wine in the evening during working days. The pregnancy was unplanned and she realized that she was pregnant when she was at week 12 of gestation. She reported that she was able to stop her drinking around week 18 when she felt the first fetal kicks. Ann's mother had no post secondary education; she had not been diagnosed with any neuropsychological impairment. She is currently working as a waiter. Ann's father had been diagnosed with specific learning impairment in reading and writing skills but had graduated as a technician and has a permanent job. Ann's parents divorced a year ago and have shared custody.

Ann comes with her father to hear the results of the neuropsychological evaluation and to plan intervention services.

On neuropsychological evaluation, Ann showed clear difficulties in executive function, memory, reading and arithmetic skills. Her social adaptive skills were 2 years below age. She had a thin upper lip and hypoplastic filtrum, her length was –1SD (standard deviation), weight –1.5SD and head circumference –1.5SD. Neither of the parents had similar facial features. The mother's head circumference was –0.5SD and the father's +0.7SD. Both parents' heights and weights were within the normal range.

The pediatric neurologist discussed the results with Ann and her father and it was decided that a meeting with the teacher and neuropsychologist should be organized to plan individual support at school. Individual intervention would be decided thereafter. A nurse was asked to play with Ann and the diagnostic assessment was discussed with the father.

The pediatric neurologist informed the father that Ann fulfills the criteria for alcohol-related neurobehavioral disorder (ARND). Ann's mother had confirmed prenatal alcohol exposure of moderate to high level at several occasions until mid-pregnancy. Owing to Ann's father's specific learning difficulties, she also has hereditary risk factors for learning difficulties. However, her profile is consistent with current knowledge on the neurocognitive deficits after prenatal alcohol exposure (at least three brain domains affected), and her facial features and growth trajectories are also in line with the diagnostic criteria for FASD. Her father disagreed with the diagnosis as he considered it to be a negative or derogatory label. Although Ann has the right to read her records when she becomes an adult, her father also disagreed that the information about prenatal alcohol exposure should be included in the electronic patient record. He did not want Ann to be aware of her mother's alcohol consumption during pregnancy. However, he was interested in hearing how the information on drinking during pregnancy or the diagnosis of FASD could be taken into account in his legal appeal to have his daughter stay with him, as he disagrees with the current arrangement on the number of days Ann can stay with him.

In clinical practice, various ethical issues arise when diagnosing children and adolescents with FASD (an umbrella term for all disorders caused by prenatal alcohol exposure). These can be encountered by biological and foster parents, and by professionals who have patients with FASD in their care. Ethical issues that are common to all countries, cultures and societies include questions about the specificity of the diagnostic process, the possibility for false-positive and false-negative diagnoses, and the possibility of stigmatization. In addition, professional and societal values have to be considered.

Is diagnosing FASD justified?

FASD is an etiological diagnosis for a multisystem disorder. It indicates that prenatal alcohol exposure is the major underlying reason for the child's multiple problems. To date, however, no uniform, internationally accepted criteria have been developed for the various subtypes of FASD. The diagnostic criteria are based on cut-off values on growth and performance values (usually at −2SD or 10%) (Astley 2006; Chudley et al. 2005; Hoyme et al. 2005; Landgraf et al. 2013). In a clinical case it is often not possible to define which neurobehavioral deficits and difficulties in psychosocial adjustment are specific to prenatal alcohol exposure and which may be due to hereditary factors or caused by adverse life events or other factors (Rangmar et al. 2015; Streissguth et al. 1996). In cases with ARND, in particular, there is a possibility of false-positive and false-negative diagnoses.

Ann has had a confirmed prenatal alcohol exposure of excessive quantity and frequency, which indicates a high risk for permanent brain damage, compromised brain development and deficit in her learning skills. Ann is already at risk for learning disabilities: her father had specific learning impairments, and her challenging home environment may have affected her ability to concentrate and develop reading skills. It is impossible to separate the effects of these various possible determinants from each other, but for clinical judgment it is justified to suspect that they have an additive effect. Ann's features and neuropsychological profile are, however, in agreement with the existing diagnostic criteria for FASD (subtype ARND).

Why give the diagnosis of FASD and not a specific learning disorder and attention deficit hyperactivity disorder (ADHD)? First, the prognosis of FASD is poorer than that of a specific learning impairment of hereditary origin, especially for social adaptation skills and executive functions (Fagerlund et al. 2012; Koponen et al. 2013). It is of clinical importance that the habilitation (intervention) plan is based not only on current difficulties, but is also designed to prevent psychosocial and behavioral problems that are common in FASD during adolescence and adulthood (Rangmar et al. 2015; Streissguth et al. 1996).

The needs of the child also require specific capabilities and parenting skills of the parents. When planning interventions, the needs of the whole family should be taken into account. Having problems with alcohol intake and with custody are both

Table 28.1 Risk and protective factors for children and adolescents with FASD during postnatal life

Risk factors	Protective factors
Neglect and maltreatment	Early instituted interventions for both the child and mother and father when needed
Witnessing domestic violence	Regular follow-up
Mental illness of parents	Psychosocial support
Alcohol or drug problem in the family	Early instituted interventions
Child protection services not available or not effective	Special education provided if needed
Taken repeatedly into custody	Child protective services accepted by parents
No individually tailored interventions	Improved parenting skills
No educational support at school	Planned and supported integration into society
Bullying	
Disrupted school	
Not accepting the diagnosis	

major risk factors that must be carefully evaluated and discussed with the parents. As for Ann, the possible risk and protective factors for her future development have to be discussed with both parents. Acknowledging these factors (Table 28.1) helps the parents to understand their role in helping Ann overcome the difficulties she faces at school.

What about a parent's fear of stigma?

FASD is one of the few diagnostic terms (e.g. human immunodeficiency virus [HIV] encephalopathy, substance abuse) that gives direct information on the link between a mother's living habits during pregnancy and the child's disorder. This is of major concern, as lay people, and some professionals too, consider it to be a stigmatizing diagnosis. When Jones and colleagues reported the syndrome (Jones et al. 1973), one aim was to inform both the public and professionals of the causal link between prenatal alcohol exposure and fetal abnormalities, which could even be fatal. At that time, FASD was thought to be an on–off phenomenon – one either had it or did not. We now know that FASD is a spectrum of disorders ranging from subtle neurobehavioral disorders to lethal malformations. Yet the message to the public and professionals is still the same – alcohol is a teratogenic agent.

The physician's task is to diagnose and identify the etiology of the neurocognitive deficit. Many professionals may consider the diagnosis of FASD to be stigmatizing, providing no direct benefit to the child. They instead may give the diagnosis ADHD and specific learning disorder for a child like Ann. However, one can ask whether it is a moral responsibility as a professional to give the diagnosis of FASD when it is evident (as in Ann's case), as we do for all disorders with a known etiology. When diagnosing FASD, one also has to consider the possibility of the current or future siblings having the same disorder – with the same or a different phenotype. A plan has to be made regarding how to proceed. In other cases the diagnosis can be much more difficult to give. What if Ann had a complex neurobehavioral disorder and confirmed prenatal alcohol exposure at a risk level, but without any facial features or traces of growth retardation, pre- or postnatal, indicating alcohol's terotegenic effects? It would be much harder to define the order of etiological factors, which could include any combination of prenatal alcohol exposure, hereditary factors, possible social deprivation, and witnessing repeated arguments at home.

It is also our professional responsibility not to blame anyone for the outcome but to discuss with the parents their fear of labeling. It is important that the parents have the opportunity to discuss with professionals the realization of the teratogenic effects of prenatal alcohol exposure in their child. It is of utmost importance that the mother is treated with respect and support. She needs to live with this information, and blaming her for the past is not helpful. The focus should be on the future – to help the child overcome the difficulties, support a safe living environment and organize the necessary support.

Societal perspective – does it play a role in individual cases?

Birth anomalies are relatively rare. In order to identify the changes in their prevalence and identify their etiology to develop a preventive strategy, many Western countries have a centralized system to register at least major birth anomalies. In Finland, it is statutory to report any identified teratogenic effects to the Birth Anomaly Register. It is generally recommended that information regarding any exposure with potential teratogenic effect, such as alcohol consumption, smoking, recreational drugs and maternal use of medication, should be documented in the patient records of both the mother and child. For alcohol intake, the child's records should document the reported dose, frequency and content of alcohol exposure, but not the reasons for drinking. These known teratogenic factors should always be carefully considered as possible etiological factors when a child presents with developmental impairments, growth retardation or malformations. When the etiological link is confirmed, it should also be recorded. However, birth anomaly registers are so far not reliable sources for the prevalence of FASD in any country, as professionals still neglect to record their suspicion of a teratogenic effect. In the future, the use of electronic patient records with structured information gathering will help to identify causal links between developmental disorders and exposure to various teratogens and adverse events during childhood. With time, structured recording of various exposures to teratogenic agents during pregnancy will also help to identify the true prevalence of various teratogenic effects, including FASD.

Alcohol is the leading cause of preventable developmental disorders. As drinking among women of reproductive age increases, so does the prevalence of FASD. In recent in-school studies, the prevalence of FASD in Western countries was as high as 2–9 per 100 (May et al. 2009, 2014). By blindfolding ourselves and giving other, more generic diagnoses (e.g. specific learning disorder and ADHD for Ann), we neglect the specific needs of the child and family due to FASD and possible alcohol problems in the family. We also miss the opportunity to make visible the specific effects of prenatal alcohol exposure. As long as FASD is not acknowledged and diagnosed by professionals, society will not provide enough resources for preventing and treating this disorder.

Many professionals continue to consider the diagnosis of FASD as stigmatizing, with no benefit for the child, and therefore hesitate to give it. From an ethical perspective, professionals who defer diagnosing FASD may unconsciously allow the prevalence of FASD to rise, as the problem remains invisible. Patients' rights vary in different countries and in different jurisdictions, often depending on the prevailing cultural and social norms (see http://www.who.int/genomics/public/patientrights/en/). In the paternalistic model, the best interests of the patient, as judged by the clinical expert, are valued above the provision of comprehensive medical information and decision-making power to the patient. The informative model, by contrast, sees the patient as a consumer who is in the best position to judge what is in her own interest, and thus views the doctor chiefly as a provider of information. Withdrawing from the information of etiology in Ann's case can be considered as a paternalistic approach. One can also question whether, by changing the name FASD to one that is less stigmatizing, this ethical dilemma would be solved.

Do I have the skills to make this diagnosis?

Despite data demonstrating its continued prevalence, the diagnosis of FASD is still rarely given. This is mainly due to three factors: it requires trustworthy information on maternal drinking during pregnancy, experienced multiprofessional teams (for children with

ARND, this requires, at a minimum, a child neurologist/developmental pediatrician and psychologist, and preferably also a speech therapist), and an acknowledgment that the diagnosis is of benefit to the child and family.

Alcohol drinking among women of reproductive age has increased up to six fold during the last 4 decades in Finland and is more common than smoking. The same holds true for many Western countries. Approximately 90% of fertile-aged women drink alcohol, and up to 50% drink it during early pregnancy (Ahlvik et al. 2006). Thus, asking about maternal drinking during pregnancy should be a customary practice by all clinicians following pregnant women and evaluating the development of children. Given these modern realities, it is important that pregnant or pre-pregnant women should be asked about their alcohol consumption.

My clinical practice has been to ask first about lifestyle prior to pregnancy, including drinking and smoking activity. I then focus on current lifestyle, and how becoming a parent may have changed the lifestyle of the parents. Then I return to pregnancy: I ask whether it was a planned pregnancy and tell people that over 50% of pregnancies are not planned in Finland. Finally, I ask when the mother noticed she was pregnant and whether and how this information affected her alcohol consumption and smoking. With this approach I obtain more reliable information about alcohol consumption during pregnancy than I would by asking directly whether the mother drank during pregnancy.

Diagnosing FASD requires expertise. This can be developed, as there are many guidelines on how to do this (Astley 2006; Chudley et al. 2005; Hoyme et al. 2005; Landgraf et al. 2013).

Clinical practice has taught me that the diagnosis of FASD is often rather welcome for foster and adoptive parents. It helps them understand the magnitude of their child's problems, and differentiates those that originate from damage to the central nervous system from those that are responses to the traumatic experiences to which they have been exposed postnatally, associated with having been removed from their biological families (see also Table 28.1). However, biological mothers also benefit from the diagnosis as they are often aware of the possibility and may be too scared to discuss it. It is helpful for them if a professional can discuss the consideration of FASD diagnosis in a respectful and supportive way. In many countries, biological mothers have founded support groups for birth mothers. National and international FASD organizations are also often founded by foster parents and birth mothers and are supported by professionals (see http://www.eufasd.org in Europe, http://www.nofasd.org.au in Australia, http://www.nofas.org in the USA, contact kachor@nofas.org and http://www.nofas-uk.org in the UK).

How to communicate the diagnosis and to whom?

When discussing the diagnosis of FASD, one has to be specific about facts and sensitive to individual reactions. The parents often have difficulties in accepting the diagnosis, and rarely do the mothers give specific and honest information on their alcohol intake. Denial and accusation are common reactions, and the professional has to explain the benefits of a FASD diagnosis for the child. In situations where the parents disagree about custody, it has to be clearly stated that the diagnosis does not inform about current drinking or the quality of motherhood or parenthood.

There is no consensus regarding the age at which the child is able to handle the diagnostic information, but it is important that the diagnosis be discussed with the child before they leave pediatric care. The diagnosis must be explained in a way that does not blame the mother but helps the child understand the unique difficulties they face. A good clinical practice is to explain the nature of alcoholism – it is not something anybody willingly chooses. The information on the risks of alcohol consumption during pregnancy has also been conflicting. This has led to situations in which the risk has been realized prior to the mother truly understanding the consequences for her child – as in Ann's mother's case. Every woman has an individual susceptibility to develop addiction to alcohol, and every fetus has individual risk factors for being permanently damaged as a result of prenatal alcohol exposure. It is also important that the young adult with FASD understands that FASD-related symptoms are not hereditary.

Diagnosing FASD may have profound consequences on an individual's self-image and behavior, and thus one has to be prepared to offer psychosocial support as long as it is needed. According to my clinical experience, adolescents and adults given the diagnosis are, in general, grateful for the diagnosis if it is discussed openly, without blame and with enough time. Many young people may, however, blame society for not offering help for their mother. Some may accuse their mother of destroying their future. At present there is only clinical experience, and no systematic research, on how a person with FASD will handle the diagnostic information. My own clinical experience suggests that the first reaction is often sorrow and grief about lost potential, and sometimes shame. Then comes anger towards those health professionals who took care of the mother while pregnant, as the mother is usually considered a victim. The professionals need to be prepared to handle these negative reactions. The next phase is adaptation to the process, relief in understanding that one's problems are based on a true organic origin and not just being 'lazy' or 'crazy'. The last phase is looking forward to a time when the patient and family develop a willingness to fight for their rights to get the support that is needed, and realize their capabilities for independent adult life. These phases are common experiences for many patients and families when receiving 'bad' or unwanted news.

The yearly congresses on FASD in Vancouver, Canada, include sessions involving adults with FASD sharing how the diagnosis of FASD changed their lives. Those adults with FASD who come forward in these congresses have expressed their thankfulness for being diagnosed correctly. They have often had lengthy diagnostic journeys with many other diagnoses, especially psychiatric ones, and many have also tried a range of pharmaceuticals. It is, however, fair to conclude that this may not be true for all persons with a diagnosis of FASD.

Diagnostic information on FASD may be of different value to different stakeholder groups. It is a moral issue to consider to whom this information must and may be communicated. Depending on the community, it may be more relevant to communicate only the identified difficulties and special needs (e.g. to the school and further education), but, in some communities, access to specific interventions requires specific diagnostic information. The societal attitude towards drinking in general (and specifically during pregnancy) or the diagnosis of FASD can be different depending on the country (Racine et al. 2015).

Is there something else to know?

Asking about drinking during pregnancy, and informing people about the detrimental and life-long consequences of drinking during pregnancy, are obligations of all health professionals meeting women with drinking problems. It is our professional responsibility to remind women of reproductive age that there is no known safety level for drinking during pregnancy. The most extreme situation involves the combination of binge drinking and accidental pregnancy, which may result in severe brain malformations and neurodevelopmental impairments and disability (Ronen & Andrews 1991).

Problematic drinking is not pregnancy-specific, but is often a life-long challenge. The health of the mother should also be a priority concern, as women who have an alcohol abuse problem during pregnancy have mortality rates over 30 times higher during the next decade (Kahila et al. 2010). They also have increased morbidity from various infectious and traumatic disorders. Consultation by a social worker and adult physicians familiar with alcohol abuse disorders should be offered.

In most cases, patients have the right to autonomy, but a child with developmental difficulties is examined with the consent of their parents. The current trend in juvenile court to screen adolescents for FASD is of some moral concern, as the value of the diagnosis is not so much for health benefit but to establish FASD as a mitigating factor (Autti-Rämö 2015). This approach has led to requests to develop FASD diagnostic centers for adolescents and adults in Canada and the USA. Screening for and diagnosing FASD requires a reallocation of human resources, funding and training. All of this raises an ethical question: Why is maternal alcohol consumption during pregnancy a more justi-fied mitigating factor than hereditary factors, preterm birth, birth asphyxia or postnatal trauma leading to neurobehavioral impairments and difficulties for understanding the consequences of one's actions? This unfortunate trend may label all people with FASD as being prone to having trouble with the law.

<hr>

Follow up

Ann's father was told that the meaning of the diagnosis and possible interventions should be discussed with both parents, preferably together. The father agreed, and both parents came to discuss the results of the neuropsychological tests, the diagnostic criteria for ARND and why this diagnosis is of benefit to Ann. In Finland there has been a lot of public information on FASD but unfortunately the media has focused on the more severe end of the spectrum and on children taken into custody. This problem can be seen worldwide.

Ann's mother was afraid of losing the custody of her child if her child received this diagnosis. This misconception was first clarified. Diagnosing FASD does not mean that the child is taken into custody; rather, postnatal maltreatment, continuous neglect in daily care and lack of par-enting skills are clear indicators for child protective services. At the moment, both parents were considered as the best caregivers of their child and the mother was relieved to hear this infor-mation. As the focus was shifted to the future, both parents were gradually able to understand what the diagnosis meant for their daily lives and the kind of personal support Ann would need both at home and at school. The necessity of having similar rules at both parents' homes was also discussed.

Neither parent was willing to reveal the diagnosis to Ann at the moment. It was decided that the timing of discussing with Ann the etiology of her difficulties would be determined later. As many teenagers seek to understand why they may be struggling at school and having problems with peers, professionals have to be prepared to give the information when they want it – and prepare the parents for the reactions that are likely to come.

Themes for discussion

- Does exposure of a fetus to alcohol constitute child abuse? Should all mothers (or indeed families) of children with FASD be reported to children's aid societies? How do our responsibilities to the many people involved in such a situation conflict?

- Does a diagnosis of FASD carry with it condition-specific management strategies? If not, what are the benefits and limitations of making such a diagnosis?

- There are many people who believe that communities should institute universal screening for FASD – while others disagree strongly. What clinical and technical elements would need to be in place for such a program to be justified, and to do more good than harm?

References

Ahlvik A, Haldorsen T, Grohol B, Lindemann R (2006) Alcohol consumption before and during pregnancy comparing concurrent and retrospective reports. *Alcohol Clin Exp Res* 30: 510–515.

Astley SJ (2006) Comparison the 4-digit diagnostic code and the Hoyme diagnostic guidlines for fetal alcohol spectrum disorders. *Pediatrics* 118: 1532–1544.

Autti-Rämö I (2015) Ethical challenges when screening for and diagnosing FASD in adults. In: Nelson M, Trussler M, editors. *Fetal alcohol spectrum disorders in adults: Ethical and legal perspectives. Int Library Ethics Law* 63: 85–97.

Chudley AE, Conry J, Cook JL, Loock C, Rosales T, LeBlanc N (2005) Fetal alcohol spectrum disorders: Canadian guidelines for diagnosis. *CMAJ* 172(Suppl. 5): S1–S21.

Fagerlund Å, Autti-Rämö I, Kalland M et al. (2012) Adaptive behaviour in children and adolescents with foetal alcohol spectrum disorders: A comparison with specific learning disability and typical development. *Eur Child Adol Psychiatr* 12: 221–231.

Hoyme HE, May PA, Kalberg WO et al. (2005) A practical clinical approach to diagnosis of fetal alcohol spectrum disorders: Clarification of the 1996 Institute of Medicine criteria. *Pediatrics* 115: 39–47.

Jones KL, Smith DW, Ulleland CN, Streissguth P (1973) Pattern of malformation in offspring of chronic alcohol mothers. *Lancet* 1(7815): 1267–1271.

Kahila H, Gissler M, Sarkola T, Autti-Rämö I, Halmesmäki E (2010) Maternal welfare, morbidity and mortality 6–15 years after a pregnancy complicated by alcohol and substance abuse: A register-based case–control follow-up study of 524 women. *Alcohol Drug Depend* 111: 215–221.

Koponen A, Kalland M, Autti Rämö I, Suominen S (2013) Socio-emotional development of children with foetal alcohol spectrum disorders in long-term foster family care: A qualitative study. *Nordic Social Work Res* 3: 38–58.

Landgraf MN, Nothacker M, Heinen F (2013) Diagnosis of fetal alcohol syndrome (FAS): German guideline version 2013. *Eur J Paediatr Neurol* 17(5): 437–446.

May P, Gossage JP, Kalberg WO et al. (2009) Prevalence and epidemiologic characteristics of FASD from various research methods with an emphasis on recent in-school studies. *Dev Disabil Res Rev* 15: 176–192.

May PA, Baete A, Russo J et al. (2014) Prevalence and characteristics of fetal alcohol spectrum disorders. *Pediatrics* 134(5): 855–866.

Racine E, Bell E, Zizzo N, Green C (2015) Public discourse on the biology of alcohol addiction: Implications for stigma, self-control, essentialism and coercive policies in pregnancy. *Neuroethics* 8: 177–186.

Rangmar J, Hjern A, Vinnerljung B, Strömland K, Aronson M, Fahlke C (2015) Psychosocial outcomes of fetal alcohol syndrome in adulthood. *Pediatrics* 135(1): e52–e58.

Ronen GM, Andrews WL (1991) Holoprosencephaly as a possible embryonic alcohol effect. *Am J Med Genet* 40: 151–154.

Streissguth AP, Barr HM, Kogan J, Bookstein FL (1996) *Final report: Understanding the occurrence of secondary disabilities in clients with fetal alcohol syndrome (FAS) and fetal alcohol effects (FAE).* Seattle, WA: University of Washington Publication Services.

Chapter 29

Growth and pubertal manipulation in children with neurodisabilities: what are the ethical implications?

M. Constantine Samaan

Prologue

As the number of people living with neurodisabilities reaches new levels (Saigal & Doyle 2008), it is apparent that long-term support is needed in several areas, including developmental interventions to promote mobility, communication abilities, and social and behavioral skills. Puberty is a maturational process through which neuronal and hormonal changes transition children to reproductive maturation and completion of physical growth. The current generally accepted age limit of normal puberty initiation is 8 years for Caucasian girls, while for African-American girls, this stands at 6 years (Nathan & Palmert 2005).

Puberty may create several challenges for care providers of children with neurodevelopmental impairment. These include unpredictable emotional and behavioral changes, and challenges in carrying out the tasks of care due to physical growth and maturation. On a healthcare systems level, there are limited resources to support parental efforts to maintain care at home, and the cost of hiring help for additional support is often quite considerable. Faced with these considerations, some parents may consider a variety of strategies to continue homecare, and one approach involves keeping bodies small and prepubertal.

Such approaches need to consider several factors, including the preferences of the person with impairment(s), their family, along with community and societal expectations and legal regulations, to ensure that the well-being of these children is secured. In this chapter, a case is presented that sparked the debate on growth and pubertal alteration in children with neurodisabilities. We then consider the parameters of ethical decision-making in light of what has been learned from this and similar cases. We also discuss the ethical principles driving the decision-making process, and propose a practical approach to address these situations.

Clinical scenario

Lisa is a 9-year-old girl with profound neurodevelopmental impairment following a hypoxic–ischemic insult at birth. She attends the endocrine clinic with her parents for discussions regarding the suppression of further growth and pubertal development. Lisa is non-ambulatory, and the family uses a wheelchair with special seating for mobilization. She has scoliosis, bilateral knee flexion contractures, and dislocation of femoral heads. She also has gastroesophageal reflux with a history of recurrent aspiration pneumonia, and receives gastrostomy tube (G-tube) feeding for all her meals and has urinary incontinence. While her parents are responsible for most of her care needs, community nursing support is provided during the daytime.

On examination, her height is congruent with her genetic potential, weight is on the 90th centile and her body mass index (BMI) is in the normal range for age and sex. Lisa has signs of early puberty, with breast buds and pubic hair development (Tanner Stage II). Her hormonal profiles confirm the clinical findings of early puberty. Her bone age is slightly advanced when compared to her chronological age.

Lisa's parents express concerns about their ability to mobilize her during routine care if she grows further, and they have been finding this an increasing challenge. They are concerned about the behavioral and physical burdens of puberty to their daughter, which they feel may lower her functioning and quality of life. They are also apprehensive about potential future pregnancies, and would like to consider options for intervention to limit growth and puberty.

The 'Ashley treatment': an approach to growth and pubertal suppression in children with neurodevelopmental impairments

Growth and pubertal attenuation in children with neurodisabilities was vigorously debated after its implementation in a child in the USA in 2006. The parents of the child, named Ashley, were concerned that her pubertal development and growth spurt would lead to limitations in their ability to continue providing care at home, and would increase her discomfort during mobilization due to the increased size of her developing breasts. They also had concerns regarding the onset of menstruation and potential dysmenorrhea. Following consultation with their physicians and an institutional ethics board, Ashley had a hysterectomy, an appendectomy and breast bud removal. In addition, high dose estrogen therapy was used to trigger premature epiphyseal closure and limit height gain (Gunther & Diekema 2006). The parents posted the details of the 'Ashley treatment' online, and argued for its benefits in their daughter's case (http://www.pillowangel.org/).

The case ignited a firestorm of debate that continues today. The decision to proceed with this treatment was criticized by many and entertained by few (Dickerson 2007; Edwards 2008; Goldworth 2010; Liao 2007; Ouellette 2008; Ryan 2008; Shannon 2007). With the publication of the case and the strong reactions it generated, Disability Rights Washington (a Washington state protection and advocacy system in the USA, where Ashley was treated) initiated an investigation into the ethics and legality of this course of action. The investigation concluded that Ashley's legal rights were violated when the treating hospital proceeded with hysterectomy without a court order, and recommendations were made to do so in the future, to which the treating hospital agreed (http://www.disabilityrightswa.org/ashley-treatment-investigation).

Dilemmas in making decisions to limit growth and puberty

If we are to contemplate a parental request for the so-called 'Ashley treatment' or a version of it for Lisa, there are several considerations when deciding on a course of action. These include the necessity, efficacy and the potential harms and benefits to Lisa and her family, as well as legal boundaries for such decisions. This is important, as there is precedence for parental requests for therapies that have not been fully evaluated, or are of questionable value, in an attempt to improve outcomes in children with neurodisabilities; therefore, careful consideration is warranted in this case (Bell et al. 2011).

First, is this intervention necessary? The limitation of growth and puberty will not improve Lisa's lifespan, and the procedures involved in administering this intervention are not being offered to manage a specific disease or health condition, but are interfering with a physiological process common to all girls. The efficacy of this intervention will be quite high in the case of applying the 'Ashley treatment' to Lisa. We can expect that the intervention will limit growth, prevent menstruation and eliminate the chance of future pregnancies. Despite the efficacy in limiting physical growth and pubertal development, questions remain as to the reasons behind pursuing such an approach. Is this treatment a 'therapeutic' choice, necessary to sustain life and well-being, or is it a 'non-therapeutic' intervention designed to enhance the ability of Lisa's parents to maintain quality homecare for as long as possible? Parental interests are very likely intertwined with Lisa's, but is this intervention designed to make the parents' lives easier for care provision, and does it take into account Lisa's needs, preferences and wishes?

From a parental perspective, this intervention may be necessary due to the potential perceived advantages of growth and pubertal attenuation. The reduced final height may improve parental ability to position Lisa more easily and more often, and this easier mobilization may allow greater frequency of social interactions with her family and care providers, and lead to improved well-being.

Lisa is likely to be unaware of her height trajectory (Erling et al. 1994). As she uses a wheelchair, other people will probably not notice the differences in height or breast development compared to other children in wheelchairs. In addition, Lisa's interactions with the world are limited to her family and caregivers, and this trend is likely to continue. Therefore, the way her caregivers view her is not likely to change if her height or pubertal status is altered (Erling et al. 1994; Wiklund et al. 1994).

If Lisa is exposed to the community beyond her immediate circle of caregivers, there is a chance that limiting growth and puberty may accentuate the stigma that surrounds neurodisability. Although this is a possibility, limiting growth and puberty may not worsen potential stigma that may emerge in dealing with the diagnosis of neurodisability (Green 2003). Lisa herself is not likely to feel stigmatized, as she will not recognize the absence of continued growth and pubertal development (Spriggs 2010).

In relation to menstruation, managing menstrual flow may be a challenge using the pads she currently wears for urinary incontinence. Period pads are designed for blood collection and chronic, low-flow situations. In contrast, urine pads are designed for a larger volume of fluid but are not suitable for managing menstrual flow. Tampons can be an alternative, but these may be more difficult to place in the presence of lower limb contractures and hip instability, and carry the risk of toxic shock syndrome if left in for prolonged periods of time (Burnham & Kollef 2015; Low 2013). Hysterectomy eliminates menstruation and the chance of pregnancy in case of non-consensual intercourse.

There are potential disadvantages of growth and puberty attenuation therapy. It can be argued that treatments of this nature are unjust, as they change the bodies of children who are unable to indicate their preferences. Another concern is that the safety of the interventions proposed should also be considered carefully. The interventions carry risks related to drugs, anesthesia and the surgical procedures themselves. The safety of high-dose estrogen in this population has been extrapolated based on data from using hormonal replacement therapy in postmenopausal women. That experience showed that the risk of clots is not increased in women on hormonal therapy, but in our case there may be a risk of thromboembolism, as Lisa is immobile. There are no specific data regarding the use of hormonal contraceptive therapies related to children with neurodevelopmental impairments (Allen et al. 2009). The risks of anesthesia may pose additional challenges in children with neurodisability. These may include positioning difficulties for intubation, altered seizure threshold and reactions to anesthetic medications. Surgical complications related to the procedures may include bleeding, pain, infection, scarring and adhesions.

The needs of people with neurodevelopmental impairments may change if their bodies are altered, and parents may find it easier to care for a smaller body, but this may be a violation of children's rights as individuals within society. This approach also raises concerns of a potential 'slippery slope', where further alterations and more invasive procedures may be justified to enable ease of care (Ouellette, 2008; Ryan 2008).

If adopted by the healthcare system, pubertal limitation by surgery and hormonal therapy has the potential to be misused in patients with neurodevelopmental impairments, as it may be perceived as an alternative to more costly management and support options. Furthermore, providing such interventions may result in the allocation of finite health-care resources to other areas, and take momentum away from lobbying for more services to provide homecare for children that may be more expensive.

Considered from a legal perspective, there may be concerns that the rights of the child have been violated. Depending on the jurisdiction, there may be wide variations in how this situation can be approached with the courts. Furthermore, constitutional, legal and societal considerations will come to bear on the decision to alter the body of a person who cannot communicate their wishes. The rights of children are intertwined with their parents' desire to care for them, and in light of the above considerations, parents are important partners in the decision-making process. Although the person with the neurodevelopmental impairment is at the center of the decision-making process, the family, community, society, policy-makers and the law may each play a role in defining the answers to this dilemma (Thomasma 1978).

Principles of ethical decision-making

Over the past several years, debate has continued on the best decision-making strategies for individuals similar to Lisa. Applying foundational ethical principles has been proposed to provide a platform for decision-making, but the potential problem with this approach is that no single paradigm is able to capture the complexity of the decision, which may thus result in limited utility (Jecker 1997).

Another approach in ethical decision-making involves comparing current cases to previous ones, to determine the limits of acceptability of decisions using different combinations of principles. This allows the evaluation of multiple approaches simultaneously, and minimizes biased conclusions when using a single principle (McCabe 1996; Tiedje et al. 2013). A description of the ethical principles used in deliberating these decisions is provided in the following.

Autonomy

The right of a patient to refuse or accept medical intervention is enshrined in law, and is accepted as a societal and ethical imperative in care provision by the medical profession. When it comes to autonomy, patients will lead, and their care team will follow. However, there are several caveats to respecting patients' autonomy. Patients' and caregivers' rights are enforced when they are deemed competent, having understood the benefits and risks in accepting or refusing an intervention, and their choices about care are considered rational. Therefore, if a person or a care provider is deemed 'irrational', given their situation, this situation may bring into question their capacity to make such decisions, and interfere with their right to challenge a treatment (Rosenbaum 2009).

This does not imply that healthcare teams should routinely dismiss refusals of therapy as evidence that people are being irrational; careful evaluation of patients' and care providers' understanding of the information, their need for more information and their right to deliberation that is free of coercion is mandatory. It should also be obvious that each situation must be considered on its own specific and individual merits rather than with some blanket policy.

One of the complexities about respecting children's autonomy is that in many cases, it is the parents who make decisions on their child's behalf. In the case presented here, it would be difficult to define what Lisa would have done if she had the capacity to understand her parents' requests and make decisions about them.

The idea of children's autonomy may be approached differently if the question is related to accepting an intervention versus refusing an intervention. In this case, the parents are considering an intervention that will irreversibly alter their daughter's body (and perhaps her mind) and does not seem to provide her with long-term benefit (such as scoliosis surgery, as discussed in Chapter 24). Although the parents very probably believe that this would be beneficial to her care, the facilitation of such a wish may impinge on Lisa's autonomy.

In this case, the physician can refuse to provide treatment due to a lack of benefit or perceived harm. However, if the physician is making the decision not to treat patients based on their own beliefs and not solely on the evidence available, then they are obliged to refer the patient to a physician who can provide the needed treatment. If the physician cannot refer the patient, they are expected to provide the treatment as long as it is within the acceptable standards of care.

Non-maleficence

Making decisions that balance risks and benefits, the 'primum non nocere' dictum, is one of the oldest principles in medicine (Gillon 2015). It drives the decision-making process in every clinical encounter, as the risk of commission or omission of interventions to treat carries the risk of potential harm to patients. This principle also applies to the relationship of parents to children. While we trust that parents are the guardians of their children's best interest, it is important to determine that an intervention is not detrimental to the child's well-being, even if sanctioned by the parents and of benefit to them.

In our case, the use of high-dose estrogen is a method to constrain growth, while limiting puberty may involve hysterectomy and breast bud removal. These interventions are associated with medication, anesthetic and the surgical risks noted above. The question might be posed as to what a reasonable family would decide in a similar situation. Would a significant proportion of parents opt for this intervention? What are the benefits and harms, and how can the latter be reduced? This situation may require a case-by-case approach to decision-making. In the overwhelming majority of cases, the expectation is that the rights of the child to bodily integrity should sway the decision.

Beneficence
This is the concept of having the welfare of the patient at the center of any decisions about their care (Goldworth 2010). Beneficence acknowledges the autonomy of the patient, yet balances this with the worthiness of the intervention, after careful consideration of the intervention's risks and benefits (Jansen 2013).

The balance between beneficence, non-maleficence and autonomy depends on the patient's competence. If a patient is deemed competent to make decisions about their health, and has the information they need to make the decision, then in this author's opinion autonomy supersedes beneficence.[1] On the other hand, if the patient or a caregiver requests interventions thought to be 'unreasonable', non-maleficence will drive the decision made by the physician to refuse to provide the intervention. In cases where there may be options requested by the patient that are deemed reasonable but not ideal, and if resources permit the provision of such interventions, then the physician may be obliged to provide the intervention at least early on in management. This may provide the patient and physician with a window to evaluate the intervention while assuring the patient that their concerns are being heard. This also allows for future reevaluation and adjustment of the intervention plans, and may increase the patient's agreement with the new approach, as they will feel that their concerns have not been ignored (Clark & Weaver 2015; Kasman 2004).

Justice
The principle of justice dictates that people are to be treated in a fair and equitable fashion. This does not mean treating everyone equally, as this may disadvantage those who are more vulnerable, and deepen the inequality. One consideration for

---

1   Editors' note: See Chapter 25 by Clarke, where the alternate view is presented that it is a mistake to frame issues as giving an overriding status to one ethical principle over another.

justice in our case is the limitation of vulnerability. Lisa is vulnerable as she has diminished capacity of self-determination, and relies on the parents to make decisions on her behalf. In addition, a critical threat to fairness involves maintaining the balance of power of parent–child and physician–family relations. In this situation, parents have enormous power over their dependent child's care decisions. The physician may also have an advantage, as parents may not fully understand the intricacies of a given care situation compared to the physician in charge of their child's care (Gillon 2015).

Clinical approach to address Lisa's case

In order to finalize the decisions needed in this case, a full evaluation is necessary. A thorough medical history should include the full family narrative, with details about the diagnosis, pregnancy and birth history, attainment of neurodevelopmental milestones, functional abilities including current and projected estimates, and family structure, finances and other biopsychosocial determinants. In addition, the input of other healthcare professionals, such as the nursing and developmental therapists involved in patient care, may provide valuable insights regarding the children and their families. These professionals are likely to have spent significant amounts of time with the patient and family, and are able to provide insights into patient function and management that can help with the decision-making process.

Detailed physical examination including anthropometric measures, current pubertal stage and evaluation of functional abilities should be done. Additional investigations may include gonadotropin testing (leuteinizing hormone, follicle-stimulating hormone), estradiol, and X-ray of the left hand and wrist for bone age to determine remaining growth potential.

If the patient is too young or the neurodevelopmental outcome remains uncertain, it is prudent to delay any decisions until more information is available to contribute to the argument for or against the intervention. Withholding the intervention may allow clarity to emerge regarding growth velocity and puberty. If there is no prospect for the patient's cognitive and communicative ability to improve to allow participation in decision-making, judgments will probably be driven by the parents with medical team support, based on what is believed to be the best interest of the child.

A practical model to reach a decision in these cases is to examine the clinical clues and quality of life predictions to determine if these procedures are feasible and provide more benefits than risks. In this case, we do not know Lisa's preferences, and there is no possibility that her ability to communicate her preferences is likely to change. Therefore, the parents make these decisions in the best interest of their child. This may have to be compared by their team to similar cases in order to deliver a solution. Importantly, the discussion needs to include the institutional ethics board, and this involves putting a summary of reasons for the consultation, the full clinical and social evaluation, and the content of discussions with the parents to the ethics board. The discussion needs to be informed by legal considerations, and the constitutional rights of the individual will have to be included in the decision-making process. There may be jurisdiction-specific rules and procedures, including legal and court procedures, that need to be taken into account for any potential action to be taken.

The role of the clinician in this scenario will vary based on how parents would like to proceed, having had a full discussion about the case. However, the clinician is the child's advocate, and should the interests of parents not align with those of the child, the clinician will be expected to support the child's issues. It is important to educate parents about the clinical, legal and ethical dimensions to enable them to make the decision to define alternative strategies for Lisa's care. Parents need to be counseled on the limited benefits and potential harms that the proposed interventions entail, and that defining alternatives to maintain care at home, or considering care in a designated facility, may be in Lisa's best interest.

If parents still want to pursue the full intervention or part thereof, this is a more challenging situation. More discussions need to be undertaken to provide information if needed, and to support the family throughout this process. Involvement of the institutional ethics board and consideration for required legal opinions are warranted if the parents still prefer to proceed with any procedures. If the physician is not supportive of the treatment, then they need to declare this to the parents, and transfer care to another physician.

Epilogue

It is possible today to manipulate pubertal and growth trajectories of children with neurodevelopmental impairments. The perceived benefits include prolongation of time the child can receive home care and improved interaction with care providers. This is coupled with retention of personal and external views of body status, and the likely absence of increased stigmatization of people with neurodevelopmental impairments who have had these procedures. The potential downside is the violation of personal rights, given the absence of a declaration by the person of their own preferences, as well as the reliance on parents as decision proxies when they may have conflicts of interest between their own needs and those of their child. Furthermore, there are medical risks attached to these interventions, as well as concern for their irreversibility. There is also a risk of justifying further interventions if these procedures become the norm. Importantly, these interventions are unlikely to result in improvements in Lisa's lifespan or quality of life.

Resolution

The approach to resolving Lisa's case involved the systematic collection of data, the performance of a full physical examination including pubertal evaluation, and review of all hormonal testing and bone age X-rays to define remaining growth potential. A detailed discussion was then undertaken with the parents to determine their views and preferences and to provide information and support of the factors that weigh on this decision. It was clear that Lisa would not clinically improve to participate in the decision-making process, and parents would remain the primary decision-makers indefinitely.

We also discussed that the alterations of body shape and size would not probably lead to improved functioning or quality of life, and that puberty is a necessary process to augment bone health as well as growth and maturation. The emphasis was then shifted to regulation of periods with hormonal therapy, should the cycles become irregular, which was not clear yet. Another alternative that was discussed is intrauterine contraceptive devices, with some having the capacity to deliver progesterone that prevents ovulation and menstruation. The parents considered the information carefully, and were comfortable allowing nature to take its course, and the consultation with the ethics board was deferred.

From the evidence available so far, the decision to alter body size and shape by interfering with growth and puberty is fraught with many challenges and difficulties. At this point, there does not appear to be a justification for using this approach in children with neurodevelopmental impairments. However, hormonal therapy seems to be justified to regulate periods after menarche similar to other children if needed.

Themes for discussion

- There are times when families request – perhaps insist on – treatments that we believe are of little benefit, but might at best do no harm. From a clinical perspective what strategies can we propose to a family to assess systematically whether the proposed intervention – something that they will do whether we agree or not – is doing more good than harm – or vice versa?

- When parents approach us with a request for a very unusual 'treatment' such as was made in this case, what can we do to 'get under the surface' of the issues and explore them with families – perhaps to find alternative 'answers'?

- In the case presented here, for whose benefit were the parents acting? How can we balance the potential indirect 'benefit' to Lisa to be 'manageable' for a longer time in the parental home, with the more immediate 'benefits' to the parents? In a climate of family-centered services and autonomy, to whom do clinicians have a primary responsibility?

References

Allen DB, Kappy M, Diekema D, Fost N (2009) Growth-attenuation therapy: Principles for practice. *Pediatrics* 123: 1556–1561.

Bell E, Wallace T, Chouinard I, Shevell M, Racine E (2011) Responding to requests of families for unproven interventions in neurodevelopmental disorders: Hyperbaric oxygen 'treatment' and stem cell 'therapy' in cerebral palsy. *Dev Disabil Res Rev* 17: 19–26.

Burnham JP, Kollef MH (2015) Understanding toxic shock syndrome. *Intens Care Med* 41: 1707–1710.

Clark CD, Weaver MF (2015) Balancing beneficence and autonomy. *Am J Bioethics* 15: 62–63.

Dickerson DP (2007) Ashley's treatment: Unethical or compassionate? *The Lancet* 369: 80.

Edwards SD (2008) The Ashley treatment: A step too far, or not far enough? *J Med Ethics* 34: 341–343.

Erling A, Wiklund I, Albertsson-Wikland K (1994) Prepubertal children with short stature have a different perception of their well-being and stature than their parents. *Qual Life Res* 3: 425–429.

Gillon R (2015) Defending the four principles approach as a good basis for good medical practice and therefore for good medical ethics. *J Med Ethics* 41: 111–116.

Goldworth A (2010) The case: The 'Ashley Treatment' revisited. Commentary: Weighing the balance. *Camb Q Healthc Ethics* 19: 415–416.

Green SE (2003) What do you mean 'what's wrong with her?': Stigma and the lives of families of children with disabilities. *Soc Sci Med* 57: 1361–1374.

Gunther DF, Diekema DS (2006) Attenuating growth in children with profound developmental disability: A new approach to an old dilemma. *Arch Pediatr Adolesc Med* 160: 1013–1017.

Jansen LA (2013) Between beneficence and justice: The ethics of stewardship in medicine. *J Med Philos* 38: 50–63.

Jecker NS (1997) Principles and methods of ethical decision making in critical care nursing. *Crit Care Nurs Clin North Am* 9: 29–33.

Kasman D (2004) The right to know – but at what cost? *Am Fam Physician* 69: 2255–2256, 2259.

Liao S (2007) The Ashley treatment: Best interests, convenience, and parental decision-making. *Hastings Center Report* 37: 16–20.

Low DE (2013) Toxic shock syndrome: Major advances in pathogenesis, but not treatment. *Crit Care Clin* 29: 651–675.

McCabe MA (1996) Involving children and adolescents in medical decision making: Developmental and clinical considerations. *J Pediatr Psychol* 21: 505–516.

Nathan BM, Palmert MR (2005) Regulation and disorders of pubertal timing. *Endocrinol Metabol Clin N Am* 34: 617–641.

Ouellette AR (2008) Growth attenuation, parental choice, and the rights of disabled children: Lessons from the Ashley X case. *Houston J Health Law Policy* 8: 207.

Rosenbaum P (2009) The quality of life for the young adult with neurodisability: Overview and reprise. *Dev Med Child Neurol* 51: 679–682.

Ryan C (2008) Revisiting the legal standards that govern requests to sterilize profoundly incompetent children: In light of the Ashley treatment, is a new standard appropriate. *Fordham L Rev* 77: 287.

Saigal S, Doyle LW (2008) An overview of mortality and sequelae of preterm birth from infancy to adulthood. *The Lancet* 371: 261–269.

Shannon E (2007) The Ashley treatment: Two viewpoints. *Pediatr Nurs* 33: 175–178.

Spriggs M (2010) Ashley's interests were not violated because she does not have the necessary interests. *Am J Bioethics* 10: 52–54.

Thomasma DC (1978) Training in medical ethics: An ethical workup. *Forum Med* 1: 33–36.

Tiedje K, Shippee ND, Johnson AM et al. (2013) 'They leave at least believing they had a part in the discussion': Understanding decision aid use and patient–clinician decision-making through qualitative research. *Patient Educ Couns* 93: 86–94.

Wiklund I, Wiren L, Erling A, Karlberg J, Albertsson-Wikland K (1994) A new self-assessment questionnaire to measure well-being in children, particularly those of short stature. *Qual Life Res* 3: 449–455.

Chapter 30

Independence in adulthood: ethical challenges in providing transition services for young people with neurodevelopmental impairments

Jan Willem Gorter and Barbara E. Gibson

Prologue

Much of the transitions literature in childhood disability focuses on enabling young people through individualized interventions and skill building. In this chapter, we reflect on how these efforts need to be tailored and timed to individual adolescents and their families, given that the greatest barriers to successful transitions to adulthood are environmental. Lack of appropriate opportunities, resources and supports hinder the ability of young people to learn to take charge of their own health, participate in their communities and exercise their citizenship. We begin by outlining some key ethical challenges in transition interventions, using a clinical case scenario. Taking the analogy of a journey, we suggest that young people in the current system are not provided enough with the opportunities to prepare for an adult life. Drawing on the notion of relational autonomy, we then present a detailed analysis of the ethical challenges inherent in a life-course approach to childhood disability. We suggest that the emphasis in the current system on independence and self-management has multiple consequences, effects and potential harms for young people, families and clinicians. We conclude by suggesting directions for managing these challenges in clinical practice.

The (composite) case we present comes from Jan Willem Gorter's clinical practice. We thus switch to the first person singular to outline the details of the case and his experience of working with the family.

It is Monday morning. I am going to see my next patient, Michael, in the teen-transition clinic. This clinic aims to assist teenagers with child-onset neurodevelopmental conditions and their families with their current health and developmental issues while helping them prepare for the future, in particular the transition from a pediatric setting to an adult healthcare setting.

Michael is 15 years old with cerebral palsy. He was born with a brain injury associated with severe perinatal asphyxia. He had overcome many medical issues as a young child, including pneumonias and feeding issues. His parents have been through many difficult situations, sometimes including threats of impending death. They have learned to speak up and to become strong advocates for their child and themselves. Now Michael is stable from a medical standpoint. He moves around on his own in a powered wheelchair and despite his significant speech and language impairments, he is able to communicate with the use of his iPad device. He enjoys hanging out with his peers. Lately, he seems to be struggling at high school, both academically and socially.

We start the clinic as usual with both Michael and his parents in the room. After 5 minutes I ask the parents to leave the room to allow Michael to have some time on his own with his doctor and his occupational therapist, who has been working with him since he was little. Michael's parents become emotional and refuse to leave the room. They want to stay during Michael's visit and express that they – as caregivers – 'need to know what's going on. After all he still is a "minor"'.

I know from previous visits that the parents will do all the talking and Michael will be quiet.

This apparent impasse brings me, as Michael's healthcare provider, to a difficult situation, and I wonder what is the right thing to do. Should I respect Michael's parents' wishes? This would mean that I cannot provide Michael with the opportunity to discuss his health and life in a private and confidential setting. Or, should I stay with the approach/philosophy of our clinic, informed by best practice guidelines, to involve Michael actively in his own care early on and help him develop the skills to take charge of his own healthcare, and more importantly accomplish a sense of competency? The latter would perhaps not respect the importance of his parents' responsibilities in the care of Michael. Although Michael does not currently have the capacity to make all healthcare decisions on his own, I know that he increasingly sees himself as an 'independent' boy who does not need to rely on his parents for everything.

And finally, I would like to provide Michael with the choice to continue in clinic with or without his parents. But it wouldn't be fair to bring this question up if the latter is not a realistic option for them. Michael's parents will likely be involved in helping him manage his health needs and life challenges for many years to come. This is true for many reasons, including that Michael's impairments will likely always limit his ability to manage his life independently, and there are extremely limited adult services in the community to support him. Moreover, there is a lack of opportunities for assisted living and employment.

The problem

Like Michael, a growing number of children and adolescents have impairments that compromise their physical, social and/or emotional health and developmental capacities. Only a few decades ago, most children with severe impairments died before reaching maturity; now the vast majority survive to adulthood. The issue of growing up with developmental conditions or complex care needs has become a new reality and has created new challenges for health and other sectors such as education, law, social and community services that provide services to young people with impairments.

Michael's case is typical in many respects. Since he was an infant, Michael and his family have been receiving healthcare from a multidisciplinary team of providers who coordinate his care needs and follow-up at regular intervals. This is about to change as Michael transitions out of pediatric care. Families often refer to this transition to adult care as 'falling off a steep cliff' (Stewart et al. 2009). They experience challenges to stay involved in the care of their child when he or she is approached as an adult person without taking into account the young person's varied capacity to make healthcare decision (Gorter & Roebroeck 2013). Moreover, they face inequity of healthcare services, and possible lifelong economic challenges. Adolescents with impairments report that they lack the opportunity to express their opinions, experience instances of lack of dignity and respect for their decisions, and may not have the ability or opportunity to discuss intimate questions with a healthcare professional, to name a few of their concerns (Racine et al. 2013, 2014). They live in a post-industrial society that valorizes self-sufficiency and expects young people to separate from their parents as they enter adulthood – to establish themselves as independent, 'contributing' citizens – yet provides few resources past childhood to help them achieve these expectations.

What should we be doing?
The ethical question of what to do in Michaels's case, and how to do it, rests on the notion of determining what processes and outcomes are in his and his family's best interests. Transitioning can be anxiety-provoking, and an emerging literature

suggests that planning well in advance has several advantages (American Academy of Pediatrics 2011; Provincial Council for Maternal and Child Health 2013). These include providing sufficient time to help the young person identify and develop the unique skills and abilities they will need to thrive (Gorter et al. 2015; King et al. 2015). Adolescents with significant neurodevelopmental impairments and complex care needs may never achieve idealized outcomes of independence, but may still benefit tremendously from individually tailored skill-building programs, opportunities and supports that build on their capacities and preferences (Kingsnorth et al. 2015). In Michael's case, supporting his developing autonomy may be helped through a gradual sharing and shifting of responsibility for healthcare decisions. How best to realize this shift requires that we weigh the family's readiness and try to determine how best to create a safe space for Michael to practice making autonomous choices. These principles are supported by research (Grant & Pan 2011), endorsed by professional organizations (e.g. American Academy of Pediatrics 2011) and have informed recent practice guidelines and recommendations (Stewart et al. 2009; Provincial Council for Maternal and Child Health report 2013) but more research is needed (Gorter et al. 2014).

Providing transitional family-centered care in the pediatric clinic
The core features of family-centered healthcare are the acknowledgement of the unique strengths, resources and needs of all family members, and the emphasis placed on partnership among the patient, the family, the doctor and other service providers (Bamm & Rosenbaum 2008). Research with transitioning young people and adults in Canada suggests that they want to be prepared well in advance for moving from pediatric to adult services (Young et al. 2009). The role of parents therefore needs to be acknowledged and supported, not only when the children are little but well into the teenage years and beyond. Although 'self-management' is often promoted as the ideal outcome of transitions, we suggest that a 'shared management' model is better able to meet these needs. Shared management involves a planned systematic process of a gradual shift in responsibilities from the healthcare provider and parents to the young person (Gorter & Roebroeck 2013). Typically, adolescents (literally meaning 'growing up') are driven to move out from the 'vertical identity' and expand/broaden their identity in a 'horizontal' direction through, for example, peer contact (to paraphrase observations made by Andrew Solomon [2012] in his book *Far from the Tree*). Having said this, parents play a key role in supporting their children's developing autonomy. To be able to provide family-centered care and to respect both child and family needs, it is essential that professionals provide families with information and support to prepare for transition and support the family as a whole while recognizing the emerging independence of the young person. The questions we explore below in relation to the case of Michael examine how to approach these challenges in clinical practice.

Recasting the ethical issues

In what follows we outline key ethical issues inherent in providing clinical care for transitioning young people; provide an analysis in relation to the case; and suggest a possible way forward.

The central challenges of transitions care that we have outlined above can be expressed as a tension between commitments to respecting and supporting family function on the one hand, and enabling greater independence of the young person transitioning to adult life on the other. In the transitions literature, including our own work, this tension is typically addressed by facilitating a gradual handing over of responsibility from parent to child. Clinicians may, for example, engage the child in skill-building programs, negotiate goals of increasing independence with children and families, and provide psychological supports. Research has demonstrated that these kinds of approaches are successful when implemented well (Kingsnorth et al. 2015). Nevertheless, very little of the literature has attended the need to unpack the *ethical* challenges inherent in these clinical processes, including conceptualizing the underlying normative principles that underpin practice, and clinicians' responsibilities in navigating these principles.

Much of the discussion about what constitutes a 'successful' transition relies on some notion of increasing a young person's autonomy and independence, but the link between naming and applying these principles, which function as clinical goals, is often not made.

To address this gap, we first do the work of critically conceptualizing 'autonomy' and 'independence', before applying the principles to the case and to transition care more broadly. What we will suggest is that a 'relational' notion of autonomy provides a nuanced version of autonomy that helps mediate the artificial division between person- and family-centered care by recasting the ethical problem in light of the particular material, social and political contexts of each young person and their family (Racine et al. 2013). We argue that because no person (child or adult) is fully independent or autonomous, goals such as self-management are not absolutes but matters of degree. Shared management models thus work to find the right balance for each family considering not only personal factors but also what the system will support. Moreover, when viewed through a relational autonomy lens, shared management acknowledges that all persons are dependent in some

"the ethical complexity of transitions extends beyond the clinic to encompass the frequent mismatch between the capacities of the young person and the available clinical, community-based and social supports they can access once they reach adulthood"

way, and does not assume ongoing dependencies are necessarily 'failures' of transition. Nevertheless, we suggest that the ethical complexity of transitions extends beyond the clinic to encompass the frequent mismatch between the capacities of the young person and the available clinical, community-based and social supports they can access once they reach adulthood.

Before diving deeper into the ethical challenges, it is necessary to say more about what we mean by 'relational' autonomy. Pervasive rights-based notions of autonomy view individuals as atomistic and capable of making independent decisions, free from outside influence (Beauchamp & Childress 2009). Children in these formulations are described in terms of their developing autonomy; that is, as they grow and mature they gradually attain the capacities to make independent choices and act as self-determining individuals. This traditional view of autonomy has been criticized for its narrow focus on individuals, and lack of consideration of broader social and political contexts in which people live (Mackenzie 2008; McLeod & Sherwin 2000). Relational autonomy addresses these critiques by considering individuals as inextricably situated in the environment, which shapes their choices and abilities to exercise their autonomy in profound ways (Mackenzie & Stoljar 2000; Sherwin 1998). The original proponents of relational autonomy were feminist scholars who were responding to the limitations of traditional autonomy in explaining and addressing women's gendered experiences of healthcare and other practices. Relational autonomy is now widely used in the literature to provide richer, context-dependent analyses of self-determination. Disability scholars, for example, have adopted relational approaches to challenge dominant views of persons as sovereign and disembodied, and instead attend to the connectedness that characterizes human experience (Reindal 1999).

A key difference between traditional and relational views of autonomy is manifested in how each considers *dependence*. Within a traditional autonomy framework, the need for assistance with completing daily activities is considered normal and acceptable for children, but problematic for adults, where it is constructed as a barrier or threat to the realization of autonomy (Dodds 2000; Sherwin 1998). A relational view instead acknowledges that dependency is inherent to the human condition, an idea that is captured by the notion of *interdependence* (Tronto 1993). Interdependence reflects the reality that the everyday lives of people are continually enmeshed in networks of mutual giving and receiving (Gignac & Cott 1998; Wendell 1996). In commenting on the ethical dimensions of care relationships, Kittay (2007; Kittay & Feder 2003) suggests that terms such as independence, dependence and interdependence should not carry any normative weight, but rather should be seen as simply descriptors of how people engage in various tasks. Relational autonomy and its focus on supporting interdependent relationships can inform an analysis of how to assist transitioning young people and their families. Independence with some tasks will no doubt be a goal of most young people's transition plans, but enhancing or modifying some forms of supports (i.e. ongoing dependencies) will also be part of goal setting in most cases.

The process of transitioning to adulthood can be approached in three phases: the preparation, the journey itself, and the landings in the adult world. The 'preparation' phase typically takes place during late childhood and early adolescence as young people begin to look ahead and prepare for adult life (Stewart et al. 2009). In this phase, children, parents and clinicians can begin to discuss options to create opportunities, and how to time these. This may include opportunities for the child to start talking privately with healthcare providers on their own before, during and/or after the clinic visit. The gradual introduction of such short visits may help create an atmosphere of trust and mutual respect. Respectful, meaningful and mutual relationships between healthcare provider, parents and the growing young person are at the core of the processes at work for the best adult outcomes (Gorter et al. 2014).

The 'journey' phase takes place during the transition from pediatric to adult care that comes with the realization that young people (typically age 16 up to 21 years) and their parents must learn to adapt to the adult care environment. This phase, in many if not most instances, can be characterized as 'disorder', meaning out of order. The child and family experience significant personal changes while concomitantly having to adjust to a new care setting, hence the dis-ordering of person–environment interactions. In our experience, it is critical that new – trustful – relationships are being established and that knowledge and skill-building continue to be supported. The final phase, 'the landing' in the adult world, hopefully reflects a new 'order' for emerging adults (typically age 20–30 years), with relative stability in their life situation, participation in society and a more or less established connection with adult healthcare and community services. Although the particulars of these phases may vary amongst families, the goals remain focused on building enabling relationships and abilities, with whatever amount of assistance works best in the context of their lives.

A relational approach helps clinicians and parents to reflect on the goals of increasing independence and provides assurances to parents and children who may not be comfortable or ready with these kinds of conversations. Easing their anxieties may be more possible with staged conversations that include simply assuring families early on why particular self-management skills are good to try, that the young person will need to develop these skills at some point, and importantly, that together you will determine how and when this might happen, taking preferences of both adolescents and their parents into account. A relational approach to ethics is always based in the particularities of the context. Thus, when and how to re-order responsibilities for care cannot be predetermined but is unique to each family and flows from their individual abilities and family dynamics. In the same vein, differences in the desires of child and parent (or other significant individuals) cannot be resolved by reducing the problem to issues of capacity that may be shifting and variable in relation to a host of factors (and tasks), and do not capture the complexity of interdependent decision-making dynamics. A relational approach also takes seriously the ethical commitment to reduce power differentials by partnering with families. This means getting to know the particularities of the personal, social and material contexts in which the transition is embedded. It involves considering multiple possible pathways, trying things out, and remaining open to other possibilities. For clinicians this might translate into letting go of a preconceived notion of the 'right' path or outcome embedded in programmatic goals, and working with the child and their significant others to explore options together.

During the actual journey – that is, the transition from the pediatric setting to the adult care setting – the young person and their family will experience the actual differences in environment and the impact these have on their own behaviors. Some young people tend to adhere to the behaviors they know well from previous experiences and 'go back' to a more dependent relationship, while others take advantage of the new environment and its expectations of independent behavior. The risks are that they cannot meet the expectations, may not follow through with professional advice, and might experience increased medical issues. More importantly, they will lack the safety net that parents used to provide. This may help explain why we typically see a phase of instability, that is, a loss of follow-up in the first years after transfer of services between pediatric and adult healthcare providers. Once young people and their families have landed in the adult healthcare system we often see a new 'order' in which both young people and their parents find their own way – with varying degrees of dependency. This is, however, determined to a great extent by a lack of opportunities to continue to foster knowledge and skills to grow and to become more autonomous. Overall with young people with impairments, we see more patterns of narrowing social interactions than widening (Gorter et al. 2014). The processes are yet to be understood, as there is very little research on the life trajectories of adults with child-onset neurodevelopmental conditions.

How a relational autonomy lens can help ethical practice

Practice

I speak with Michael's parents (at first separately and then along with Michael) about how they envision their son gradually taking over some of the decision-making about his care. They agree that this will be important at some time but do not feel comfortable doing so yet. I acknowledge and respect this choice but also introduce the idea that at a later visit, perhaps next time, I would like to meet with Michael briefly to discuss a particular issue. I frame this in terms of skill building, and emphasize the parents' continued involvement while he learns the skills. The goal of this approach is to provide Michael with the opportunity to practice articulating his experiences, and deciding what he wants to share, or not, with his parents.

Process

I give an outline of the structure of our next meeting. I suggest that first we start with a group discussion to bring everyone on the same page, and discuss how we will approach Michael's privacy and confidentiality. The middle part of the visit will entail Michael meeting me on his own, while his parents meet with Michael's occupational therapist in an adjacent room. The last part of the visit is planned as a group discussion where Michael is invited to share what he wants with his parents. I suggest that this is not only a good opportunity for him to practice, but it also allows Michael to exercise control over the information being shared, and his parents to experience this control and voice any concerns.

Content

The issue for discussion could be anything, but for the first meeting, in order to build trust, it might be something that is not particularly sensitive or pressing. I typically use the domains of the Rotterdam Transition Profile as a structure/guide for discussion: school, finances, housing (including chores), relationships (with family and friends), transportation and leisure (Gorter & Roebroeck 2013). From this list I would suggest we focus on something that has not raised too many issues within the family to date. Agreeing on the initial topic builds trust with the parents and may also decrease Michael's anxiety about having his first private meeting with the health professionals. Importantly, in this planning discussion I would acknowledge the importance of the parents' ongoing role in Michael's life, and assure them that they will always be included in his circle of care. I will be clear that the goal is not to begin separating Michael from his family, but to help him learn a skill that he may need and value, if not now, then in the future.

Future directions

Our approach to the case provides an example of how a relational autonomy lens can help guide ethical practice. Strategies like the one we have suggested here do not construct the goals of transitioning in terms of a vague notion of global 'independence'; rather the focus is on developing achievable capacities that are negotiated and individualized for each young person with their family, and take into account the young person's abilities and impairments, family styles and dynamics, their access to resources, and their preferences. The focus on skill-building acknowledges that the aptitude for exercising autonomy is not an inherent capacity but one that is developed with practice. Young people require exposure to

> *"The focus on skill-building acknowledges that the aptitude for exercising autonomy is not an inherent capacity but one that is developed with practice"*

safe opportunities to develop the level of self-trust that is necessary to gain and use these skills effectively. Simply inviting Michael to assert his preferences or make choices might set him up for failure if he has not had the opportunity to learn to exercise choices responsibly (McLeod & Sherwin 2000). Parents may also have these concerns and may face the consequences of their child's choices in terms of health risk, financial implications and so on, which may underpin comments like 'he is still a minor'. Framing the discussion and the transition plan in terms of incremental and individualized skill-building may go far towards alleviating these concerns and building trust while helping Michael to develop capacities for articulating and exercising autonomous choices, as well as inviting him to increase his participation in decisions.

The proverbial elephant in the room in the case we have presented is the paucity of supports and services that will be available to Michael once he transitions to adult care. Pediatric clinicians are well aware that parents will often be placed in a position of having to provide ongoing financial, social and physical supports to their adult children. Helping young people to learn to articulate and manage their healthcare and other needs will arm them with the skills needed to function within environments with limited supports, but it will often not be enough. For many young people with lifelong impairments, environmental mastery of these skills will not meet all their needs. Clinicians cannot solve this systemic problem on their own, but are often positioned as the bearers of this 'bad news'. Here we have few solutions to offer, other than ongoing engagement with research and political advocacy efforts to improve services for adults with child-onset impairments. At the clinical level, we suggest that it is important to be transparent so that families know what to expect and can prepare financially and otherwise. Moreover, young people and their families need to know what services are available, including how to 'work the system' to access these services when it is not readily apparent how to do this.

We also hope that this chapter will encourage healthcare providers to reflect on their own roles and competencies, including but not limited to medical expertise, communication and advocacy, as transitions is as much about us as it is about 'them' (Gorter et al. 2011). Also, it is important to consider the concept of shared agency, which implies shared intentions, reciprocal exchange of information, experience of being heard and respected, joint decision-making, and an agreement of mutual responsibilities in implementing the plan for which all require practice. Much of this learning happens through interprofessional education, interactions, collaborations and working closely with colleagues from, for example, social work and occupational therapy who have expertise working through psychosocial challenges with young people and their families (Reeves 2013). Once the challenges and tensions associated with the shift required to share or let go of control are understood, healthcare providers require support to identify strategies for forming partnerships with patients/families. Strategies that have been found to be helpful include dedicating time to practice reciprocity in communication style, peer support and self-reflection (Mudge et al. 2015). The case scenario could also be presented to both emerging and experienced healthcare providers to ground discussions of the ethical challenges of transitions and how 'to do good' in clinical practice.

Although the notion of supporting transitions is becoming more common in pediatric practice, it is still in its infancy in adult healthcare. We hope that this chapter will find its way into the education of healthcare providers and will contribute to raising awareness, building capacity and developing collaborative partnerships between young people, families and healthcare providers in both pediatric and adult settings.

Epilogue

In transitions care, as in all healthcare practices, clinicians are motivated by a question of 'what to do' for their patients – a question that is always both normative and practical. What is best and how can it best be achieved? Annemarie Mol states that doing good – that is, ethical – practice '... does not follow on finding out about, but is a matter of indeed doing' (Mol 2002 p. 177). Given the many ways that transitions care and its aims are 'enacted' in the doing (to use Mol's term), reconfiguring the goals of transitions along the lines of encouraging some forms of independence while also enabling 'useful dependencies' (Gibson 2014) seems to us a fruitful direction for ethical practice across pediatric and adult healthcare settings.

Relational autonomy provides a principle for individualizing transitions goals that make sense in the context of the young person's and family's lives. Moreover, it provides an ethical mooring for a shared management approach that gradually introduces supported autonomous choice without pitting the needs of child against the wishes of parents. Shared management acknowledges ongoing involvement and roles for parents/families of young people once they have transitioned out of pediatric services. Our suggestions for how to apply these principles in practice are not meant to be prescriptive; indeed this would be contrary to the context-based and particularized approach we have outlined. 'What to do', we suggest, is worked out through the everyday doings of clinical practice. What we hope we have contributed is a point of reflection regarding the limits of reducing transitions care to the promotion of independence. Considerations of the best mix of independence (skills) and dependence (supports) provide an ethically supportable framework for practice.

Themes for discussion

- In Chapters 30 (Gorter & Gibson), 20 (Reddihough & Davis) and 19 (Blasco), all the authors raise important questions concerning the scope and limits of our (clinical) responsibilities to children with impairments and their families. What are the historical bases for 'traditional' biomedically focused approaches; what are our clinical and ethical responsibilities in the 'modern' era of neurodisability; and should we/can we change the nature of our approaches to these issues?

- It is increasingly being argued that as health care professionals we should start our conversations with families about transition to adulthood when their children are 'young' (even before the adolescent years). Given the paucity of services for adults with child-onset impairments, what are the ethical implications of doing this?

- What are the responsibilities – and opportunities – for child-and-adolescent focused professionals to 'till the soil' in the world of 'adult' care in order to smooth the path for transition to adulthood of young people with neurodisabilities?

References

American Academy of Pediatrics, American Academy of Family Physicians, American College of Physicians (2011) Supporting the health care transition from adolescence to adulthood in the medical home. *Pediatrics* 128: 182–200.

Bamm EL, Rosenbaum P (2008) Family-centered theory: Origins, development, barriers and supports to implementation in rehabilitation medicine. *Arch Phys Med Rehabil* 89: 1618–1624.

Beauchamp T, Childress J (2009) *Principles of biomedical ethics* 6th edn. New York, NY: Oxford University Press.

Dodds S (2000) Choices and control in feminist bioethics. In: Mackenzie C, Stoljar N, editors. *Relational autonomy: Feminist perspectives on autonomy, agency, and the social self*, pp. 213–235. New York, NY: Oxford University Press.

Gibson BE (2014) Parallels and problems of normalization in rehabilitation and universal design: Enabling connectivities. *Disabil Rehabil* 36: 1328–1333.

Gignac MAM, Cott C (1998) A conceptual model of independence and dependence for adults with chronic physical illness and disability. *Soc Sci Med* 47: 739–753.

Gorter JW, Roebroeck M (2013) Transition to adulthood: Enhancing health and quality of life for emerging adults with neurological and developmental conditions. In: Ronen G, Rosenbaum P, editors. *Life quality outcomes in children and young people with neurological and developmental conditions: Concepts, evidence and practice*, pp. 306–317. London: MacKeith Press.

Gorter JW, Stewart D, Woodbury-Smith M (2011) Youth in transition: Care, health and development. *Child Care Health Dev* 37: 757–763.

Gorter JW, Stewart D, Woodbury-Smith M et al. (2014) Pathways toward positive psychosocial outcomes and mental health for youth with disabilities: A knowledge synthesis of developmental trajectories. *Can J Commun Ment Health* 33: 45–61.

Gorter JW, Stewart D, Cohen E et al. (2015) Are two youth-focused interventions sufficient to empower youth with chronic health conditions in their transition to adult healthcare: A mixed-methods longitudinal prospective cohort study. *BMJ Open* 5: e007553.

Grant C, Pan J (2011) A comparison of five transition programmes for youth with chronic illness in Canada. *Child Care Health Dev* 37: 815–820.

King G, McPherson A, Kingsnorth S et al. (2015) Residential immersive life skills programs for youth with disabilities: Service providers' perceptions of change processes. *Disabil Rehabil* 37: 971–980.

Kingsnorth S, King G, McPherson A, Jones-Galley K (2015) A retrospective study of past graduates of a residential life skills program for youth with physical disabilities. *Child Care Health Dev* 41: 374–383.

Kittay EF (2007) Beyond autonomy and paternalism: The caring transparent self. In: Nys T, Denier Y, Vandevelde T, editors. *Autonomy & paternalism: Reflections on the theory and practice of health care*, pp. 23–70. Leuven: Peeters Publishing.

Kittay EF, Feder EK (2003) *The subject of care: Feminist perspectives on dependency*. Lanham: Rowman & Littlefield Publishers.

Mackenzie C, Stoljar N (2000) Introduction: Autonomy refigured. In: Mackenzie C, Stoljar N, editors. *Relational autonomy: Feminist perspectives on autonomy, agency, and the social self*, pp. 3–34. New York, NY: Oxford University Press.

Mackenzie C (2008) Relational autonomy, normative authority and perfectionism. *J Soc Philos* 39: 512–533.

McLeod C, Sherwin S (2000) Relational autonomy, self-trust and health care for patients who are oppressed. In: Mackenzie C, Stoljar N, editors. *Relational autonomy: Feminist perspectives on autonomy, agency, and the social self*, pp. 259–279. New York, NY: Oxford University Press.

Mol A (2002) *The body multiple: Ontology in medical practice*. Durham and London: Duke University Press.

Mudge S, Kayes N, McPherson K (2015) Who is in control? Clinicians' view on their role in self-management approaches: A qualitative metasynthesis. *Br Med J* 5: e007413.

Provincial Council for Maternal and Child Health (2013) *Transition to adult healthcare services work group report*; http://www.pcmch.on.ca/.

Racine E, Larivière-Bastien D, Bell E, Majnemer A, Shevell M (2013) Respect for autonomy in the healthcare context: Observations from a qualitative study of young adults with cerebral palsy. *Child Care Health Dev* 39: 873–879.

Racine E, Bell E, Yan A et al. (2014) Ethics challenges of transition from paediatric to adult health care services for young adults with neurodevelopmental disabilities. *Paediatr Child Health* 19(2): 65–68.

Reeves S (2013) Interprofessional education and collaboration: Key approaches for improving care. In: Ronen G, Rosenbaum P, editors. *Life quality outcomes in children and young people with neurological and developmental conditions: Concepts, evidence and practice*, pp. 282–292. London: Mac Keith Press.

Reindal SM (1999) Independence, dependence, interdependence: Some reflections on the subject and personal autonomy. *Disabil Soc* 14: 353–367.

Sherwin S (1998) A relational approach to autonomy in health care. In: Sherwin S, coordinator. *The politics of women's health: Exploring agency and autonomy*, pp. 19–47. Philadelphia, PA: Temple University Press.

Solomon A (2012) *Far from the tree. Parents, children, and the search for identity.* New York, NY: Scribner.

Stewart D, Freeman M, Law M et al. (2009) The best journey to adult life for youth with disabilities: An evidence-based model and best practice guidelines for the transition to adulthood for youth with disabilities; www.canchild.ca.

Tronto JC (1993) *Moral boundaries: A political argument for an ethic of care.* London: Routledge.

Wendell S (1996) *The rejected body: Feminist philosophical reflections on disability.* New York, NY: Routledge.

Young NL, Barden WS, Mills WA, Burke TA, Law M, Boydell K (2009) Transition to adult-oriented health care: Perspectives of youth and adults with complex physical disabilities. *Phys Occup Ther Pediatr* 29: 345–361.

Chapter 31

Conservatorship in emerging adults: ethical and legal considerations[1]

Henry G. Chambers

Prologue

In the USA, at age 18 years, a teenager is considered an adult. They may vote, they can make decisions concerning their healthcare, their education, whom they may marry, where they spend their money, where they live and other life decisions. Adolescents with chronic developmental conditions who turn 18 have the same rights as typically developing adults. However, there are many situations in which – for a myriad of reasons – this granting of adult privileges may not be recommended for young adults with developmental disabilities.

Clinical scenario: Alex

Alex is a 21-year-old young man with cerebral palsy, Gross Motor Function Classification System (GMFCS) Level II. He has a trust fund of several hundreds of thousands of dollars after winning a lawsuit against his obstetrician. He is currently attending a state university and carrying a full load of classes, majoring in history. He is living with his parents and he has a scholarship that pays for college. He has mild epilepsy that is managed well with antiseizure medication, but he

---

1   Editor's note: Dr Hank Chambers and his wife Jill both reviewed a late draft of this book, and commented specifically on the need for people to recognize the legal as well as ethical dilemmas that can arise as young people make their life journey across the divide between 'childhood' and 'adulthood', at least as these are defined in law. This chapter was invited by the editors to bring these issues into sharp focus.

has to go to see his neurologist occasionally to get his blood drawn and to get prescription refills. His mother has taken him to all of his doctor's appointments since he was an infant, and has been involved in all aspects of his life, education and healthcare.

Alex is now in love with a young woman and after dating for several years, they have decided to get married. They have begun looking for an apartment and are setting a wedding date. His parents are against the marriage and refuse to allow him to get married as they are sure that this young lady is after the money in his trust.

Clinical scenario: Mary

Mary is a 19-year-old woman with cerebral palsy, GMFCS Level IV. She is in community college and living with her parents. She has had eight orthopedic surgeries to keep her hips in place, to fuse her spine for scoliosis and to lengthen her tendons to enable her to stand in a stander and walk in a gait trainer. Her dystonia has become worse over the years, and as a consequence she is experiencing significant pain and discomfort on a daily basis. She has been treated with oral baclofen and has had intramuscular botulinum toxin injections. She has a friend who has baclofen pump and would like to consider it to help with her movement disorder. Her parents are against it and refuse to let her get the surgery.

Commentary

These are not unusual case scenarios for a physician who deals with transitioning emerging adults; they happen on an almost weekly basis. The most common scenario involves a young adult in his or her twenties, perhaps a patient who is at GMFCS Level IV or V, whose parents still sign the consent for procedures and surgeries. However, there are several ethical and legal aspects of these case scenarios that challenge the patient, the family and the physician.

In the USA, an 18-year-old has all of the rights of an adult. In order for the parents, a guardian, a ward or another family member to make decisions for that person, a legal process must be followed to essentially take these rights away. This process is called *guardianship* in most states and *conservatorship* in California. Because each state has different, though similar, laws, I will use my home state of California as an example of how this system is structured (California Courts n.d.; Erickson 2014; NBRC n.d.; Shea n.d.).

There are two types of *conservators* (*guardians* in other states): *Limited Conservator of the Person* and *Limited Conservator of the Estate*. The seven 'powers' that are in question are (1) where the conservatee can live; (2) who can access their medical records; (3) whether and to whom they can marry; (4) whether they can enter into financial contracts; (5) who can give or withhold medical consent on behalf of the conservatee; (6) who can select the conservatee's social and sexual contacts and relationships; and (7) who makes decisions regarding the conservatee's education.

In our state, the adult in question will have a lawyer (court appointed if necessary) and the person filing for conservatorship must also have a lawyer. The case is then heard before a judge who may grant the conservator all, some, or none of the seven rights above. This is obviously a solemn question as someone (parent, sibling, other adult) is suing to abrogate or at least limit one of the disabled adult's essential rights and assume responsibility for them in this area.

Courts take this assumption of rights very seriously and have investigators interview both parties before the first hearing and at regular intervals afterwards to determine if anything has changed. Several advocacy groups, such as the Association of Retarded Citizens (ARC), have grave misgivings about how this process is implemented, feeling that some adults have had their rights withheld in an inappropriate manner (NBRC n.d.).

How does a legal system determine competency and capacity? These are, at the best of times, very difficult determinations, especially if the person is not verbal or has other communication or intellectual impairments. This is a legal decision rather than a medical one. Most parents and their families have only the best interests of their child (now adult) in mind. They have been devoting their lives to managing their myriad medical and social problems from birth and are not prepared, out of love and concern, to turn these decisions over to their now legally adult children. However, there are also some parents who do not have what we as healthcare providers would consider the best interests of their adult son or daughter in mind. An 'adult' has a right to make eccentric or unusual choices. Although a parent may not, for example, like a series of tattoos and piercings, or a young person's sexual orientation, they have no right to intervene on their typically developing adult offspring's decisions or actions.

Healthcare providers have a role in this very important matter, and discussion of this legal issue should be raised early in transition planning. Most families have never heard of this process and need a good deal of education. As professionals we have a legal obligation to ensure that, for our procedures, the correct person understands and signs the informed consent and that health information is not released to those who do not have the right to view it. The ethical question is always present when caring for an adult who has not yet been 'conserved' but where one is uncertain whether they have the competency or capacity to make an informed decision. In these situations, in California, the clinicians have to obtain a court order to perform any procedure on someone who is over 18 years old who has not gone through this legal process. There cannot be a 'wink-wink, just sign here' relationship with the parents. In essence, if the physician does not perform this due diligence, they can be cited for assault.

Our legal and ethical obligations to our adult patients are to ensure that they are treated with dignity and respect, that we respect their legal rights such as privacy and confidentiality, that we are aware of the limits of the conservatorship (guardianship), that we provide both the patient and the conservator with all of the information to make informed decisions, and that we understand the implications of these legal imperatives.

Clinical scenario: Kim

Eight months ago, I saw Kim, a young 17-year 10-month old adolescent girl with cerebral palsy (GMFCS Level II), who had a several-year history of bipolar disorder that was severely affecting her life. She was taking advanced placement classes in high school, but had bursts of rage altering with days where she could not get out of bed, and these were affecting her grades and of course all other aspects of her life. Her mother refused to allow the young woman's psychiatrist to give her any medication as the mother believed in 'natural treatments'. I spent 20 minutes trying to convince the mother to consider the treatment, but then this very intelligent girl told me to stop wasting my time, because in 2 months she was going to be an adult and did not need her mother's permission to start taking the medications. Currently, her mental health is much more stable as she is taking the medication and has been accepted to several universities.

References

Arc Tennessee (2015) Conservatorship and alternatives to conservatorship; https://www.thearctn.org/Assets/Docs/Conservatorship_Handbook.pdf.

California Courts (n.d.) What is a Limited Conservatorship?; www.courts.ca.gov/partners/documents/SelfHelpManualconser.doc.

Erickson Y (2014) Limited conservatorship guide. Los Angeles, CA: Bet Tzedek; http://www.bettzedek.org/wp-content/uploads/2011/04/BetTzedek2014LtdConservGuide.pdf.

NBRC (n.d.) Conservatorship, trusts and wills for people with developmental or other disabilities – a guide for families; http://nbrc.net/wp-content/uploads/CONSERVATORSHIP-BOOKLET-FOR-FAMILIES-2.pdf.

Shea J (n.d.) Limited conservatorship in California; www.allenshea.com/limited.html.

Epilogue

Looking back to the future

Bernard Dan

This book has taken readers on a journey into some of the ethical dimensions of practice in developmental disability. With the authors providing a wide variety of scenarios and experiences, writing with sensitivity and offering modes of reasoning, we hope that the journey has resonated with familiarity for most readers who have a clinical background. From a different perspective, the stories and issues may also sound familiar to many individuals with neurodisability and their families (Chapter 1). The scenarios draw their substance from real encounters between clinical professionals and families, and from some of the most challenging questions that occur in this interaction when discussing diagnosis, prognosis or intervention (Chapter 2). Collectively – with a wide array of topics, from development from fetal life (Chapter 4) to transition to adulthood (Chapter 30) – the essays are replete with rich material.

The chapters present and cover a broad range of opinions and sources of ethical discourse that reflect the diversity that exists in clinical settings and practice. Yet, the general analytical framework adopted by most of the authors in their efforts to disentangle the ethical complexity of the scenarios includes principles that are widely applied in healthcare, such as respect for autonomy, beneficence, non-maleficence and justice (Beauchamp & Childress 2001), and they exemplify how these concepts can be used as guides in childhood neurodisability. These principles do not impose attitudes or provide rules; rather, they can help in organizing reflections on the moral issues that often arise in clinical practice. In several chapters, the line between good clinical practice and ethics is faint. This is most obvious in scenarios dealing with issues such as the clinicians' knowledge or skills, partnership with parents or professional team members, communication and trust. In truth, the primary message of the book is that ethical questioning and deliberation are always an essential part of good practice.

The authors have thus shown how ethical reflections emerge from features that they strived to identify in individual situations. This is perhaps the second implication of this book: clinical encounters are inherently *particular*, both humanly and contextually. This is not an original observation, but it forms the premise to the approach developed throughout the book, which considers the essential singularity of the situations and at the same time provides us, hopefully, with useful clues to address other more or less related situations. These individual situations and their 'resolution' cannot act as precedent cases do in legal discussion, where a principle established in a previous legal case becomes binding or at least a persuasive argument when deciding on subsequent cases with similar issues. This is because of their irreducible singularity, which includes the clinical notion that similar facts do not reliably yield predictably similar outcomes. Ethical reasoning cannot *a priori* identify what is 'good' as a principle for judgment and what is 'bad' (Chapter 3). Yet, the scenarios in the book are informative of how principles can be usefully handled. From the recognized paramount importance of individual situations, ethics of singular 'truths' can be approached – such as that of Kaeko's parents' hope (Chapter 21), Nicole's family turmoil (Chapter 17) or Carter's neurologist's knowledge of the possibility of sudden death in epilepsy (Chapter 27).

By being attentive to those singular truths, the authors also illustrate that any individual clinical situation needs to be seen as being composed of multiple realities; these in turn account for differently informed viewpoints and mindsets as well as projections into the possible evolution of the situation in the future. The views and projections of each of the implicated individuals should not be expected to coincide. They may (in fact often do) come into conflict with each other; indeed, they may even fail to have enough in common to foster communication unless special efforts are made towards resolving this conflict by creating a space for respectful thinking with different subjective perspectives. Respect and trust are instrumental to articulating the different ways of reasoning. Within such a space, singular truths coexist and need not be unified but, as is apparent, consensus can be reached on critical issues.

"The authors have shown how ethical reflections emerge from individual situations ... clinical encounters are inherently particular, both humanly and contextually."

Each chapter presents aspects of how the relationships that underlie the situation form the basis for this multiplicity. This is another practical conclusion of the book: the need to recognize stakeholders and characterize those relationships. This is why concepts such as trust, honesty, commitment and also paternalism or observation of 'tension in the room' recur in the book. Chapter 7 focuses explicitly on the link between professionalism and humanism, with particular emphasis on integrity, humility, respect, empathy and generosity. These attitudes rest on the recognition of the complexity of issues as well as on the conviction of stakeholders' competences. As illustrated in many scenarios, attention to the aforementioned characteristics should promote the emergence of an ethical decision from interaction. The implied ethical construct underscores the importance of being open to, and responsible for, the 'other'. In this way, it calls for specific reflection on the tension between identity and difference (Levinas 1961): to what extent can we regard ourselves as the same in our experiences, views and projections, and to what extent are we not? This appears to be particularly relevant to developmental neurodisability. It promotes the ethical experience as an empathic experience of 'otherness' through consciously crossing the distance between oneself and the other, that is, of essential non-identity: *What would you do if you were me or the other way around?*

This is, however, a difficult exercise. One of the pitfalls underlined here is the danger of alienation through cultural relativism, based on the assumption that an individual's beliefs and attitudes are determined by the specifics of his or her culture. Cultural aspects are decoded in a number of scenarios (e.g. Chapters 6, 15, 16 and 18), not only where different geographic origins seem to call for this, but based on the recognition that *every* individual relates to his or her own culture. Cultural factors contribute to 'singular truths' and thus appear to result in divergences in understanding, opinions or expectations, but the authors also underline that cultural factors, together with other social factors (Chapter 5), should not overshadow non-specific issues such as communication, lack of adaptiveness of the system, or uncertainty in diagnosis, outcome, management planning and so on – factors that are often at the very core of problems. Against a vision of cultural relativism that surmises that ethical thinking is confined within cultural borders, the authors in this book favored a theoretical premise of inclusiveness in the evaluation of situations associated with disability. The same premise was previously discussed with regard to the World Health Organization's International Classification of Functioning, Disability and Health (ICF; Bickenbach 2012), the framework of which is used by many of the authors in this book. In the ICF, the inclusive approach denies that people with disabilities are discreet and insular minorities. On the contrary, it implies that disability is a universal human trait rather than 'something that happens to some people' (Bickenbach 2012). This has been termed the universal vulnerability and interdependence of people (Fineman 2008), calling for (ethical) respect for humanity. Therefore, the approach does not isolate a specific aspect, either in the human population (e.g. a minority) or in an individual (e.g. health), but promotes a holistic view.

Similarly, the alliance of stakeholders described by the authors as specifically organized for each situation incorporates the interdisciplinary approach championed in the ICF. On key aspects, a common language should be adopted, as exemplified by a recent project that engaged families and professionals (Cross et al. 2015) on the basis of Rosenbaum and Gorter's list of important F-words of childhood disability, namely Function, Family, Fitness, Fun, Friends and Future (Rosenbaum & Gorter 2012). Within the team of stakeholders, good communication is required, based on appropriate communication context and clear language. The relational approach that is suggested in this book invites us to appraise how features in a given situation are named by the stakeholders – child, each parent, each professional and so on – as this naming process is often related to values. This is particularly sensitive when disclosing information (Chapter 8), suggesting diagnoses with potential moral implications (Chapter 28), or when using terminology with social connotations (Chapter 14) (Dan & Abramowicz 2009). More subtly, phrases such as 'shortened life expectations', 'quality of life', 'all life [is] sacred', 'this machine [...] keeping Espérance alive', are but a few examples of word choices on the theme of the representation of life stemming from specific values. These values largely determine the singular truths mentioned above. They thus modify the very logic of the situation.

In this interdisciplinary communication, specific role boundaries may get blurred, because practical consensus, beyond moral distress, tension and eventual conflict, does not rely strictly on specialty with respect to a problem or an approach. Complexity in management and relationships in the system in which this is offered (Chapter 23) or in the alliance itself between the family and professionals (Chapter 22) may call for creative discussion of Humpty Dumpty's (im)pertinent remark in Lewis Carroll's *Through the Looking-Glass* that 'The question is [...] which is to be master'. In the scenarios, this communication was often supported by sharing and weaving together a narrative (Chapter 10), a story in which *the patient is the hero* (Chapter 6). At times, this allows for envisaging alternative stories (Chapter 29) and processes by which the possibilities of a situation can be considered.

The narratives of most of the chapters in this book are based on observed signs, facts and empirical data, and they must also deal with incomplete knowledge, conjecture and situational judgment (Dan 2014). In a number of chapters, the focus of such judgment appears to be placed on decisions between options of action, as though this were the crux of ethical thinking. Under Dewey's influence, the scope of ethics may have shifted from Kantian reflection on principles for judgment of people's practices towards those that would more directly affect decision-making, but it would be inaccurate to accept that ethics consists essentially of immediate decision-making (Chapter 3). Rather, the chapters in this book insist on the necessity of recognizing that decision-making is a gradual, stepwise *process* that must be inscribed in time. The complexity of the process demands the setting of priorities (Chapter 9). This may imply postponing difficult questions later along the unfolding of the situation. It also implies that one should not be tempted or expected to 'understand too quickly', because each individual has their own 'singular time' along their own logic, and differences should be recognized through dialog. Barriers between the stakeholders should be identified and specifically addressed. They may concern fundamental issues in the team alliance, such as trust (Chapter 18): when mistrust occurs, for example, it appears important to name it, to share one's own difficulty explicitly, and address it together.

In sum, this book deals with an aspect of the practical art of clinical experience, starting from case stories relating to childhood disability, as in 'real-life' practice. We are guided in an organized, didactic but non-prescriptive fashion as to how the ethical questions that arise from these cases can be identified and addressed based on principles that apply widely in healthcare. This approach can deal with contingencies, complexities and the singularities of individual situations. In spite of uncertainty, which commonly occurs, healthcare professionals must aim for the best in every case while running the risk of failure because of reliance on practical judgment. While stretching the limits of knowledge, we have much to learn from our own experience, whether successful or not, and from the experiences and reflections of others, such as are described and analyzed in this book.

References

Beauchamp TL, Childress JF (2001) *Principles of biomedical ethics*. New York, NY: Oxford University Press.

Bickenbach J (2012) Ethics, disability and the ICF. *Am J Phys Med Rehabil* 91(Suppl.): S163–S167.

Cross A, Rosenbaum P, Grahovac D, Kay D, Gorter JW (2015) Knowledge mobilization to spread awareness of the 'F-words' in childhood disability: Lessons from a family–researcher partnership. *Child Care Health Dev* 41: 947–953.

Dan B (2014) Medical rhetoric and rhetoric medicine. *Dev Med Child Neurol* 56: 916.

Dan B, Abramowicz M (2009) Le statut du discours scientifique. In: Thanassekos Y, Danblon E, Javeau C et al., editors. *Les lumières contre elles-mêmes: Avatars de la modernité*, pp. 74–89. Paris: Kimé.

Fineman M (2008) Vulnerable subject: Anchoring equality in the human condition. *Yale J Law Feminism* 20: 1–20.

Levinas E (1961) *Totalité et infini: Essai sur l'extériorité*. The Hague: Martinus Nijhof.

Rosenbaum P, Gorter JW (2012) The 'F-words' in childhood disability: I swear this is how we should think! *Child Care Health Dev* 38: 457–463.

Index

Recent titles from Mac Keith Press www.mackeith.co.uk

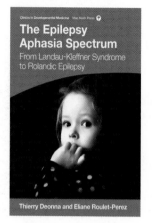

The Epilepsy Aphasia Spectrum: From Landau-Kleffner Syndrome to Rolandic Epilepsy
Thierry Deonna and Elaine Roulet-Perez

Clinics in Developmental Medicine
Winter 2016 ▪ 200pp ▪ hardback ▪ 978-1-909962-76-7
£50.00 / €62.94 / $75.00

Landau-Kleffner syndrome (LKS) is a rare childhood epilepsy, now considered to be at the severe end of the 'epilepsy-aphasia spectrum'. This book is aimed at the large range of professionals involved in the diagnosis, therapy and rehabilitation of children on the spectrum. The authors discuss work-up and management strategies and the reader will find chapters on topics such as the link between LKS and developmental language and communication disorders.

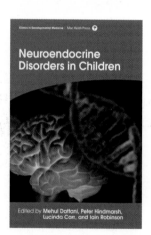

Neuroendocrine Disorders in Children
Mehul Dattani, Peter Hindmarsh, Lucinda Carr and Iain Robinson (Editors)

Clinics in Developmental Medicine
2016 ▪ 424pp ▪ hardback ▪ 978-1-909962-50-7
£74.95 / €105.90 / $120.00

Impairments in the endocrine system can lead to a number of disorders in children including diabetes mellitus, Addison's disease, growth disorders, and Graves' disease among others. This book provides a comprehensive examination of these disorders from infancy to adolescence. This text will be indispensable reading for paediatric endocrinologists, trainee paediatricians, neurologists and adult neurologists.

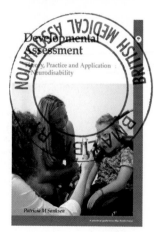

Developmental Assessment: Theory, Practice and Application to Neurodisability
Patricia M. Sonksen

A practical guide from Mac Keith Press
2016 ▪ 384pp ▪ softback ▪ 978-1-909962-56-9
£39.95 / €56.50 / $65.00

This handbook presents a new approach to assessing development in preschool children that can be applied across the developmental spectrum. The reader is taught how to confirm whether development is typical and if it is not, is signposted to the likely nature and severity of impairments, with a plan of action. The author uses numerous case vignettes from her 40 years' experience to bring to life her approach with clear summary key points and helpful illustrations.